Creation and Procreation

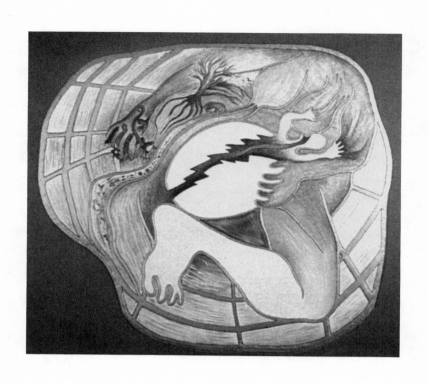

Creation
and Procreation

Feminist Reflections on Mythologies of Cosmogony and Parturition

Marta Weigle

University of Pennsylvania Press
Philadelphia

Publications of the American Folklore Society
New Series

General Editor, Patrick Mullen

FRONTISPIECE: "Egg/Her." Painting: Judy Chicago, © 1984. Embroidery on antelope skin: Pamella Nesbit. 34" × 34". Part of The Birth Project (1980–1985), the piece is pictured and discussed by Judy Chicago (1985:88–89) under the heading "*Hatching the Universal Egg* and the *Tree of Life*." Note too the spider and earth mother imagery.

Library of Congress Cataloging-in-Publication Data

Weigle, Marta.
  Creation and procreation: feminist reflections on mythologies of cosmogony and parturition / Marta Weigle.
    p. cm. — (Publications of the American Folklore Society. New series)
  Bibliography: p.
  Includes index.
  ISBN 0-8122-8096-2. — ISBN 0-8122-1264-9 (pbk.)
    1. Creation. 2. Human reproduction—Mythology. 3. Women—Mythology. I. American Folklore Society. II. Title. III. Series.
BL226.W45 1989
291.2'4'082—dc20   89-40401
                                                                       CIP

To
Amadea
Barbara
Beverly
Jane
Kay
Mary
—fine gossips and midwives all

Contents

List of Illustrations   ix

Preface   xi

1   Introduction: Notes on Cosmogony and Creativity   1
2   Spiders and Spinsters in Creation Mythology   17
3   Creator and Procreator   39
4   Impregnation and Conception   63
5   Construction and Gestation   95
6   Couvade and Parturition   121
7   Midwifery and the Dialogue of *Mythos* and *Mundus*   147

Appendix: Selected Texts of Creation and Procreation   177

Notes   247

Bibliography   263

Permissions   279

Index   285

List of Illustrations

Judy Chicago, "Egg/Her," 1984   ii

Creation *ex nihilo* as depicted by Johann Theodore de Bry in
Robert Fludd, *Utriusque cosmi,* 1617–21   2

"God as Architect of the Universe," in an Old Testament *Bible
moralisée,* France, thirteenth century   12

Navajo Indian women, ca. 1915   18

Navajo cat's cradle depicting the Pleiades   28

Prehistoric Hopi pottery with sun and spider symbols   34

God, Nature, and Art as depicted by Johann Theodore de Bry in
Robert Fludd, *Utriusque cosmi,* 1617–21   40

Sandpainting of Navajo creation chant, 1969   54

Tlingit crest hat and shamans' masks   64

Bartel Bruyn, "Annunciation," Cologne, sixteenth century   78

Acoma Pueblo Indian altar sandpainting   90

Our Lady of Guadalupe, by the Truchas Master, New Mexico,
1780–1840   92

"Ichnographia operis Philosophia alia," in Libavius, *Alchymia,*
1606   96

Hermes Trismegistus, in Michael Maier, *Atalanta fugiens,* 1618   106

Venus of Lespugue, France, ca. 24,000 B.C.   112

Navajo sandpainting of the Earth Mother, 1928   116

Philosophia with the World Disk, miniature in manuscript of St.
Augustine, *De civitae Dei,* Flanders, ca. 1420   118

Aztec goddess Tlazolteotl giving birth   122

Athena being born from Zeus's head, in Michael Maier,
Atalanta fugiens, 1618   136

Birth scene, early Greek relief   148

Yggdrasill, the World Tree, in *Elder Edda,* Finnur Magnusson
edition, eighteenth century   158

Judy Chicago, "Creation of the World," 1982   168

Preface

Mythology—that is, the study of myth or mythos—has for the most part been defined androcentrically. Much mythology, like much theology, philosophy, psychology, and aesthetics, elaborates a fundamental premise: that procreation poses an antithesis to creation; to be procreant is not to be creative; parturition cannot be considered the symbolic equivalent of cosmogony. Procreation is thus relegated to elemental or physical or biological status, while spiritual or metaphysical or symbolic creation becomes the valued paradigm for ritual, custom, art, narrative, and belief systems.

Thus, for example, when Henry Miller (1941, in Ghiselin 1952:185) describes his writing in mythic earth-diver terms as "a still deeper plunge into the brackish pool [of everyday reality]—. . . to the source where the waters were being constantly renewed," he exalts himself through association with a much-reported and often-studied myth/metaphor, one which Alan Dundes (1962) calls the "creation of the mythopoeic male." A "mythopoeic female" artist like Judy Chicago (1985) cannot readily claim such empowerment for her Birth Project. To present images of the creation of the world (including cosmogonic eggs), birth, and crowning in needlepoint, macramé, smocking, quilting, maternity clothes, and birth garments is discomfitting—somewhat trivial, too physiological, and not particularly aesthetic.

The feminist reflections in this volume are an attempt to establish a dialogue between myth as generally defined and women's mythology, a relatively unexplored domain that I have earlier suggested involved "appreciating the mundane" (Weigle 1982:285–98). I contend that "mythographers, folklorists, ethnographers, and others need to re-value the mundane, *mundus,* this world, as a more feminist complement and counterpart to the usual, largely sexist definitions of *mythos* as numinous, *ganz andere,* other and other worldly" (Weigle 1987a:433). In developing this appreciation, interpreters must encompass childbirth, gossip, and midwifery in their mythology.

The first two chapters review the typical androcentric definitions, classifications, and analyses of cosmogony, creation mythology, and creativity. They are surveyed in the introduction and elaborated with other, more feminist, perspectives in Chapter 2, "Spiders and Spinsters in Creation

Mythology." The remaining five chapters are structured with a sense of the dialogue set up by the book's title, *Creation and Procreation:* "Creator and Procreator" (3), "Impregnation and Conception" (4), "Construction and Gestation" (5), "Couvade and Parturition" (6), and "Midwifery and the Dialogue of *Mythos* and *Mundus*" (7). The first term of each pair is usually associated with the traditional, androcentric view of pro/creation.

These feminist reflections are not argued but narrated—woven, perhaps, in the manner of the spider creations discussed in the second chapter. This is a deliberately chosen midwifery, a collaborative storying or gossip in the sense suggested in the final chapter. Various mythologists' usual theoretical concerns are noted throughout but are always treated as part of the story narrated (the myth performed) by a range of extensively quoted, fully contextualized myth and interpretive texts. Their texture and narrative sense, not their internal logic or systemic validity, is at issue here, or is itself the issue.

The purpose of storytelling in this way recalls that voiced to folklorist Barre Toelken by the Navajo Yellowman when asked about the "pretty languages" in his humorous Coyote tales:

> Why, then, if Coyote is such an important mythic character (whose name must not even be mentioned in the summer months), does Yellowman tell such funny stories about him? Yellowman's answer: "They are not funny stories." Why does everyone laugh, then? "They are laughing at the way Ma'i does things, and at the way the story is told. Many things about the story are funny, but the story is not funny." Why tell the stories? "If my children hear the stories, they will grow up to be good people; if they don't hear them, they will turn out to be bad." Why tell them to adults? "Through the stories everything is made possible."

The final idiom is translated literally and "may also mean, 'They make things simple, or easy to understand'" (Toelken and Scott 1981:80, 114). It is hoped that these pro/creation stories will empower a woman's mythology, balancing the androcentric with a gynocentric so that all children may "grow up to be good people" who sense and begin to understand all the mysteries.

Among the many collections of creation and other myths (see Chapter 1), there are few that devote much (if any) attention to the complex symbolic systems of procreation, as, for example, does David Meltzer's

Birth: An Anthology of Ancient Texts, Songs, Prayers, and Stories (1981).
Creation and Procreation sets up the dialogue of pro/creation by combining
the two kinds of texts and thus becomes an anthology like Rosemary
Radford Ruether's *Womanguides: Readings Toward a Feminist Theology*
(1985) or the one proposed later in Chapter 7.

In the seven chapters that follow, a range of sources—theoretical,
mythological, historical, ethnographic, linguistic, psychological, aesthetic,
narrative, and so on—are extensively quoted, complemented by a broad
spectrum of illustrations. Like the sources similarly arrayed in *Spiders &
Spinsters: Women and Mythology* (Weigle 1982), these are primarily "New
World": Native American and the transplanted classical and Judeo-
Christian mythologies. The story fabric of the seven chapters is retold in the
appendix, which is organized according to the book's sequence of interwoven myths. It "reweaves" the book in a different (con)text(ure) and can
serve as a primary resource in myth and women studies.

The psychoanalytic work of Alan Dundes clearly has been seminal, if
not exasperating. In a way, what I present here is an attempt to counter or at
least balance his 1962 article, "Earth-Diver: Creation of the Mythopoeic
Male," with the likes of the trickster spider, the co-creative world parents,
the cosmogonic womb, emergence, and the gossip of participants in birthing. I hope my kind of midwifery in presenting this dialogue of mythos and
mundus will suggest aspects of the "pro/creation of the mythopoeic female."

Many of the germinal ideas for this book were planted during my
tenure as editor of the *Folklore Women's Communication* (1977–79), a time
when I also served as consulting editor for a special "cluster" of articles on
women as verbal artists for *Frontiers: A Journal of Women Studies* (vol. 3, no.
3, fall 1978). The women I worked with on these ventures and my students
in Mythology, Women and Folklore, and Women and Oral Tradition
classes in the Departments of American Studies, Anthropology, and English at the University of New Mexico have contributed much to the book's
conception and gestation.

In 1979 my English Department colleague David Johnson and I received a grant from the Exxon Education Foundation, Educational Research and Development Program, to develop an undergraduate curricu-
lum entitled "Mythology of the Americas: An Interdisciplinary Approach
to Cultural Identity." The funding enabled us to coauthor *Lightning &
Labyrinth: An Introduction to Mythology* (1979) and *At the Beginning: Ameri-*

can Creation Myths (1980), both of which have influenced this volume. The Exxon grant also made it possible for me to write the first version of *Spiders & Spinsters: Women and Mythology* in 1980, subsequently revised and published by the University of New Mexico Press in 1982.

Creation and Procreation explores more fully parts of *Spiders & Spinsters*. However, its major impetus comes from my colleague and friend at Indiana University, Beverly J. Stoeltje. She invited me to participate in a panel, "Feminist Revisions: Scripts and Acts," that she had organized as part of the day-long Folklore and Feminism program during the 1986 Annual Meeting of the American Folklore Society in Baltimore. Some of those papers, including mine (Weigle 1987a), became part of a special Folklore and Feminism issue of the *Journal of American Folklore,* a centennial number (vol. 100, no. 398) that culminated a century of continuous publication.

A version of the emergence myth discussion appeared in the newly revived *New Mexico Folklore Record* (Weigle 1987b), for which opportunity I thank editor Rowena Rivera. Some of the last section of Chapter 4, "Earth Mother, Virgin Mother: Empowering in Emergence and Marian Apparition Mythologies," was delivered at the 1987 Annual Meeting of the American Folklore Society in Albuquerque. My colleagues on that panel, "Women of Power: Image, Myth, Ritual"—Mari Lyn Salvador, Barbara Babcock, and Jane Caputi—have contributed much to this book. I would also like to thank Judy Chicago, Mary Ross Taylor, and Elizabeth Kay for making it possible for me to include two images from The Birth Project.

I count myself fortunate indeed to have enjoyed and benefitted from the myth/play of the six fine gossips and midwives to whom this pro/creation is dedicated, with trepidation.

1

Introduction: Notes on Cosmogony and Creativity

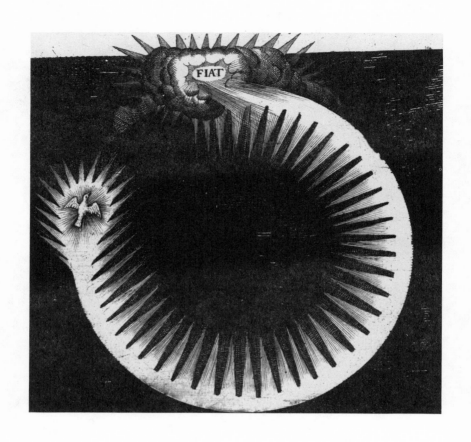

Creation *ex nihilo* as depicted by Johann Theodore de Bry in *Utriusque cosmi, maioris scilicet et minoris, metaphysica atque technica historia* (Oppenheim, 1617–21), vol. I, p. 49, by the English Hermetic philosopher Robert Fludd (1574–1637).[1] Courtesy, The Bancroft Library, University of California, Berkeley.

In the beginning God [Elohim] created the heavens and the earth. The earth was without form and void, and darkness was upon the face of the deep; and the Spirit of God was moving over the face of the waters.

And God said, "Let there be light"; and there was light. And God saw that the light was good; and God separated the light from the darkness. God called the light Day, and the darkness he called Night. And there was evening and there was morning, one day. (Genesis 1:1–5 [RSV])[2]

Cosmogonies, especially those resembling Judeo-Christian creation myths, are accorded elevated status in mythology. Often considered the measure of a culture's theological and philosophical speculation, cosmogonic myths are marked by anthologists as exemplary. Many scholars view them as fundamental metaphors in religious, psychological, and aesthetic studies—paradigmatic for collective ritual and individual creativity. Both androcentrism and ethnocentrism figure in such discussions, and a critical examination of mythologists' definitions, classifications, evaluations, and analyses of creation myths is thus crucial to a feminist mythology.

"True" Creation Myths

> First of all there came Chaos,
>   and after him came
> Gaia of the broad breast . . .
> and Tartaros the foggy in the pit
>   of the wide-wayed earth,
> and Eros, who is love. . . .
> From Chaos was born Erebos, the dark,
>   and black Night. . . .
> —Hesiod, *Theogony*, 116–23 (trans. Richmond Lattimore, in Lattimore 1959:130)

The identification of "genuine" cosmogonic myths and their classification and comparison has concerned many mythographers. Mircea Eliade (1969:76) claims that, in any mythology, there is always a *primordial history* and this history has a *beginning:* a cosmogonic myth proper, or a myth that describes the first, germinal stage of the world. This beginning is always implied in the sequence of myths which recounts the fabulous events that took place after the creation or the coming into being of the universe, namely, the myths of the origin of plants, animals, and man, or of the origin of marriage, family, and death, etc.

Eliade (1969:75) concedes: "Certainly, the myth of the creation of the world does not always look like a cosmogonic myth *stricto sensu,* like the Indian or Polynesian myth, or the one narrated in *Enuma elish* [Babylonian]. In a great part of Australia, for example, such cosmogonic myths are unknown. But there is always a central myth which describes the beginnings of the world."

In a 1914 article on "Mythology and Folk-Tales of the North American Indians," Franz Boas makes similar distinctions, maintaining that most Indian "origin myths" assume the existence of "the mythical world, earth, water, fire, sun and moon, summer and winter, animals and plants."

The idea of creation, in the sense of a projection into objective existence of a world that pre-existed in the mind of a creator, is also almost entirely foreign to the American race. The thought that our world had a previous existence only as an idea in the mind of a superior being, and became objective reality by a will, is not the form in which the Indian conceives his mythology. There was no unorganized chaos preceding the origin of the world. Everything has always been in existence in objective form somewhere. (Boas 1940:468; also Parsons 1939:210)

Stith Thompson echoes Boas in the introduction to his 1929 collection, *Tales of the North American Indians:* "The true creation myth, as Professor Boas points out, is almost wholly lacking, but origin myths of a sort are found over a large territory" (1966:xvii; also Erminie Wheeler-Voegelin in Leach 1972:259).

One Southwest emergence myth does qualify as a true creation myth, according to Thompson—Frank Hamilton Cushing's outline of a Zuni creation narrative collected in various versions during the 1880s.[3] The first paragraph of "The Genesis of the Worlds, or The Beginning of Newness" reads: "Before the beginning of a new-making, Áwonawílona (the Maker and Container of All, the All-father Father), solely had being. There was nothing else whatsoever throughout the great space of the ages save everywhere black darkness in it, and everywhere void desolation" (Cushing 1896:379). This sanctioned text apparently resembles Hesiod's *Theogony* (ca. 700 B.C.), in which the male Chaos is first to come into being. "The Greek word *Chaos* means a 'yawning.' For Hesiod, then, Chaos is a void," from which comes "Gaea, or Ge (Earth), Tartarus (a dim place in the depths of the ground), Eros (Love), Erebus (the gloom of Tartarus), and dark Night" (Morford and Lenardon 1985:30).

Dennis Tedlock points out the ethnocentrism in Boas's and Thompson's assertions about "'true creation myths' in North America, by which they apparently meant origin myths on the metaphysical model of Genesis 1, John 1, and, for that matter, Aristotle's *Metaphysics*" (1983:338). He thus highlights two strong Western biases in the mythology of creation: the premium on so-called *ex nihilo* creation by spirit, breath, dream, speech, and the like—especially as exemplified in Judeo-Christian tradition—and the fascination with Greek mythology and philosophy.

Androcentrism also influences these and other mythographers. Much of *Theogony*, for example, concerns "the holy stock / of the everlasting immortals / who came into being out of Gaia / and starry Ouranos," Gaia's firstborn (Lattimore 1959:129). But this "female" procreation has been given far less consideration than Gaia's coming into being out of the nothingness of the male Chaos. The hierogamy of earth and sky and her bearing the Titans and others by so-called elemental creation has been of less interest mythologically than the "male," so-called *ex nihilo*, creation.

Classifying Cosmogonic Myths

The main groupings for this anthology [*Origins: Creation Texts from the Ancient Mediterranean, A Chrestomathy*] are *creation through word* and *elemental creation*. These seemed the ones our material suggested, not our willful imposition. . . . These categories seem to hold up about as well as any, and, more importantly, do least damage to the stories and even tell us something about creation story itself, over and beyond narrative summaries of individual tales. (Doria and Lenowitz 1976: xxiii)

In *From Primitives to Zen: A Thematic Sourcebook of the History of Religions*, Mircea Eliade (as rpt. 1974:83) proposes the following classification for "the great variety of cosmogonic myths":

1. creation *ex nihilo* (a High Being creates the world by thought, by word, or by heating himself in a steam-hut, and so forth)

2. the Earth Diver Motif (a God sends aquatic birds or amphibious animals, or dives, himself, to the bottom of the primordial ocean to bring up a particle of earth from which the entire world grows)

3. creation by dividing in two a primordial unity (one can distinguish three variants: a. separation of Heaven and Earth, that is to say of the World-Parents; b. separation of an original amorphous mass, the "Chaos"; c. the cutting in two of a cosmogonic egg)

4. creation by dismemberment of a primordial Being, either a voluntary, anthropomorphic victim (Ymir of the Scandinavian mythology, the Vedic Indian Purusha, the Chinese P'an-ku) or an aquatic monster conquered after a terrific battle (the Babylonian Tiamat).

With one exception, this is basically the scheme used by Eliade's student, Charles H. Long, in his anthology, *Alpha: The Myths of Creation* (1963). Long adds emergence myths to categories of world-parent myths, creation from chaos and from the cosmic egg, creation from nothing, earth-diver myths, creation and sacrifice, and the ancestors as creators. Neither historian of religions includes as cosmogonic the *Deus faber* motif, identified by Jungian analyst Marie-Louise von Franz (1972:87) as "a technical term which characterizes God as the craftsman or artisan, who as an architect, carpenter, smith, etc., creates the world on the analogy of some skill or craft." Additional categories are also suggested in folklorist Anna Birgitta Rooth's comparative study (1957) of eight types of North American Indian creation myths: Earth-Diver, World-Parent, Emergence, Spider, Fighting or Robbery, Ymir, Two Creators and their contests, and Blind Brother.

These and most other classifications of cosmogonic myths and motifs may be operationalized as follows:

1. *Accretion* or *conjunction,* like the mingling of waters or fire and frost, the cosmic mountain rising from the sea, random or accidental joining of elements.

2. *Secretion,* like vomit, sweat, urination, defecation, masturbation, web-spinning, parthenogenesis.

3. *Sacrifice* of self or other.

4. *Division* or *conjugation,* the former usually associated with discriminating primal matter or a cosmogonic egg, the latter usually with the consummated marriage of earth and sky.

5. *Earth-diver,* who brings the seed or mud of earth from beneath primal or flood waters.

6. *Emergence* into this world by journeying through lower or other worlds, domains, or wombs.

7. *Two creators,* cooperating or competing.

8. *Deus faber,* the architect/artisan/craftsperson or "making" deity.

9. *Ex nihilo,* through "spirit"—dream, thought, breath, laughter, or speech.

Both ethnocentrism and androcentrism bias such etic classifications.[4] Generally discernible are implicit distinctions between "higher," metaphysical or spiritual, or *ex nihilo* creation and "lower" or "lesser" physical, natural, or elemental creation through accretion, excretion, copulation, division, dismemberment, or parturition. The former are too readily regarded as male and more highly valued, especially when they can be associated with the monotheism of a supreme (preferably masculine) deity; the latter are often considered female and less valuable for being related to nature and animism. In these analytic schemes, creation by a *Deus faber* is more equivocally valued, influenced by sociocultural notions of art and artists, with concomitant gender considerations.

Creativity as Compensation and Transformation

Diotima, a Mantinean wise woman, to Socrates: "You'll see how right I am if you only bear in mind that men's great incentive is the love of glory. . . .

". . . Those whose procreancy is of the body turn to woman as the object of their love, and raise a family, in the blessed hope that by doing so they will keep their memory green. . . . But those whose procreancy is of the spirit rather than of the flesh. . . conceive and bear the things of the spirit. And what are they? you ask. Wisdom and all her sister virtues; it is the office of every poet to beget them, and of every artist whom we may call creative." (Plato, *Symposium,* 208c,e-209 [trans. Michael Joyce, 1935, in Hamilton and Cairns 1961:560])

Ordinary English language usage supports Diotima's contention. Linguist George Lakoff and philosopher Mark Johnson (1980:74–75) propose that the following sentences "are all instances of the general metaphor CREATION IS BIRTH":

Our nation was *born out of* a desire for freedom.

His writings are products of his *fertile* imagination.

His experiments *spawned* a host of new theories.

Your actions will only *breed* violence.

He *hatched* a clever scheme.

He *conceived* a brilliant theory of molecular motion.

Universities are *incubators* for new ideas.

The theory of relativity *first saw the light of day* in 1905.

The University of Chicago was the *birthplace* of the nuclear bomb.

Edward Teller is the *father* of the hydrogen bomb.

These predominantly masculine examples cannot be matched with an equivalent set using words like *project, penetrate, erect,* and *ejaculate* to form a predominantly feminine, "general metaphor" CREATION IS PROJECTION. Women, it would seem, do not have "projects" in the way men have "babies," unless, perhaps, they cannot or do not have children.[5]

Folklorist Alan Dundes (1962:1038) summarizes the psychoanalytic view of male creativity thus: "Whether it is called 'parturition envy' (Boehm) or 'pregnancy envy' (Fromm), the basic idea is that men would like to produce or create valuable material from within their bodies as women do. . . . A number of psychoanalysts have suggested that man's desire for mental and artistic creativity stems in part from the wish to conceive or produce on a par with women." As psychoanalyst Karen Horney (1967:61; also in Strouse 1974:177) asks in her 1926 article, "The Flight from Womanhood: The Masculinity-Complex in Women as Viewed by Men and by Women": "Is not the tremendous strength in men of the impulse to creative works in every field precisely due to their feeling of playing a relatively small part in the creation of living things, which constantly impels them to an overcompensation in achievement?"[6]

Psychoanalysts have identified penis envy as women's compensatory mechanism similar to men's "womb envy." However, Horney (1967:62; also in Strouse 1974:177, 178) wonders "why no corresponding impulse to

compensate herself for her penis envy is found in woman." According to
her:

> There is much to be said in favor of the view that women work off their
> penis envy less successfully than men, from a cultural point of view. We
> know that in the most favorable case this envy is transmuted into the
> desire for a husband and child, and probably by this very transmuta-
> tion it forfeits the greater part of its power as an incentive to sublima-
> tion. In unfavorable cases, however, . . . it is burdened with a sense of
> guilt instead of being able to be employed fruitfully, while the man's
> incapacity for motherhood is probably simply felt as an inferiority and
> can develop its full driving power without inhibition.

Jungian psychologists suggest a more teleological perspective, viewing
cosmogonic myths as purposive and essential for women and men alike, not
merely compensatory for anatomical and cultural deficiency. Analyst Sheila
Moon calls her study *A Magic Dwells: A Poetic and Psychological Study of the
Navaho Emergence Myth* "a book about a myth—the Navaho creation
myth—about meanings of myth, and about the relevance of myths and
their meanings to the psychological-religious growth of the individual
personality" (1970:3). She defines myths as "tries for understanding; when
really alive and functional they are more satisfactory tries than most intellectual systems." Her interpretive stance is summed up as follows:

> Cosmic myths such as the Navaho creation are, as Dr. Jung indi-
> cated, dreams of mankind. They contain symbols and symbolic situa-
> tions relating to man's spiritual search for himself. . . . While cultural
> evolution, as well as personal development chronologically viewed, is
> reflected in such cosmic myths, my conviction grows that the myths
> touch levels of meaning more basic than personal or cultural, that they
> speak to contemporary man as articulately as to his forebears of su-
> prapersonal realities and of ultimate destinies. We can assume that
> man's needs for individual meaning and value are expressed in his
> myths as in his outer social strivings and, further, that myths can be
> psychologically "explained" as man's symbolization of processes which
> seek to re-establish harmonies both within himself and between him-
> self and others. (Moon 1970:4)

In *Patterns of Creativity Mirrored in Creation Myths* Jungian analyst
Marie-Louise von Franz (1972:11) asks, "Where do we see creation myths

nowadays, or elements, or typical motifs of creation myths in our practical analytical work and in dreams?" Her crucial answer: "You find creation myth motifs *whenever the unconscious is preparing a basically important progress in consciousness*" (1972:13). Significant psychic transformation—whether an important decision, critical insight, creative task, schizophrenic break, or change in consciousness—is heralded and expressed by cosmogonic myths and motifs in dreams and various verbal and visual creations.

Von Franz's approach is consonant with that in Jungian analyst Heinz Westman's 1961 study, *The Springs of Creativity*. Westman relates biblical imagery to the creative process of psychic development in therapy and art. He interprets both the case of his artist-patient Joan and the book of Genesis, which he calls "an astonishingly accurate poetic revelation of the psyche's ontogenesis." Cosmogonic myths and images like Elohim's *ex nihilo* creation, and like poetry itself, "must have emerged out of personal night," the poet/mythmaker depending "not at all upon cool observation of the world around him, but only upon the warmth of his own imagination searching his own darkness."

> There are as many myths about the creation of the cosmos as there are peoples. Science has shown these myths of the origins of the material world to be at best charmingly naive, yet they keep their beauty and power. This is not only because of the grandeur of their language; they are all, I believe, variations on a single, much deeper theme: The creation of the cosmos and the drama of its slow unfolding is a symbol of the poet's experience of his own inner creation and his own slow opening to the light. On their deepest level all these myths are really concerned with the ontogenesis of the psyche itself. (Westman 1986:x, 75, 23)

Creation as Ritual Paradigm

> In India, before a single stone is laid, "The astrologer shows what spot in the foundation is exactly above the head of the snake that supports the world. The mason fashions a little wooden peg from the wood of the Khadira tree, and with a coconut drives the peg into the ground at this particular spot, in such a way as to peg the head of the snake securely down. . . . If this snake should ever shake its head really violently, it would shake the world to pieces" [Stevenson 1920:354]. A

foundation stone is placed above the peg. The cornerstone is thus situated exactly at the "center of the world." But the act of foundation at the same time repeats the cosmogonic act, for to "secure" the snake's head, to drive the peg into it, is to imitate the primordial gesture of Soma (*Rg-Veda*, II, 12, 1) or of Indra when the latter "smote the Serpent in his lair" (VI, 17, 9), when his thunderbolt "cut off its head" (I, 52, 10). The serpent symbolizes chaos, the formless and non-manifested. Indra comes upon Vṛtra (IV, 19, 3) undivided (*aparvan*), unawakened (*abudhyam*), sleeping (*abudhyamānam*), sunk in deepest sleep (*suṣupaṇam*), outstretched (*aśayānam*). The hurling of the lightning and the decapitation are equivalent to the act of Creation, with passage from the nonmanifested to the manifested, from the formless to the formed. (Eliade 1971:19)

Mircea Eliade (1961:80) claims that *illud tempus*, the original mythic time when the world first came into being, serves as exemplar for all rituals and significant human activities. "*In illo tempore* the gods had displayed their greatest powers. *The cosmogony is the supreme divine manifestation*, the paradigmatic act of strength, superabundance, and creativity. Religious man thirsts for the real. By every means at his disposal, he seeks to reside at the very source of primordial reality, when the world was *in statu nascendi*." Myths and ritual acts of foundation, consecration, inauguration, and renewal recreate that time symbolically.

The cosmic architect's creation is ritually repeated by humans whenever a settlement or city is founded or a sanctuary or house built. Both the circular trench Romulus dug with his plow around the square altar, when founding the city walls of Rome, and the universe itself were called *mundus*, or world (Eliade 1958:373–74). Anthropologist Frank G. Speck's description of the Delaware Indian Big House illustrates the homology between cosmic and terrestrial architecture:

The Big House stands for the universe, its floor, the earth; its four walls, the four quarters; its vault, the sky dome, atop which resides the Creator in his indefinable supremacy. . . . The center post is the staff of the Great Spirit with its foot upon the earth, its pinnacle reaching to the hand of the Supreme Deity. The floor of the Big House is the flatness of the earth upon which sit the three grouped divisions of mankind, the human social groupings . . . in their appropriate places. . . . The ground beneath the Big House is the realm of the underworld

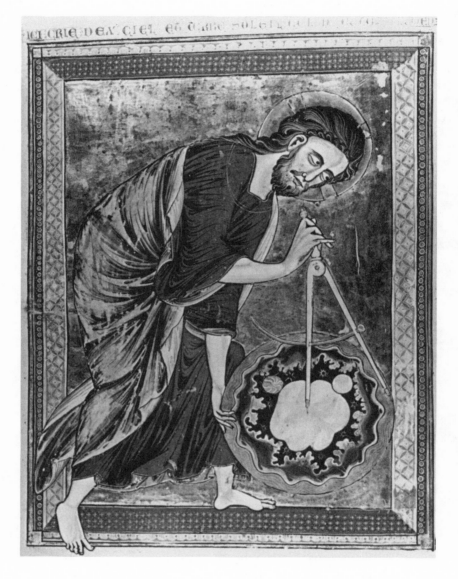

"God as Architect of the Universe" ("Gott als Architekt des Universums"), miniature from the manuscript of the Old Testament *Bible moralisée,* France, thirteenth century, Cod 2554 fol IV. Courtesy Österreichische Nationalbibliothek Bild-
Archiv und Porträt-Sammlung. This *Deus faber* image suggests the Lord's questioning Job "out of the whirlwind": "Where were you when I laid the foundation
of the earth? . . . Who determined its measurements . . . or who stretched the line
upon it?" (Job 38:4–5).[7]

---

while above the roof lie the extended planes or levels, twelve in number, stretched upward to the abode of the "Great Spirit, even the
Creator" as Delaware form puts it. (Speck 1931:22–23)

Domestic architecture is no less sacred, as Eliade (1976:27) makes clear:

> Exactly like the city or sanctuary, the house is sanctified, in whole or in
> part, by a cosmological symbolism or ritual. This is why settling
> somewhere—by building a village or merely a house—represents a
> serious decision, for the very existence of man is involved; he must, in
> short, create his own world and assume the responsibility of maintain-
> ing and renewing it. Habitations are not lightly changed, for it is not
> easy to abandon one's world. The house is not an object, a "machine to
> live in"; *it is the universe that man constructs for himself by imitating the
> paradigmatic creation of the gods, the cosmogony.* . . . Even in modern
> societies, with their high degree of desacralization, the festivity and
> rejoicing that accompany settling in a new house still preserve the
> memory of the festive exuberance that, long ago, marked the *incipit
> vita nova.*

New Year's celebrations provide occasion for renewing cosmogonic
myth and ritual. The "Enuma elish," the Babylonian creation epic, was
recited several times during the twelve-day *akitu,* or New Year's festival
(Heidel 1951:16–17; Johnson 1977). During "world renewal" (New Year's)
rites of the California Karok, Hupa, and Yurok Indians, events that happened "in the beginning" according to mythology are periodically re-
enacted. This "strengthening of the World is accomplished by ritually
rebuilding the steam cabin, a rite that is cosmogonic in structure" (Eliade
1963:44).

Likewise, the installation or consecration of a new ruler—essentially, a
new reign or age—often requires the reiteration of the creation myth. The

Hawaiian *Kumulipo,* or "Beginning-in-deep-darkness," a lengthy cosmo-gonic and genealogical prayer that was never sung casually, usually was used to consecrate and name a chief's son. "This prayer chant . . . traced the family's divine origin by genealogical pairs through great rulers, heroes, and primary gods back to the first spark of life in the universe [and] it linked the family with the spiritual representatives of all phenomena, great and small, on the earth, in the sea, in the heavens, in the spirit world, and in the world of living men" (Katharine Luomala in Beckwith 1972:xiv).

Christianity, too, employs symbols and liturgy from the creation myth in Genesis for the Sacrament of Baptism, the traditional rite (for infants and adults) of entrance into the mysteries and membership in the Christian church. Alan Watts (1968:177–78) describes the blessing of the baptismal font in the Roman Catholic Church of the thirteenth century:

> Arrived at the Font, the priest or bishop proceeds to the solemn consecration of the baptismal waters, singing an invocation . . . :
> O God, whose Spirit in the very beginning of the world moved over the waters, that even the nature of water might receive the virtue of sanctification. . . .
> . . . As God with his "compass" divided the waters of Chaos in the beginning of time, the priest now with his hand divides the water of the Font in the form of a cross, singing:
> Who makes this water fruitful for the regeneration of man by the arcane admixture of his Divine Power, to the end that those who have been conceived in sanctity in the immaculate womb of this divine Font, may be born a new creature, and come forth a heavenly off-spring: and that all who are distinguished either in sex or in body, or by age in time, may be born into one infancy by grace, their mother.

Clearly a male-authorized rite of simulated parturition, the sacrament apparently does not have an equivalent female-authorized rite of midwifery that derives its power from a paradigmatic, primordial procreation.

Knowledge of cosmogony constitutes and validates knowledge of this world. Sam Gill (1977:6–7) describes how, at a meeting to discuss public education programs for Indians, a Papago elder stood and spoke formally and deliberately:

> He began with the creation of the Papago world, by telling how Earthmaker had given the Papago land its shape and character. He

identified the features of that creation with the land on which he had always lived, as had his father and all his grandfathers before him. Pausing in his story, he asked how many of us could locate our heritage so distinctly. . . .

It was perhaps fifteen minutes before he began to speak directly to the subject of education, but the old man had been talking about education all along. He was demonstrating to his audience a basic principle in education: knowledge has meaning and value only when placed within a particular view of the world. He was utilizing the way of his people by consulting the stories of the creation for the proper perspective from which to speak.

The question to be explored in the following chapters is whether the perspective of women, of parturition and procreation, can be equally primary, paradigmatic, and empowering.

2

*Spiders and Spinsters
in Creation Mythology*

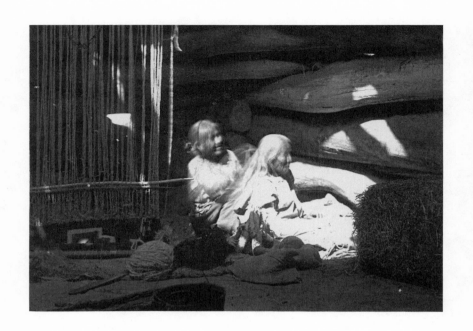

Navajo Indian women combing hair beside loom in hogan, ca. 1915. (Neg. no. 21635, courtesy Photo Collections, Museum of New Mexico, Santa Fe.)

In the beginning Tse che nako, Thought Woman [Old Spider Woman],[1] finished everything, thoughts, and the names of all things. She finished also all the languages. And then our mothers, Uretsete and Naotsete said they would make names and they would make thoughts. Thus they said. Thus they did. (Laguna Pueblo creation myth [Purley 1974:29])

In her historic-geographic analysis of some three hundred versions of North American Indian creation myths, Anna Birgitta Rooth (1957:503—4) identifies one of the eight types as myths with a spider as "creator or first being."

Spider weaves an umbrella-like foundation for the earth, or he fastens with his web or thread the rushes which will be the earth. This motif is interwoven in a secondary manner in the deluge myths where the Spider weaves not the earth but the scaffold which saves people from drowning. In some versions Spiders of different colours fasten down the world at the four world corners.

Such myths are centered in the southern part of North America, with some found northward in the Plains area, and are connected to Mexican tradition, with parallels in the Pacific Islands, East Asia, and India.

Åke Hultkrantz (1979:31) also notes: "In scattered parts of western North America the Supreme Being or another deity occurs as a spider whose web constitutes the foundation of the earth (the Arapaho Indians use a name for the Supreme Being which may be translated 'spider')." His claim, "that the belief in the creator as a spider is an expression of the idea of creation out of nothing [ex nihilo] . . . : the spider weaves his web out of himself," challenges Alan Dundes's psychoanalytic interpretation of these as elemental (and compensatory) cosmogonic myths:

Another anal creation myth which does occur in aboriginal North America has the spider as creator. The Spider myth . . . is reported primarily in California and the Southwest . . . [and] is also found in Asia and Africa. . . . Without going into primitive Spider creation myths in great detail, it should suffice to note that, as in other types of male myths of creation, the creator is able to create without any reference to women. Whether a male creator spins material, molds clay, lays an egg, fabricates from mucus or epidermal tissue, or dives for fecal mud, the psychological motivation is much the same. (Dundes 1962:1045–46)

Few *Deus faber* cosmogonies involving weavers are included in studies of cosmogonic myths. In part, this may be attributed to the androcentrism (and ethnocentrism) implicit in interpretations like the following by Marie-Louise von Franz (1972:88–89):

> Another craft sometimes mentioned in connection with cosmogonic myths is weaving, where the God weaves the whole world on a loom.[2] . . . Weaving is not so often used as an image because it is naturally attributed more to a Goddess, weaving having always been a more feminine activity. . . .
>
> Spinning and weaving activities are connected with the idea of nature. The Goddess of nature is the loom into which God throws the shuttle so as to weave the world. One of the pre-Socratic Greek philosophers, Pherekydes, has the same image: in the beginning there were Zeus and Chthonia, the Earth-Goddess; the Sky-God married the Earth-Goddess, and he wove the whole world as a big mantle and spread it over an oak. . . . But whenever the weaving element is implied, the thing tends towards being more the affair of a Goddess of nature and not of a Creator-God.

When weaving is "the affair" of a male *Deus faber* "Creator-God," Alan Dundes claims, the creation resembles that described in Walt Whitman's "A Noiseless Patient Spider," from the 1891–92 edition of *Leaves of Grass:*

A noiseless patient spider,
I mark'd where on a little promontory it stood isolated,
Mark'd how to explore the vacant vast surrounding,
It launch'd forth filament, filament, filament, out of itself,
Ever unreeling them, ever tirelessly speeding them.

And you O my soul where you stand,
Surrounded, detached, in measureless oceans of space,
Ceaselessly musing, venturing, throwing, seeking the spheres
       to connect them,

Till the bridge you will need be form'd, till the ductile
      anchor hold,
Till the gossamer thread you fling catch somewhere, O my
      soul.

Dundes (1962:1046) calls this spider "the perfect symbol of male artistic creativity . . . detached and alone in 'measureless oceans of space' launching forth filament out of itself."

In contrast is the "woman's work" of the female spider in "Arachne," Rose Terry Cooke's 1860 poem (in Pearson and Pope 1976:208–9):

I watch her in the corner there,
As, restless, bold, and unafraid,
She slips and floats along the air
Till all her subtile house is made.

     . . .

Poor sister of the spinster clan!
I too from out my store within
My daily life and living plan,
My home, my rest, my pleasure spin.

I know thy heart when heartless hands
Sweep all that hard-earned web away:
Destroy its pearled and glittering bands,
And leave thee homeless by the way.

I know thy peace when all is done.
Each anchored thread, each tiny knot,
Soft shining in the autumn sun;
A sheltered, silent, tranquil lot.

I know what thou hast never known,
—Sad presage to a soul allowed;—
That not for life I spin, alone,
But day by day I spin my shroud.

This spider purposefully builds a "subtile house" in a corner and does not endlessly launch filament into "the vacant vast surrounding." Her craft produces a shroud and not a bridge or "ductile anchor" of "gossamer thread" to connect the spheres. Unlike Whitman's isolated spider and poet's soul, Cooke and her "sister" belong to a "spinster clan." An examination of this "clan"—of spiders and spinsters in poems, beliefs, rituals, and myths, especially from non-Western cultures—helps balance and extend notions of cosmogony and female "artistic creativity."

Elemental or Excretory Creation

In the early 1900s, Henriette Rothschild Kroeber collected narratives from Juan Dolores, a trilingual, "educated full-blood member" of the Papago Indian tribe in southern Arizona. One myth contains elemental creation motifs of "natural" accretion and conjunction (of water, darkness, and air), "instinctual" creating by earthworms and spiders, and possibly a *Deus faber* in Older-Brother.

> In the beginning there was nothing but darkness and water. The darkness, the water, and the air composed the whole universe. As they came together, wherever they met, the friction of these bodies, the darkness and the water, finally produced a living being, which lay upon the water and was carried from place to place. Whatever formed this being also fed it, and it grew until it became a great man. He became our "Older-Brother," the first-born.
>
> After he became a man, he saw that there was a substance gathering around him, the bubbles or scum which always gather around an object in the water. He took some of that and made it into earthworms. He sent them around to gather up the stuff he had seen and had already gathered around himself. They went about and gathered and gathered, and left it all around him. They kept on piling up and piling up. Finally he found himself on a little piece of dry land. . . .
>
> After the earth was made, it kept on floating. It had no steady place. So Older-Brother made spiders, and sent them all around to tie the earth down. So they went around and made their web, and tied the earth and left it on the water. Then the earth had a steady place. (Kroeber 1912:95–96)[3]

The Papago helper-spiders' cosmogonic contributions, like the earthworms', seem to be "lesser"—"merely" instinctive, virtually excretory.

Empirical observation of spiders would quite easily give rise to the notion of the spider as a self-sufficient creator who appeared to excrete his own world, and a beautiful and artistic world at that. Although psychoanalysts have generally tended to interpret the spider as a mother symbol . . . , Freud noted at least one instance in folklore where the thread spun by a spider was a symbol for evacuated feces. In a Prussian-Silesian tale, a peasant wishing to return to earth from heaven is turned into a spider by Peter. As a spider, the peasant spins a long thread by which he descends, but he is horrified to discover as he arrives just over his home that he could spin no more. He squeezes and squeezes to make the thread longer and then suddenly wakes up from his dream to discover that "something very human had happened to him while he slept." (Dundes 1962:1045–46; citing Freud and Oppenheim 1958:45)

"Empirical observation" need not be confined to the excretory, however. For example, William K. Powers (1986:155–56) reports that

the Lakota regard the spider as the wisest of all creatures, and part of this reasoning is based on observations of real spider behavior.

According to Lakota medicine men with whom I have spoken, the spider is the most knowledgeable of creatures because he is the most ubiquitous; he lives and travels everywhere. Ellis Chips, the grandson of the well-known Yuwipi man, Horn Chips, told me that spiders walk on the ground and walk underground. They can fly, and they can also swim. They can be found anywhere even in the most remote places, and there is nowhere a person can go without being seen or heard by spiders.

Because of their ability to traverse the four important planes of Lakota cosmology—the sky, the place between the sky and the clouds, the earth, and beneath the earth—they are particularly knowledgeable about sacred things.

These Lakota beliefs recall Mircea Eliade's interpretation of lunar, ritual spider imagery: "Not for nothing is she [Moon] envisaged in myth as an immense spider—an image you will find used by a great many peoples. For to weave is not merely to predestine (anthropologically), and to join together differing realities (cosmologically) but also to *create,* to make something of one's own substance as the spider does in spinning its web" (Eliade 1958:181). Essence, not excreta, is symbolically and ritually crucial. Making "something of one's own substance" is essential—sacrificial and sacramental, not simply the expulsion and/or manipulation of wastes.

In the tenth part of her 1977 poem "Natural Resources," Adrienne Rich (1978:64–65) captures this sense of substance and sacrament in the female spider's passionate, intentioned creativity:

> *This is what I am:* watching the spider
> rebuild—"patiently," they say,
>
> But I recognize in her
> impatience—my own—
>
> the passion to make and make again
> where such unmaking reigns
>
> the refusal to be a victim
> *we have lived with violence so long*
>
> Am I to go on saying
> for myself, for her
>
> *This is my body,*
> *take and destroy it?*

Spiritual or Ex Nihilo *Creation*

In his 1924 lecture, "Monotheism among Primitive Peoples," Paul Radin discusses an *ex nihilo,* masculine, dream-creation myth published by Konrad T. Preuss (1921:166–68). As translated literally by Renate Lewis from Preuss's literal German text, the beginning of this Colombian Uitoto Indian cosmogony reads:

> 1. A phantasm. Nothing else was. A phantasm touched the Father. He grasped something mysterious. Nothing existed. Through a dream, the Father Nainuema (He who has or is the vision) held on and explored it. 2. Not even a tree existed. He held the phantasm with a dream-thread, with breath. . . . 3. Then the Father again sought the bottom of this thing, touched the base of the empty phantasm. The Father tied the dream-thread, pressed it on the emptiness with magic glue. Thus he dreamed, and the magic adhesive held it like tobacco smoke or a fluff of raw cotton. (Weigle and Johnson 1979:1)[4]

Radin (1954:13, 14) calls this a "poetic account" by a Uitoto "monotheist" and "religious man" that "represents an attempt to solve the riddle of creation by postulating something that existed before the beginning, and our primitive philosopher and theologian has quite logically assumed that the appearance of things preceded their actual existence . . . an admirable solution."

What Radin and the anthologists (e.g., Astrov 1962:325–26; Rothenberg 1968:27; Bierhorst 1976:40–41) who tout this text as a prime example of *ex nihilo* "spiritual" cosmogony fail to note is the similarity between the Father's creation by dream-thread or breath and the spider's creation. Rather than comparing (usually unfavorably) Father Nainuema to Elohim and other male supreme deities of "high culture" religions, then, it might be more hermeneutically appropriate to compare him with other male and female "spider" creators like those in Southwest Pueblo and Navajo Indian cultural beliefs.

According to Hamilton A. Tyler (1964:82),

The beginning goddess of the Keres Indians is "Thinking Woman," or to use the spelling of Sia pueblo, Sus'sistinako. She seems to belong to the underworld, but her creative capacity for "thinking outward into space," a kind of silent Logos which brings everything into existence, indicates a close relationship with the upper, if not the heavenly, world. There is some ambivalence about the sex of Thinking Woman, as at Sia she is male.

Tyler himself displays some ambivalence in his implicitly sexist devaluation of the underworld and earth goddesses, his preference for the upper or heavenly worlds, and his unease about a female's *ex nihilo* creation via "a kind of silent Logos." He also cites:

Another view from the Western Keres . . . from a curious man of the last century, John M. Gunn,[5] who wrote a book [1917] on the many things he knew about Acoma and Laguna. Unfortunately he made no literal transcriptions, but he has this to say of Thinking Woman: "Their theory is that reason (personified) is the supreme power, a master mind that has always existed, which they call Sitch-tche-na-ko. This is the feminine form for thought or reason. She had one sister, Shro-tu-na-ko, memory or instinct. Their belief is that Sitch-tche-na-ko is the creator of all, and to her they offer their most devout prayers."

However lofty a conception this goddess may be, it seems that when she has a form it is that of a spider, and in the popular mind she is often equated with Spider Grandmother. (Tyler 1964:90–91)

To suggest that such theriomorphic manifestation compromises a seemingly "lofty" creator goddess seems a gratuitous, if not sexist, qualification.

No such reservations vitiate Paula Gunn Allen's feminist description of Thought Woman in her Keresan Pueblo tradition at Laguna:

> The Keres conceptualize the supreme being as a puzzling figure commonly referred to as Old Spider, Grandmother Spider, or Spider Woman. Spider Woman's Keres name is translated as Thought Woman (it can be better understood if translated as Creating-through-Thinking Woman). She is the Dreamer, the ritual center, who sang her sister goddesses Uretsete and Naotsete into life and taught them the rituals they used to sing everything in their baskets, their medicine bundles, into being. Among the things in their baskets were the heavens, the waters, the mountains, the earth, the katsina (spirit messengers and protectors), the creatures, and the plants. (Allen 1986:98–99)

Comparable creative omnipotence and omnipresence is attributed to Thought Woman by Leslie Marmon Silko (like Allen of part Laguna Pueblo ancestry) in the epigraph to her novel *Ceremony* (1977:1):

> Ts'its'tsi'nako, Thought-Woman,
>   is sitting in her room
> and whatever she thinks about
>   appears.
>
>   She thought of her sisters,
>   Nau'ts'ity'i and I'tcts'ity'i,
> and together they created the Universe
>   this world
> and the four worlds below.
>
> Thought-Woman, the spider,
>   named things and
> as she named them
>   they appeared.
>
> She is sitting in her room
> thinking of a story now
>
> I'm telling you the story
>   she is thinking.

Artificial or Artisan Creation

In 1908 Father Berard Haile, O.F.M., recorded from Gishin Biye' a version of the Navajo creation myth associated with the healing ceremony variously known as Upward-moving-way, Moving-up-way, Upward-reaching-way, and Emergence-way. At the Place of Emergence into this (herein, the fourth) world, on the "Eleventh Speech" Level, just below the "Twelfth Speech" Level of our world, scouts Mountain Sheep and Hunch-eye have descended to escape the terrible noise of rushing waters separating in the world above. They report to the people assembled below:

> "It's frightful up there," they said, and after they had told what they had done, the people turned to Spider Man and Woman for help. The Spider Man then blew a dark web to the mouth of the opening and followed this with a yellow one, while the Spider Woman furnished a blue and white one so that there were four webs covering the opening. And these hung over it as four curtains, a black, yellow, blue and white one so that no water might pass through it. And this prevented the water from rushing upon the people below, for even today you do not observe water passing through a spider's web.
>
> The noise and rush of the water above lasted something like four days—after which it ceased. The Spider Man and Spider Woman then inhaled their webs again and the light shone through the opening. (Haile 1981:121)

This "spidery" form of the word is discussed in Gary Witherspoon's study of Navajo culture, "Creating the World through Language." He (1977:39) explains his intellectual Navajo friends' conceptions of ritual language as "the means of transforming chaos into cosmos [in healing ceremonies], but it can also be used to reduce cosmos to chaos [in witchcraft]." According to Witherspoon (1977:17), "Thinking and singing the world into existence attributes a definite kind of power to thought and song to which most Westerners are not accustomed. It is rather obvious that the Navajo ontological conception of thought and speech is very different from our own."

A concept of wind is fundamental to that ontology, as James Kale McNeley (1981:1) maintains:

> Nilch'i, meaning Wind, Air, or Atmosphere, as conceived by the Navajo, is endowed with powers that are not acknowledged in West-

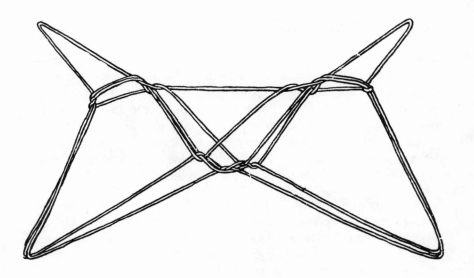

---

ern culture. Suffusing all of nature, Holy Wind gives life, thought, speech, and the power of motion to all living things and serves as the means of communication between all elements of the living world. As such, it is central to Navajo philosophy and world view.

This power is evident in a version of the emergence recorded on August 5, 1885, by Alexander M. Stephen from Guisheen Bige (Gishin Biye'), then a Navajo priest at Keams Canyon, Arizona. Bige tells how, in the underworld, the people

> made a hole in the reed in the side of the shaft and the people got inside and Old Man went in last, but Wunustcinde (locust) got up to the top of the reed and sat upon a leaf. As the reed began to move upward [from the underworld] Wunustcinde began to make a noise through the holes in his thorax and as he did so the reed began to shake like wind. Black Wind shook it at the roots and made it move. The reed grew up higher and higher. The water now covered all the earth, everything except this reed which kept growing and Wunustcinde was always on the leaf at the top. As the reed grew, the water continued to rise; as Wunustcinde made his noise, the reed kept growing and Black Wind kept blowing at the roots and the people became aware that they were close to the roof of the world and did not know what to do as there was no space left for them between the surface of the water and the under side of this earth. Wunustcinde stopped his noise and Black Wind stopped blowing, and the reed stopped growing. They did not know what to do . . . [and] they could not find a hole anywhere nor any way to get out. They were frightened and thought they would all die there. But the Spider Woman wove a web on the surface of the water. It floated like a raft and all the people got out and sat upon it. (Stephen 1930:94)

Spider Woman's crafted, cosmogonic contribution is not relegated to a remote, mythic world; her beneficent web is recreated every time a Navajo woman weaves—or when any Navajo makes the string figures known in

Anglo tradition as cat's cradle. Barre Toelken reports that a teenage Navajo woman in southeastern Utah told him: "The Spider Woman taught us all these [string] designs as a way of helping us think. You learn to think when you make these. And she taught us about weaving, too." Her father demonstrated a number of string figures, some related to stellar constellations, and explained their significance:

> "These are all matters we need to know. It's too easy to become sick, because there are always things happening to confuse our minds. We need to have ways of thinking, of keeping things stable, healthy, beautiful. We try for a long life, but lots of things happen to us. So we keep our thinking in order by these figures and we keep our lives in order with the stories. We have to relate our lives to the stars and the sun, the animals, and to all of nature or else we will go crazy, or get sick." (Toelken 1979:95, 96; also Reichard 1974:467–69)

Clearly, Spider Woman's discipline is paradigmatic for the continual, ritual recreation of cosmic and human harmony.[6]

Weaving, spinning, and the sheep's growing wool are also integral cosmological processes. According to Toelken (1976b:19),

> The Navajos explain the relationship there not in terms of the rug, the end product—which, of course, is what our culture is interested in—but in terms of the relationship with the yarn and with the sheep, and with the spinning of the yarn, which has to be done in a certain direction because it goes along with everything else that is spinning. . . . Thus, the yarn itself becomes a further symbol of man's interaction with the animal on the one hand, and with the whole of the cosmos on the other. When one works with yarn one is working with something that remains a symbol of the cyclic or circular interaction with nature.

This is a far cry from the female plaiter and weaver's compensatory "interaction with nature" proposed by Sigmund Freud in "Femininity," lecture 33 of his 1933 *New Introductory Lectures on Psycho-Analysis*:

> It seems that women have made few contributions to the discoveries and inventions of the history of civilization; there is, however, one technique which they may have invented—that of plaiting and weav-

ing. If that is so, we should be tempted to guess the unconscious motive for the achievement. Nature herself would seem to have given the model which this achievement imitates by causing the growth at maturity of the pubic hair that conceals the genitals. The step that remained to be taken lay in making the threads adhere to one another, while on the body they stick into the skin and are only matted together. If you reject this idea as fantastic and regard my belief in the influence of lack of a penis on the configuration of femininity as an *idée fixe,* I am of course defenceless. (Strouse 1974:90–91)

Navajo women, in stark contrast to Freud's ludicrous contention, view their creation as an important healing discipline. In spinning,

the spindle must be turned in one direction ("clockwise") . . . , for it represents the direction of the sun's movement; to spin the yarn by turning the spindle "backward" would be to produce yarn which represents the reverse of the normal state, yarn which will "come unravelled," "won't stay in the rugs" and "might cause sickness." It matters little whether the yarn might really physically come unravelled, for Navajo health beliefs are ritual and psychosomatic: the *idea* of unravelling is a greater reality and therefore a greater threat to health and stability than mere physical "fact." (Toelken 1976a:33–34)

Weaving, according to Gary Witherspoon (1977:161), is for Navajo women "an effort in creative transformation":

Navajo women develop and create designs in their minds, and then project them onto the world of external reality through the art of weaving. The intricate and often complex patterns created by Navajo weavers are generated in the mind and kept there through the whole process from dyeing through weaving. She must know exactly how much dye to use or exactly what amounts of black and white wool to mix in order to get the very exact color combinations and contrasts she has in her mind. In carrying out the design on the loom, she must keep the design in her mind in two ways:

The weaver must keep the composition of the entire rug surface in her mind, but she must see it as a huge succession of stripes only one weft strand wide. It matters not how ideal her general conception may be, if she cannot see it in terms of the narrowest stripe, meaning a row, of properly placed wefts, it will fail of execution (Reichard, 1968:86).

This is what is necessary for the weaver to maintain control of her composition, and to carry it out effectively. Weaving thus requires a unique combination and coordination of conceptual and manual skills. A woven rug is a product of the mind and the body. The inner form of the rug is in the mind; the outer form of the rug is projected onto the loom.

Among the Pueblos, weaving is generally a male activity, but no less transformative than in Navajo culture. Spider Woman's cosmogonic sacrament is a powerful paradigm for her spinster progeny of both sexes, as evident in Paula Gunn Allen's 1977 poem, "Grandmother" (1978:50):

Out of her body she pushed
silver thread, light, air
and carried it carefully on the dark, flying
where nothing moved.

Out of her body she extruded
shining wire, life, and wove the light
on the void.

From beyond time,
beyond oak trees and bright clear water flow,
she was given the work of weaving the strands
of her body, her pain, her vision
into creation, and the gift of having made it,
to disappear.

After her,
the women and the men weave blankets into tales of life,
memories of light and ladders,
infinity-eyes, and rain.
After her I sit on my laddered rain-bearing rug
and mend the tear with string.

Spinster as Trickster Creator

While doing fieldwork at Zia Pueblo in the fall of 1928, Leslie A. White discovered that "the most important deity in Sia [*sic*] cosmology is

Tsityosti·nako, 'Prophesying Woman' . . . [so-called] because 'she knows (rather than deciding, or determining) what is going to happen'; one informant added 'when a person is thinking about doing something that is Tsityostinako expressing herself in him.'" Those informants also told him that the creator deity "had the shape of a certain kind of spider." A Zia man recounted a commonly known version of the "creation and emergence" myth, which began as follows:

> In the beginning were Tsityostinako and her daughters, Utctsiti and Naotsiti. There were clouds and fog (he.yac) everywhere. There were four worlds. The bottom world was Yellow. Above this was a Blue-green world. Above that was a Red world. And on top was the White world. Tsityostinako and her daughters were in the Yellow world.
>
> Utctsiti and Naotsiti had a naback' (a "manta," or blanket) and a Djacoma (cane) to create things with. Utctsiti created tiamunyi (cacique) first. She told him that he would have to take care of the people and love them as a mother loves her children. Tsityostinako and her daughters were sitting like tcaiyanyi (medicinemen) in a ceremonial house. Tsityostinako was sitting between her daughters. They spread the naback'(manta) on the floor in front of them and put the cane (Djacoma) on top of it. Then, with magic and songs, they created things under the manta. Then they would pick up the manta and see what they had created. Tsityostinako could not be seen, but she was there, and it was she who put ideas into Utctsiti's and Naotsiti's heads. After they had created something, Tsityostinako would explain why it had been created. The daughters would take turns: first Utctsiti would create something, then Naotsiti would. (White 1962:113, 115)

The cooperative and caring turn-taking in the Zia ritual creation contrasts with the competitive, combative testing-contesting in male creation myths like those Rooth (1957:503) identifies as The Two Creators, The Blind Brother, and "some myths where the Spider praises his ability to stand on the water or float in the air as he did in the beginning of the world . . . [or] in a contest with other boasting competitors the Spider wins." Nevertheless, there is an element of surprise and a kind of trickery in Utctsiti and Naotsiti's creations under the manta. They do not recognize their productions until their mother explains them. In this respect Tsityostinako resembles the Lakota spider trickster Inktomi, who led the people from the earth during their emergence.

In his study of "supernatural discourse in Lakota," based on fieldwork

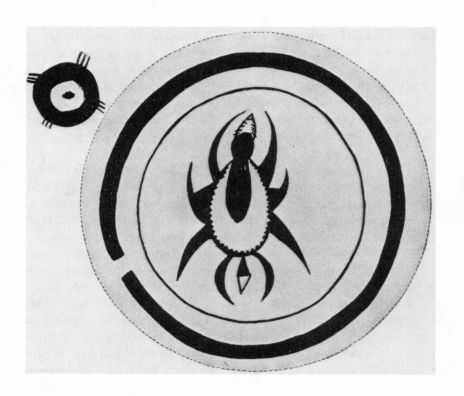

Sun and spider symbols on prehistoric Hopi pottery. "In Hopi mythology the spider and the sun are associated, the former being the symbol of an earth goddess" (Fewkes 1973:150; plate 87c).

---

during the 1960s and 1970s, William K. Powers discusses "the paradox of Inktomi" in a chapter entitled "Naming the Sacred." According to Powers (1986:153):

> Although the creation of the universe is seen by most people as a theological statement about first causes, one may look at the same stories profitably from the point of view of classification. The creation story in any culture is an attempt to put the chaotic universe that surrounds humans into some kind of order, and part of the mechanism used to accomplish this is the simple act of naming everything.

The culture hero Inktomi performs this creation.

> And it was by the act of naming that Inktomi differentiated all natural phenomena. He is given the credit for having not only named all species, but for having assigned them their distinctive colorations, configurations and behaviors. He also is credited for having taught humans how to obtain and prepare food and how to make clothing and shelters from otherwise natural phenomena. But Inktomi himself, important as he was to the establishment of Lakota culture, remains a paradox. He who served to distinguish between all living things as well as inanimate forms was destined never to have his own distinguishable features. Inktomi, one might say, in the process of naming the constituent elements of the entire Lakota universe, never named himself. As a matter of fact, the term Inktomi refers to only one of his many shapes and forms that he is capable of assuming, the spider, and it is a term that he never uses when he addresses himself. (W. K. Powers 1986:154)

As trickster, Inktomi "can change himself into virtually anything or anybody" (Powers 1986:155)—of any nature or gender. This ability suggests the classical Greek notion of *mētis,* what Ann L. T. Bergren (1983:73) calls the "intellectual counterpart" of weaving:

> As Detienne and Vernant [1978:27–53] have shown, *mētis* denotes throughout Greek thought the power of transformation, the power to

change shape continuously or to imitate the shape of your enemy and defeat him at his own game. It is both a strategy of deception, the plot itself, and the mental ability to devise one. The connection between the woman, weaving, and *mētis* is explicit in two divine figures, the goddess Metis and her daughter Athena, goddess of weaving and as she herself says, "famous among all the gods for *mētis*" (*Od.* 13.299).

A key text for this is the myth of Tereus, Procne, and Philomela.[7]

> When Tereus, the husband of Procne, rapes her sister Philomela, he cuts out the woman's tongue to keep her silent, but Philomela, according to Apollodorus (3.14.8), *huphēnasa en peplōi grammata* "wove pictures/writing (*grammata* can mean either) in a robe" which she sent to her sister. Philomela's trick reflects the "trickiness" of weaving, its uncanny ability to make meaning out of inarticulate matter, to make silent material speak. In this way, women's weaving is, as *grammata* implies, a "writing" or graphic art, a silent, material representation of audible, immaterial speech. (Bergren 1983:72)

In classical Greek culture, according to Bergren (1983:71), "Greek women do not speak, they weave. Semiotic woman is a weaver. Penelope is, of course, the paradigm." Thus, Herodotus (2.35) could remark on critical inversions in Egyptian culture:

> The Egyptians themselves in their manners and customs seem to have reversed the ordinary practices of mankind. For instance, women attend market and are employed in trade, while men stay at home and do the weaving. In weaving the normal way is to work the threads of the weft upwards, but the Egyptians work them downwards. Men in Egypt carry loads on their heads, women on their shoulders; women pass water standing up, men sitting down. (trans. Aubrey de Selincourt, in Burn 1972:142)

In Herodotus's own society, these reversals were enacted metaphorically, for "Greek culture inherits from Indo-European a metaphor by which poets and prophets define themselves as 'weaving' or 'sewing' words . . . [and] describe their activity in terms of what is originally and literally woman's work *par excellence*" (Bergren 1983:72).

That kind of "woman's work," however, is both cosmogonic and creative. It is a creation like that of the spinster trickster in Apache/Comanche Judith Mountain Leaf (Ivaloo) Volborth's 1979 poem, "Self-Portrait":

> Crooked Old Woman
> sits, composes shadows,
> weaves tapestries
> of dust and cobwebs,
> sings to the lines
> in her face.

3

Creator and Procreator

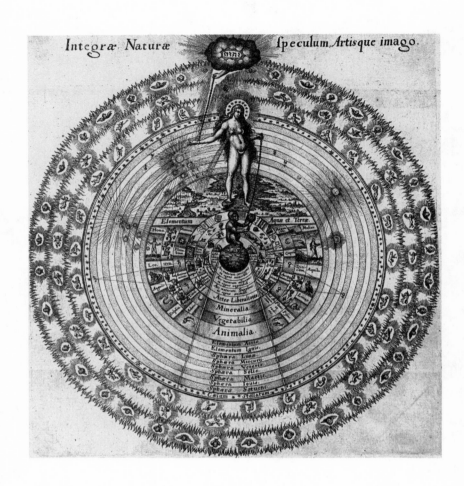

Engraving by Johann Theodore de Bry from Robert Fludd's *Utriusque cosmi* (Oppenheim, 1617–21), vol. I, frontispiece (see Chapter 1, note 2). Courtesy, The Bancroft Library, University of California, Berkeley.

Emile Grillot de Givry (1973:215, fig. 179) entitles this "Nature and her Ape, Art, according to the Adepts." It is related to another de Bry/Fludd engraving, "The Universe wholly Created" (fig. 178), which shows earth surrounded by water (with fishes), air (with birds), fire, "the circles of the seven planets, the heaven of the fixed stars, and lastly the empyrean, or Abode of the Blessed." The present engraving of "the Mirror of Nature and the image of Art" shows the same arrangement with Nature and Art added. "Nature . . . is represented by a woman crowned with stars, like the Virgin, and bearing the crescent moon of Diana upon her body. She holds her power directly from the Lord, one of Whose arms is seen extended from a cloud. The Divine name in four letters shines on the surface of the cloud. The Lord keeps Nature in his power by a chain fastened to her arm, but she in her turn holds the Art of mankind . . . by another chain. Art is wholly subject to her, and is represented by an ape, in order to show that man, with all his wise and subtle knowledge, will never be more than the ape of Nature. Art is seated upon the terrestrial globe, which he has made his own; he is measuring a small copy of it with a pair of callipers. The whole of his surroundings show the results of the sophistications by which he has transformed the elements and altered the surface of the globe. The four elements have become the animal, vegetable, and mineral kingdoms; animals and plants have been classified, metals extracted from the bowels of the earth. Man has discovered geomancy, mathematics, music, painting, and the art of fortification; he has measured time and constructed clocks, 'improved Nature in the mineral kingdom' by employing retort and cucurbit distillation, 'helped Nature in the vegetable kingdom' by cultivating the soil and grafting, and 'supplemented Nature in the animal kingdom' by the art of medicine and the rearing of bees and domestic poultry" (de Givry 1973:212, 214).[1]

Our Father who art in heaven,
Hallowed be thy name. (Matthew 6:9)

Our mother of the growing fields, our mother of the streams, will have
pity upon us. For to whom do we belong? Whose seeds are we? To our
mother alone do we belong. (Kagaba Indian prayer collected by Konrad T. Preuss [in Radin 1954:15])

One of Roland Barthes' 1957 *Mythologies,* "Novels and Children,"[2] is a
photograph posed for the French women's weekly *Elle.* Pictured are seventy women novelists who have produced both books and babies. *Elle* has
thus captured specimens of a mythic creature, "the woman of letters . . . a
remarkable zoological species: she brings forth, pell-mell, novels and children" (Barthes 1972:50).

At first glance this seems a mythology of parthenogenetic, fecund, and
potent great mothers. "At a pinch, and by dint of seeing seventy times
books and kids bracketed together, one would think that they are equally
the fruits of imagination and dream, the miraculous products of an ideal
parthenogenesis able to give at once to women, apparently, the Balzacian
joys of creation and the tender joys of motherhood." But this is illusory, for,
like a supreme deity who has withdrawn from his creation to the heavens,
man is "nowhere and everywhere, like the sky, the horizon, an authority
which at once determines and limits a condition." As the empyrean encir-
cles the cosmos, or the Lord chains Nature, "Man is never inside, . . .
but . . . everywhere around, he presses on all sides, he makes everything
exist; he is in all eternity the creative absence, that of the Racinian deity: the
feminine world of *Elle,* a world without men, but entirely constituted by
the gaze of man, is very exactly that of the gynaeceum" (Barthes 1972:51).

The world of *Elle* is a natural, chthonic, and material one of earth,
pillars, nursery, and gynaeceum walls; the world of *Il* is ethereal, spiritual,
celestial, and metaphysical. The two are not far from the cosmos imagined
by philosopher Hartley Burr Alexander in the interpretations of the "great
mysteries of the North American Indians" that he was preparing for publication before his death in 1939:

Man is of the sky, woman is of the earth: Zeus is $\pi\alpha\tau\dot{\eta}\rho$, Gē is
$\mu\dot{\eta}\tau\eta\rho$, and from their union issues the Birth, which the Hellenes
named the *Physis,* and we, after the Latins, call *Nature.* There is
something chill and austere and battlefree in the wind-swept blue; the
squadrons of the clouds are there, and the birds of war, with their

flashes of levin and their heavy bolts; and there the Sun, *Invictus,* is chieftain, and leads his war-bands in the seasonal Titanomachies of the heavens; thence also descends the bearded rain of *Pluvius,* whereby recipient Earth is made fertile and life-productive. The green, on the other hand, is a warmer and more intimate and sedentary being; it is she who is the nourisher of life, she who gives breast to her children, she, too, who cherishingly receives back into herself the bodies of her brood . . . , so that they may be born again, and nature be ever renewed. . . . Quite directly this is the image which underlies cosmogonies—procreation and birth, parents and child—where with an understanding deeper than has perhaps been surmised, men have everywhere mythically divined that nothing less than a *vital* force could have produced a world wherein man himself vitally stands, the conscious offspring of Sky and Earth. (Alexander 1953:80)

Whatever the parental "*vital* force," however, it still "grounds" women, and Alexander might well concur with Barthes' *Elle* that the nature of women (if not of Nature herself) is procreation. This is both a biological and a biblical condition, a primary imperative. If obeyed, then women may, like men, attempt "the superior status of creation," but only if they "always remember that man exists, and that you are not made like him" (Barthes 1972:51). If that dogma is not compromised, then the woman pro/creator may become, in alchemist Robert Fludd's terms, both the Lord's handmaiden and her own ape's ape:

Women, be therefore courageous, free; play at being men, write like them; but never get far from them; live under their gaze, compensate for your books by your children; enjoy a free rein for a while, but quickly come back to your condition. One novel, one child, a little feminism, a little connubiality. Let us tie the adventure of art to the strong pillars of the home: both will profit a great deal from this combination: where myths are concerned, mutual help is always fruitful. (Barthes 1972:50)

Such mythic pro/creator women are anomalous, curious, and finally, perhaps, inconsequential as creators, culture heroines, or trickster/transformers. For the mythological domain, in theory at least, is peopled with supreme deities measured by the standards of "high" cultures' monotheism and nature deities dismissed as exemplifying "primitive" cultures' animism, and women are more often associated with the latter.[3] In what follows these domains are viewed through the "mythologies" of their early "photographers"—an outline of the nineteenth-century mythographers' gynaeceum.

Supreme Deities and Monotheism

All the Lenape [Delaware] so far questioned, whether followers of the native or of the Christian religion, unite in saying that their people have always believed in a chief *Mani 'to,* a leader of all the gods, in short, a Great Spirit or Supreme Being, the other *mani 'towuk* for the greater part being merely agents appointed by him. His name, according to present Unami usage is *Gicelĕmû 'kaong,* usually translated "great spirit," but meaning literally, "creator." Directly, or through the *mani 'towuk* his agents, he created the earth and everything in it, and gave to the Lenape all they possessed, "the trees, the waters, the fire that springs from flint,—everything." To him the people pray in their greatest ceremonies, and give thanks for the benefits he has given them. Most of their direct worship, however, is addressed to the *mani 'towuk* his agents, to whom he has given charge of the elements, and with whom the people feel they have a closer personal relation, as their actions are seen in every sunrise and thunderstorm, and felt in every wind that blows across woodland and prairie. Moreover, as the Creator lives in the twelfth or highest heaven above the earth, it takes twelve shouts or cries to reach his ear. (Harrington 1921:18–19)

Naturist Daniel G. Brinton is an American proponent of comparative philologist Max Müller's European school of solar mythology.[4] In his 1868 study, *The Myths of the New World: A Treatise on the Symbolism and Mythology of the Red Race in America,*

a work reprinted for the remainder of the century [3d rev. ed. 1896], Brinton compared the origin and creation myths and culture-hero legends of North and South American Indian tribes, to ascertain their inner meanings. The tropes of language and rites of worship offered him clues, and before long he had found the answer. "As the dawn brings light, and with light is associated in every human mind the ideas of knowledge, safety, protection, majesty, divinity, as it dispels the spectres of night, as it defines the cardinal points, and brings forth the sun and the day, it occupied the primitive mind to an extent that can hardly be magnified beyond the truth."

Primeval man worshipped no brutes, but his own dim perception of the One, construed as lightness and whiteness. Hence the first White men were regarded as gods. (Dorson 1965:48)

According to Brinton (1976:46–47), this celestial hegemony informs notions of supreme deities.

The heavens, the upper regions, are in every religion the supposed abode of the divine. What is higher is always the stronger and the nobler; a *superior* is one who is better than we are, and therefore a chieftain in Algonkin is called *oghee-ma*, the higher one. Proud, in Latin *superbus,* is in Dakota *wakanicidapi,* etymologically the same. There is, moreover, a naif and spontaneous instinct which leads man in his ecstasies of joy, and in his paroxysms of fear or pain, to lift his hands and eyes to the overhanging firmament. There the sun and bright stars sojourn, emblems of glory and stability. Its azure vault has a mysterious attraction which invites the eye to gaze longer and longer into its infinite depths. Its color brings thoughts of serenity, peace, sunshine, and warmth. Even the rudest hunting tribes felt these sentiments, and as a metaphor in their speeches, and as a paint expressive of friendly design, blue was in wide use among them.

So it came to pass that the idea of God was linked to the heavens long ere man asked himself, are the heavens material and God spiritual, is He one, or is He many? Numerous languages bear trace of this. The Latin Deus, the Greek Zeus, the Sanscrit Dyaus, the Chinese Tien, all originally referred to the sky above, and our own word heaven is often employed synonymously with God.

Brinton's formulations, like most of his mythographer contemporaries', are ethnocentric and androcentric. In "Monotheism among Primitive Peoples," the Arthur Davis Memorial Lecture delivered to the Jewish Historical Society in 1924,[5] Paul Radin (1954:3) emphasizes the ethnocentrism, if not the androcentrism, in most accounts of supreme deities and monotheism, since "many of our best works on the subject come from priests and missionaries who naturally and understandably begin with certain preoccupations which often make their data and their conclusions somewhat biased."[6]

To most men [sic] monotheism is intimately bound up with the Hebrew Scriptures and with those religions manifestly built upon its foundation—Judaism, Christianity and Mohammedanism. Because of the definite association with these three historic faiths of the last three thousand years, and of the integral part it plays in those civilizations which, rightly or wrongly, we regard in many ways as representing the highest cultural expressions to which man has hitherto attained, monotheism has come to have a very specific meaning and has been given a special evaluation. (Radin 1954:5; also 1957a:342)

Radin refers to an earlier address by C. Buchanan Gray, part of the 1922–23 proceedings of the Oxford Society of Historical Theology, on three stages in the historical evolution of Hebrew monotheism: "monolatry, i.e. a belief in a Supreme Being but the persistence of the worship of other deities at the same time; implicit monotheism, i.e. a belief in a Supreme Deity yet no definite denial of the existence of other gods, and lastly explicit monotheism, a belief in a Supreme Deity and a denial of the existence of other gods" (Radin 1954:22). It is only "the last stage, that of Deutero-Isaiah, [that] gives us the definite formulation that there is no God but one," and that belief "cannot be definitely traced back beyond the sixth century" (Radin 1954:27; also 1957a:368).

Monotheism is also found "among practically all primitive peoples," and the only appropriate question is ethnographic: "whether we find a pure monotheism and not some form of monolatry or henotheism and whether it is the belief of a comparatively small number of individuals, a special group, or of the tribe as such" (Radin 1954:3).

Explicit monotheism, it is true, is rare among primitive peoples, but it is possibly not quite so uncommon as the literal reading of the facts might seem to indicate. Knowing the tremendous part symbolism plays in the interpretation of religious phenomena, particularly the Godhead in our own civilizations, what right have we to assume that it played an inferior role in avowedly similar temperaments among primitive peoples especially when it is universally admitted that symbolism permeates every aspect of primitive man's culture? What the facts really are it is admittedly difficult to ascertain, but from my own experience I am inclined to assume that a limited number of explicit monotheists are to be found in every primitive tribe that has at all developed the concept of a Supreme Creator. (Radin 1954:28–29; also 1957a:371–72)

Monotheists in any culture, Radin claims, "have sprung from the ranks of the eminently religious individuals." These individuals, apparently, are men.

> I feel quite convinced that the idealist and the materialist, the dreamer and the realist, the introspective and the non-introspective man have always been with us. . . . If individuals with specific temperaments, for instance the religious-aesthetic, have always existed we should expect to find them expressing themselves in much the same way at all times. . . . The pagan polytheistic religions are replete with instances of men—poets, philosophers, priests—who have given utterance to definitely monotheistic beliefs. It is characteristic of such individuals, I contend, always to picture the world as a unified whole, always to postulate some First Cause. (Radin 1954:25; also 1957a:365–66)

The envisioned First Cause is generally male,[7] and Radin identifies only one female supreme deity, from the Kagaba of northern Colombia. He quotes the following "profession of faith" from Konrad Theodor Preuss's 1922 *Die hochste Gottheit bei den kulturarmen Volkern:*

> "The mother of our songs, the mother of all our seed, bore us in the beginning of things and so she is the mother of all types of men, the mother of all nations. She is the mother of the thunder, the mother of the streams, the mother of trees and of all things. She is the mother of the world and of the older brothers, the stone-people. She is the mother of the fruits of the earth and of all things. She is the mother of our younger brothers, the French and the strangers. She is the mother of our dance paraphernalia, of all our temples and she is the only mother we possess. She alone is the mother of the fire and the Sun and the Milky Way. . . . She is the mother of the rain and the only mother we possess. And she has left us a token in all the temples . . . a token in the form of songs and dances." (Radin 1954:15; also 1957a:357–58)[8]

It would seem, according to Radin, that this might "satisfy even the most exacting monotheist," being a supreme creator as defined by Andrew Lang in his 1898 *The Making of Religion:* "Such a deity had no cults; prayers were only infrequently directed to him and he rarely intervened directly in the affairs of mankind." He was "Creator of all things, beneficent and ethical, unapproachable directly and taking but little interest in the world after he has created it" (Radin 1954:8; also 1957a:346, 347). But the Kagaba deity is somewhat suspect for two reasons: (1) "there are traces, however faint they may be, of a direct intervention of the All-Mother of the Kagaba in the ordinary affairs of man," and (2) "no origin myth has been recorded" (1954:15; also 1957a:358–59).

Supreme creator deities untainted by hints of the first suspicion are the Pawnee of Oklahoma's Tirawa, who "rules from his position beyond the clouds and has both created and governs the universe by means of commands executed by lesser gods who are subject to him," and the Winnebago of Wisconsin's Earthmaker, who "never holds direct communion with men . . . [and] acts only through his intermediaries, the deities and the Culture-heroes he has created" (Radin 1954:15, 18; also 1957a:359, 362). The "ordinary affairs of man" are not the concern of such male deities.

> These Supreme Beings are not meant to be worshipped. When they are, then we see them transferred almost immediately into the highest gods of a polytheistic pantheon and they lose much of their abstract character as well as those traits that set them off as Supreme Beings. . . . The moment it left the protecting atmosphere of its [elite] creators it became something else, something entirely different. The priest-thinkers, with that intellectual arrogance which their later colleagues have inherited, seem to have sensed this and to have looked with commiserating contempt upon their less intellectual fellowmen who vitalized their idealistic and static construct but who destroyed its abstract qualities in the process. (Radin 1957b:266–67)

When Everyman gets hold of the elite philosophical speculations (or, for that matter, scholarly constructs), he derives definitions like the following for monotheism: "To the average man it signifies the belief in an uncreated, Supreme Deity, wholly beneficent, omnipotent, omniscient and omnipresent: it demands the complete exclusion of all other gods. The world in its most minute details is regarded as His work, as having been created out of nothing in response to His wish" (Radin 1954:5; also 1957a:342–43). This creation *ex nihilo* is not possible for the Kagaba supreme deity, for, as Radin (1954:15; also 1957a:358) reluctantly admits, "Here we have pure pantheism and the recorder of the above data [Preuss] may perhaps be quite right when he insists that we can hardly expect an origin myth, for the All-Mother is obviously nature personified." Hers would not be a "true" creation myth, presumably.

Purely pantheistic, the Kagaba All-Mother is neither abstract nor remote enough to enjoy the exalted status of male "otiose deities" like the Wichita of Texas's *Man-never-known-on-earth,* who creates first the earth and then bestows a "divine impulse" to create further in the first couple he brings into being (Radin 1954:12–13; also 1957a:354–55). Clearly, mother-creators theoretically cannot overcome their ordinariness, their mundaneness, and their pantheistic nature to be worthy of the truly abstract conceptualization of the primarily male priest-thinker. Animism and not monotheism is their lot—to be procreators and not to act as creators.

Nature Deities and Animism

You ask me to plow the ground! Shall I take a knife and tear my mother's bosom? Then when I die she will not take me to her bosom to rest.

You ask me to dig for stone! Shall I dig under her skin for her bones? Then when I die I can not enter her body to be born again.

You ask me to cut grass and make hay and sell it, and be rich like white men! But how dare I cut off my mother's hair?

It is a bad law, and my people can not obey it. I want my people to stay with me here. All the dead men will come to life again. Their spirits will come to their bodies again. We must wait here in the homes of our fathers and be ready to meet them in the bosom of our mother. (Wanapûm prophet, priest and chief Smohalla to Major J. W. Mac-Murray, June 1884, while the latter was interviewing Indians along the Columbia River who were angered by the homestead laws and the Northern Pacific Railroad's usurpation of their lands. [Mooney 1896:721])[9]

Evolutionist Sir Edward B. Tylor develops the concept of animism in his 1871 classic of anthropology, *Primitive Culture.* According to Marvin Harris (1968:202), animism is

Tylor's minimum definition of religion. Animism exists wherever there is a belief in souls, ghosts, demons, devils, gods, or similar categories of phenomena. The root of all these concepts is traced by Tylor to the belief in the human soul. This belief, which is found in almost every culture, results from the universal subjective experience of dreams and visions. In dreams and visions one sees phantom people, doubles, who detach themselves from their bodies and move about independently of material conditions: one sees "a thin unsubstantial human image, in its nature a sort of vapour, film or shadow" (1958 II:12, orig. 1871).

The key notion in *Primitive Culture* is that "the conception of human soul once attained to by man, served as a type or model on which he framed not only his ideas of other souls of lower grade, but also his ideas of spiritual beings in general, from the tiniest elf that sports in the long grass up to the heavenly Creator and Ruler of the world, the Great Spirit" (Tylor 1958 II:196). In the "theology of the lower races," these beliefs are elaborated by "the powers of the low-culture mind to reason out, [and] the low-culture imagination to deck with mythic fancy." It is Tylor's famous contention that "among these races, Animism has its distinct and consistent outcome, and Polytheism its distinct and consistent completion, in the doctrine of a Supreme Deity" (1958 II:422).

In the Malinowski Memorial Lecture delivered to the London School of Economics and Political Science, Percy S. Cohen (1969:338–39) counts Tylor's as the first of "seven types of theory of myth: [one,] that which treats myth as a form of explanation and, in particular, a form which occurs at a certain stage in the development of human society and culture." Cohen claims Tylor views myths as "peculiar explanations: for him, the chief peculiarities are that myths make use of the language of metaphor and that metaphor is used by primitive man to *personalise* the forces of the natural world which he seeks to understand and control." As Tylor maintains in his 1881 introduction, *Anthropology,*

> When to the rude philosopher the action of the world around him was best explained by supposing in it nature-life like human life, and divine nature-souls like human souls, then the sun seemed a personal lord climbing proudly up the sky, and descending dim and weary into the under-world at night; the stormy sea was a fearful god ready to swallow up the rash sailor; the beasts of the forest were half-human in thought and speech; even the forest-trees were the bodily habitation of spirits, and the woodman, to whom the rustling of their leaves seemed voices, and their waving branches beckoning arms, hewed at their trunks with a half-guilty sense of doing murder. The world then seemed to be "such stuff as dreams are made on"; transformation of

body and transmigration of spirit were ever going on; a man or god might turn into a beast, a river, or a tree; rocks might be people transformed into stones, and sticks transformed snakes. Such a state of thought is fast disappearing, but there are still tribes living in it, and they show what the men's minds are like who make nature-myths. (Tylor 1960:239)

In Tylor's terms, myths like the Okanagan one told to James A. Teit in the early 1900s by Red-Arm, an old Nespelim (western division of the Sanpoil) man related to the Okanagan, are both animistic and etiological.

> Old-One, or Chief, made the earth out of a woman, and said she would be the mother of all the people. Thus the earth was once a human being, and she is alive yet; but she has been transformed, and we cannot see her in the same way we can see a person. Nevertheless she has legs, arms, head, heart, flesh, bones, and blood. The soil is her flesh; the trees and vegetation are her hair; the rocks, her bones; and the wind is her breath. She lies spread out, and we live on her. She shivers and contracts when cold, and expands and perspires when hot. When she moves, we have an earthquake. (Boas 1917:80)[10]

Åke Hultkrantz calls such creation myths "an 'emanatistic' speculation: from himself a primal being provides material for the whole universe. The earth, the forests, the seas, and so forth are created from the parts of his body. Thus everything created is here represented as parts of the god." In some societies, creation is from the dead body of the goddess (Hultkrantz 1979:31, 55). This corporeality is symbolically problematic, whatever the corpse's gender.

Bruce Lincoln (1986:16–20) has analyzed nine basic, recurring homologies in Indo-European cosmogonies and anthropogonies—"a system of natural philosophies, a system of stunning elegance and infinite subtlety" found in sources spanning more than three thousand years: Flesh/Earth, Bone/Stone, Hair/Plants, Blood (or other bodily fluids)/Water, Eyes/Sun, Mind/Moon, Brain (or thoughts)/Cloud, Head/Heaven, and Breath/Wind. Of particular interest here is an observation about "the homology of earth and flesh—or, more broadly, the body—. . . one of the most firmly established":

> In certain Christianized versions of the anthropogony, this homology is denigrated to the advantage of other "loftier" or more spiritual

homologies. Thus, the "Discourse of the Three Saints" calls the portion of the body formed from the earth the "lowliest" (*xužď'ši*) of all,
and whereas most texts use a neutral term to denote the earth (ON
jǫrð, OFris *erthe*, OE *fold*, OIr *talam*, ORuss *tělo*, Pahl *zamїg*, OCS
and ORuss *zemlja*), certain others refer to "mud," "soil," "clay," or
"loam," as the source of the base flesh (Lt *limus*, OE *lām*, MHG *leim*,
Rum *pǎmântu*). (Lincoln 1986:16)

The ideologically debased "base flesh" of an animistic or emanatistic
earth is, however, quite unlike what Mircea Eliade describes as the "cosmic
structure" of religious persons' "elemental intuitions" about the earth.
"With all that it supports and contains, [it] has been seen from the first as an
inexhaustible fount of existences, and of existences that reveal themselves
directly to men."

> The mere *existence* of the soil was seen as significant in the religious
> sphere. The earth, to the primitive religious consciousness, was some-
> thing immediately experienced and accepted; its size, its solidity, its
> variety of landscape and of vegetation, formed a live and active cosmic
> unity. The first realization of the religious significance of the earth was
> "indistinct"; in other words, it did not localize sacredness in the earth
> as such, but jumbled together as a whole all the hierophanies in nature
> as it lay around—earth, stones, trees, water, shadows, everything. The
> primary intuition of the earth as a religious "form" might be formu-
> larized thus: "The cosmos—repository of a wealth of sacred forces."
> (Eliade 1958:242–43)

Like Gaia in Greek cosmogony, "one of the first theophanies of the
earth as such, and particularly of the earth as soil, was its 'motherhood', its
inexhaustible power of fruitfulness. Before becoming a mother goddess, or
divinity of fertility, the earth presented itself to men as a Mother, *Tellus
Mater*" (Eliade 1958:245).[11] In this belief system humans are not earthly in
the sense of dust returning to dust or putrefying corpses.

> The connection between *homo* and *humus* must not be understood
> simply to mean that man is earth because he is mortal but also that the
> fact that man can live is due to his being born of—and returning to—
> the *Terra Mater*. Not long ago, Solmsen explained *mater* from *mate-
> ries*; and although this is not in fact the true etymology (the original

meaning of "matter" was, apparently, something like "heart of wood"), yet it has a place in a mythico-religious outlook: "matter" does the work of a mother, for it unceasingly gives birth. What we call life and death are merely two different moments in the career of the Earth-Mother as a whole: life is merely being detached from the earth's womb, death is a returning "home." The wish so many people feel to be buried in their own country is simply a profane form of this mystical love of one's own earth, of this need to return to one's own home. (Eliade 1958:253)

This supremely sacred sense of autochthony is part of a worldview that was transformed in Western culture during the scientific revolution of the sixteenth and seventeenth centuries. In *The Death of Nature,* Carolyn Merchant (1980:2) shows how the machine then came to replace the organism as the dominant or root metaphor "binding together the cosmos, society, and the self into a single cultural reality—a world view."

Central to the organic theory was the identification of nature, especially the earth, with a nurturing mother: a kindly beneficent female who provided for the needs of mankind in an ordered, planned universe. . . . The metaphor of the earth as a nurturing mother was gradually to vanish as a dominant image as the Scientific Revolution proceeded to mechanize and rationalize the world view.

Carl G. Jung laments the twentieth-century's spiritual legacy of this drastic revolution.

Today, for instance, we talk of "matter." We describe its physical properties. We conduct laboratory experiments to demonstrate some of its aspects. But the word "matter" remains a dry, inhuman, and purely intellectual concept, without any psychic significance for us. How different was the former image of matter—the Great Mother— that could encompass and express the profound emotional meaning of Mother Earth. In the same way, what was the spirit is now identified with intellect and thus ceases to be the Father of All. It has degenerated to the limited ego-thoughts of man; the immense emotional energy expressed in the image of "our Father" vanishes into the sand of an intellectual desert.

These two archetypal principles lie at the foundation of the contrast-

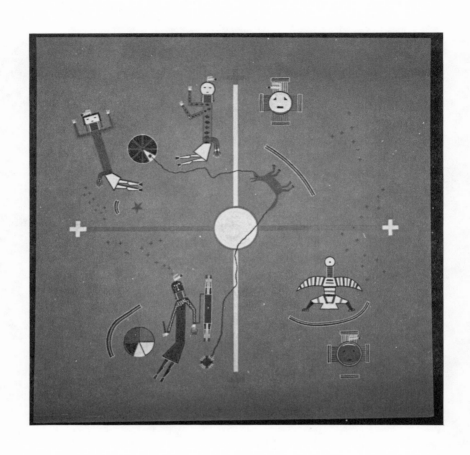

Sandpainting of Navajo creation chant made by Fred Stevens, 1969. (Museum of New Mexico Artifact no. 18553/12. Photo by Arthur Taylor. Neg. no. 21635, courtesy Photo Collections, Museum of New Mexico, Santa Fe.)

The powerful divinities depicted (clockwise from upper left)—First Man and First Woman, Moon, Coyote, Thunderbird, Sun, Fire (Dark) God—are within the worlds, probably in the dark First World, the farthest from the present Fifth World of human habitation (cf. Appendix 11). The sandpainting is thus the inverse of the de Bry/Fludd engraving with its terrestrial, elemental, planetary, and empyrean realms. This immanent Earth Mother is no less powerful than the imperial supreme creator deity whose right arm extends from his divinely lettered cloud.

Also striking is the similarity between Coyote with his path and Nature with her golden chains. A truly versatile and vital deity, as Karl W. Luckert (1984:7) claims, Coyote defies classification: "The most a commentator can inflict on this archaic all-person is to recognize him as such a one and to construct a larger name for him, one which identifies most status levels over which he is said to have roamed. Coyote is Excrement-corpse-fool-gambler-imitator-trickster-witch-hero-savior-god." So too Nature, perhaps.

---

ing systems of East and West. The masses and their leaders do not realize, however, that there is no substantial difference between calling the world principle male and a father (spirit), as the West does, or female and a mother (matter), as the Communists do. Essentially, we know as little of the one as of the other. In earlier times, these principles were worshiped in all sorts of rituals, which at least showed the psychic significance they held for man. But now they have become mere abstract concepts. (Jung et al. 1968:84–85; cf. also Spretnak 1987)

Creator Versus Procreator

The gods Quetzalcoatl and Tezcatlipoca brought the earth goddess down from on high. All the joints of her body were filled with eyes and mouths biting like wild beasts. Before they got down, there was water already below, upon which the goddess then moved back and forth. They did not know who had created it.

They said to each other, "We must make the earth." So saying, they changed themselves into two great serpents, one of whom seized the goddess from the right hand down to the left foot, the other from the left hand down to the right foot. As they tightened their grip, she broke at the middle. The half with the shoulders became the earth. The remaining half they brought to the sky—which greatly displeased the other gods.

Afterward, to compensate the earth goddess for the damage those two had inflicted upon her, all the gods came down to console her, ordaining that all the produce required for human life would issue from her. From her hair they made trees, flowers, and grasses; from her skin, very fine grasses and tiny flowers; from her eyes, wells and fountains, and small caves; from her mouth, rivers and large caves; from her nose, valleys and mountains; from her shoulders, mountains.

Sometimes at night this goddess wails, thirsting for human hearts. She will not be silent until she receives them. Nor will she bear fruit unless she is watered with human blood. (Aztec myth of the earth goddess Coatlicue, Lady of the Serpent Skirt, who wears a necklace of human hands and hearts [Bierhorst 1976:50–51])[12]

One of the more farfetched "mythologies" of the nineteenth-century evolutionists was proposed by John Lubbock, a contemporary of Sir Edward B. Tylor. As Marvin Harris (1968:200) observes: "Two thirds of *The Origin of Civilizaton* (1870) is dedicated to a sketch of the stages of religious belief. Reaffirming his earlier view that the most primitive savages lack anything which could be called religion, Lubbock displays an infuriating certainty concerning the doctrinal superiority of his own brand of superstition. . . . If there is 'one fact more certain than another,' he proclaims, it is 'the gradual diffusion of religious light, and of nobler conceptions as to the nature of God' (1870:349)." Harris reprints Lubbock's scheme (1870:119) verbatim:

> *Atheism;* understanding by this term not a denial of the existence of a Deity, but an absence of any definite ideas on the subject.
>
> *Fetichism;* the stage in which man supposes he can force the Deity to comply with his desires.
>
> *Nature-worship,* or *Totemism;* in which natural objects, trees, lakes, stones, animals, &c. are worshipped.
>
> *Shamanism;* in which the superior deities are far more powerful than man, and of a different nature. Their place of abode also is far away, and accessible only to Shamans.
>
> *Idolatry,* or Anthropomorphism; in which the gods take still more completely the nature of men, being, however, more powerful. They

are still amenable to persuasion; they are a part of nature, and not creators. They are represented by images or idols.

In the next stage the Deity is regarded as the author, not merely a part, of nature. He becomes for the first time a really supernatural being.

The last stage to which I will refer is that in which morality is associated with religion.

Notable in this bizarre evolutionary scale is not only the low status of "Nature-worship" but the change from "Idolatry," in which the increasingly anthropomorphic gods "are a part of nature, and not creators," to "the next stage" and the "really supernatural" deity "regarded as the author, not merely a part, of nature."

The denigration of the natural is even more apparent in another fanciful nineteenth-century "mythology." In his 1861 *Das Mutterrecht; eine Untersuchung über die Gynaikokratie der alten Welt nach ihrer religiösen und rechtlichen Natur* ("Mother Right: An Investigation of the Religious and Juridical Character of Matriarchy in the Ancient World"), Johann Jakob Bachofen finds in myths evidence for three main evolutionary stages: "unregulated hetaerism," Demetrian matriarchy, and patriarchy. The first two exhibit "the homogeneity of a dominant idea," that of "the primacy of motherhood." Bachofen presents the two as the symbolic inversion of the paternal system's high spirituality and philosophical speculation, especially that of "the Greek classical period."

> This homogeneity of matriarchal ideas is confirmed by the favoring of the left over the right side. The left side belongs to the passive feminine principle, the right to the active masculine principle. The role played by the left hand of Isis in matriarchal Egypt suffices to make the connection clear. . . . Another no less significant manifestation of the same basic law is the primacy of the night over the day which issued from its womb. The opposite relation would be in direct contradiction to matriarchal ideas. Already the ancients identified the primacy of the night with that of the left, and both of these with the primacy of the mother. . . . Extension of the same idea permits us to recognize the religious preference given to the moon over the sun, of the conceiving earth over the fecundating sea, of the dark aspect of death over the luminous apsect of growth, of the dead over the living, of mourning over rejoicing, as necessary characteristics of the predominantly matriarchal age. (Bachofen 1967:77)

Moreover,

> Like childbearing motherhood, which is its physical image, matriarchy
> is entirely subservient to matter and to the phenomena of natural life,
> from which it derives the laws of its inner and outward existence. . . .
> Obedient in all things of physical existence, they fasten their eyes upon
> the earth, setting the chthonian powers over the powers of uranian
> light. They identify the male principle chiefly with the tellurian waters
> and subordinate the generative moisture to the *gremium matris* (ma-
> ternal womb), the ocean to the earth. . . . No era has attached so much
> importance to outward form, to the sanctity of the body, and so little
> to the inner spiritual factor; . . . and none has been so given to lyrical
> enthusiasm, this eminently feminine sentiment, rooted in the feeling
> of nature. (Bachofen 1967:91–92)

The first two stages on Bachofen's evolutionary scale are distinguish-
able only in "the degree of closeness to nature with which they interpret
motherhood." Hetaerism is characterized by "the full, unrestricted natural-
ism of pure tellurism, . . . the *iniussa ultronea creatio,* the unbidden wild
growth of mother earth, manifested most abundantly and luxuriantly in the
life of the swamps." In Demetrian matriarchy, that wild profusion is culti-
vated in "the tilled fields" of the orderly agriculturalist, and that matriarchal
system "reveres the ear of grain and the seed corn, which become the most
sacred symbols of its maternal mystery" (Bachofen 1967:97).

In either of the first two stages, it is thought, "the mother's connection
with the child is based on a material relationship, it is accessible to sense
perception and remains always a natural truth." Higher spiritual truths are
possible only when the father's invisible relationship to the child, "remoter
potency," and "immateriality" are recognized.

> The triumph of paternity brings with it the liberation of the spirit from
> the manifestations of nature, a sublimation of human existence over
> the laws of material life. While the principle of motherhood is com-
> mon to all spheres of tellurian life, man, by the preponderant position
> he accords to the begetting potency, emerges from this relationship
> and becomes conscious of his higher calling. Spiritual life rises over
> corporeal existence, and the relation with the lower spheres of exis-
> tence is restricted to the physical aspect. Maternity pertains to the
> physical side of man, the only thing he shares with the animals: the

paternal-spiritual principle belongs to him alone. Here he breaks through the bonds of tellurism and lifts his eyes to the higher regions of the cosmos. Triumphant paternity partakes of the heavenly light, while childbearing motherhood is bound up with the earth that bears all things; the establishment of paternal right is universally represented as an act of the uranian solar hero, while the defense of mother right is the first duty of the chthonian mother goddesses. (Bachofen 1967:109–10)

Neither the authorship of nature that Lubbock welcomes nor the triumph of paternity that Bachofen hails is strictly procreative. Both mythographers in this respect anticipate Simone de Beauvoir, who asserts "the key to the whole mystery":

On the biological level a species is maintained only by creating itself anew; but this creation results only in repeating the same Life in more individuals. But man assures the repetition of Life while transcending Life through Existence; by this transcendence he creates values that deprive pure repetition of all value. In the animal, the freedom and variety of male activities are vain because no project is involved. Except for his service to the species, what he does is immaterial. Whereas in serving the species, the human male also remodels the fact of the earth, he creates new instruments, he invents, he shapes the future. (de Beauvoir 1961:58–59)[13]

These and countless other "mythologies" express the same fundamental premise: procreation is the antithesis of creation; to be procreant is not to be creative; and parturition is not symbolically equivalent to cosmogony. The *Oxford English Dictionary* (1933) definitions illustrate the differences:

Create . . . , *v.* . . . 1. *trans*[itive]. Said of the divine agent: To bring into being, cause to exist; *esp.* to produce where nothing was before, "to form out of nothing" (J. [quotation from Johnson]). . . . 2. *gen*[erally]. To make, form, constitute, or bring into legal existence (an institution, condition, action, mental product, or form, not existing before). . . .

Procreate . . . , v. Now *rare*. . . . *trans*[itive]. To beget, engender, generate (offspring). . . . b. *absol*[ute] or *intr*[ansitive]. To produce offspring. . . . c. *trans*[itive] (*trans*[ferred sense] and *fig*[urative]). To bring into existence, produce; to give rise to, occasion.[14]

In Judeo-Christian tradition, the polarity has its mythic charter in scripture in the book of Genesis,[15] according to Gerda Lerner. By eating of the fruit of the tree of the knowledge of good and evil, when "the eyes of both were opened, and they knew that they were naked" (Genesis 3:7), the first couple gained sexual knowledge. As part of the curse,

> God puts enmity between the snake and the woman (Gen. 3:15). In the historical context of the times of the writing of Genesis, the snake was clearly associated with the fertility goddess and symbolically associated with her. Thus, by God's command, the free and open sexuality of the fertility-goddess was to be forbidden to fallen woman. The way her sexuality was to find expression was in motherhood. Her sexuality was so defined as to serve her motherly function, and it was limited by two conditions: she was to be subordinate to her husband, and she would bring forth her children in pain. (Lerner 1986:196)

The knowing couple is then banished from the Garden of Eden, "lest he put forth his hand and take also of the tree of life, and eat, and live for ever" (Genesis 3:22). "Once and forever, creativity (and with it the secret of immortality) is severed from procreativity. Creativity is reserved to God; procreativity of human beings is the lot of women. The curse on Eve makes it a painful and subordinate lot" (Lerner 1986:197). As a result, only "god-like" men and extraordinary *Elle* pro/creator women can aspire to creativity.

On the other hand, Adam's transgression means that "cursed is the ground because of you; / in toil you shall eat of it all the / days of your life . . . / till you return to the ground, / for out of it you were taken; / you are dust, / and to dust you shall return" (Genesis 3:17, 19). Lerner (1986:197) notes that, "in the very next line Adam re-names his wife Eve 'because she was the mother of all living,' [expressing] . . . the profound recognition that in her now lies the only immortality to which human beings can aspire—the immortality of generation." She concludes:

> The development of monotheism in the Book of Genesis was an enormous advance of human beings in the direction of abstract thought and the definition of universally valid symbols. It is a tragic accident of history that this advance occurred in a social setting and under circumstances which strengthened and affirmed partiarchy. Thus, the very process of symbol-making occurred in a form which marginalized women. For females, the Book of Genesis represented

their definition as creatures essentially different from males; a redefinition of their sexuality as beneficial and redemptive only within the boundaries of patriarchal dominance; and finally the recognition that they were excluded from directly being able to represent the divine principle. The weight of the Biblical narrative seemed to decree that by the will of God women were included in his covenant only through the mediation of men. Here is the historic moment of the death of the Mother-Goddess and her replacement by God-the-Father and the metaphorical Mother under patriarchy. (Lerner 1986:198)

This powerful symbolic redefinition in Western myth and culture has meant that procreation is reduced to elemental or physical or biological status, to reproduction, while creation—viewed as spiritual or metaphysical or symbolic—is exalted as the valued paradigm for important rituals, customs, narratives, and belief systems. Consequently, there remains scant mythological power in what Eliade (1958:261, 262) calls "the activity of motherhood, of an inexhaustible power of creation, [even] creation . . . of a monstrous kind, as in Hesiod's myth of Gaia." He terms this Earth divinity a "universal procreatrix" and concludes:

All divinities tend to become *everything* to their believers, to take the place of all other religious figures, to rule over every sphere of the cosmos. And few divinities have ever had as much right or power to become *everything* as had the earth. But the ascent of the Earth-Mother to the position of the supreme, if not unique, divinity, was arrested both by her hierogamy with the sky and by the appearance of the divinities of agriculture. . . . But the Earth-Mother never entirely lost her primitive prerogatives of being "mistress of the place," source of all living forms, keeper of children, and womb where the dead were laid to rest, where they were reborn to return eventually to life, thanks to the holiness of Mother Earth.

4

Impregnation and Conception

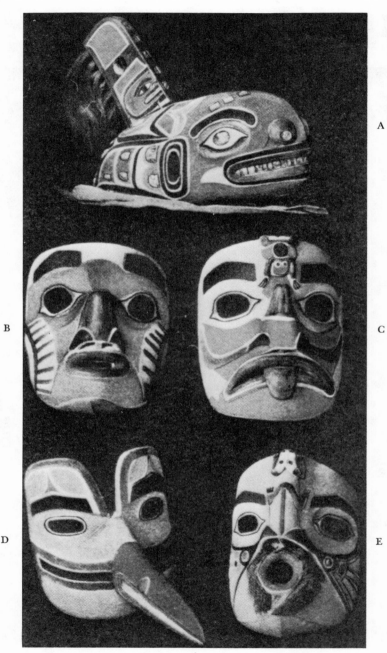

Earth-diver creation myths are often associated with shamanic beliefs in North American Indian and northern Eurasian traditions. This grouping of Northwest Coast Tlingit crest hat (*A*) and copies of shamans' masks (*B–E*) is plate LVIII (in color; this copy reproduced from Naylor 1975:71) of John R. Swanton's Bureau of American Ethnology Annual Report paper (1908). The top is a clan emblem hat, "which is painted in blue, red, and black and set with abalone shell, . . . [and] represents the killer whale, . . . but was not used many times" (Swanton 1908:419–20). Tlingit shamans were "powerful and influential," and "each . . . was guarded by a number of helpers and possessed a number of masks." Swanton says that the copies in *B–E* "are said to be models of masks used by a Luqā'xAdî shaman at Alsek river, called Weasel-wolf (Goteda'), and represented his spirits (yek): *B* represents a spirit known as Cross Man (AnAxłxa'), called by the makers of this model 'the strongest spirit that ever was'; *C* was called Spirit-put-on (Ada'oli-yēk), because it (the mask) was put on in time of war. The tongue is represented as hanging out, because the spirit gets tired in war time. The frog on the forehead represents another spirit; *D* represents the Raven; *E* represents Land-otter-man Spirit (Kū'cta-qa-yēk), while the lines on each cheek represent starfishes, which are also spirits" (Swanton 1908:463, 467–68).

In the beginning, Eurynome, the Goddess of All Things, rose naked from Chaos, but found nothing substantial for her feet to rest upon, and therefore divided the sea from the sky, dancing lonely upon its waves. She danced towards the south, and the wind set in motion behind her seemed something new and apart with which to begin a work of creation. Wheeling about, she caught hold of this north wind, rubbed it between her hands, and behold! the great serpent Ophion. Eurynome danced to warm herself, wildly and more wildly, until Ophion, grown lustful, coiled about those divine limbs and was moved to couple with her. Now, the North Wind, who is also called Boreas, fertilizes; which is why mares often turn their hind-quarters to the wind and breed foals without aid of a stallion. So Eurynome was likewise got with child.

Next, she assumed the form of a dove, brooding on the waves and, in due process of time, laid the Universal Egg. At her bidding, Ophion coiled seven times around this egg, until it hatched and split in two. Out tumbled all the things that exist, her children: sun, moon, planets, stars, the earth with its mountains and rivers, it trees, herbs, and living creatures. (Pelasgian creation myth [Graves 1975:27])[1]

The so-called facts of life are generally thought to be misconstrued by children, "primitives," and the ignorant. In 1908, influenced in part by the case history of Little Hans, Sigmund Freud proposed that children's misconceptions were prompted by the advent of siblings, either actual or in fantasy, since "at a rather later age, if no small brother or sister has appeared, the child's wish for a playmate, such as he has seen in other families, may gain the upper hand."

> The elder child expresses unconcealed hostility towards his rival, which finds vent in criticisms of it, in wishes that "the stork should take it away again" and occasionally even in small attacks upon the creature lying helpless in the cradle. . . .
>
> At the instigation of these feelings and worries, the child now comes to be occupied with the first, grand problem of life and asks himself the question: *"Where do babies come from?"*—a question which, there can be no doubt, first ran: "Where did this particular, intruding baby come from?" We seem to hear the echoes of this first riddle in innumerable riddles of myth and legend. The question itself is, like all research, the product of a vital exigency, as though thinking were entrusted with the task of preventing the recurrence of such dreaded events. (Freud 1959:212–13)

Sir James George Frazer, one of Freud's contemporaries, begins his 1909 survey of "Some Primitive Theories of the Origin of Man" with a sketch about standing on the hill of Panopeus in Phocis, where, "if Greek story-tellers can be trusted . . . , the sage Prometheus created our first parents by fashioning them, like a potter, out of clay." At the bottom of the glen,

> I found a reddish crumbling earth, a relic perhaps of the clay out of which the potter Prometheus moulded the Greek Adam and Eve. In a volume dedicated to the honor of one [Charles Darwin] who has done more than any other in modern times to shape the ideas of mankind as to their origin it may not be out of place to recall this crude Greek notion of the creation of the human race, and to compare or contrast it with other rudimentary speculations of primitive peoples on the same subject, if only for the sake of marking the interval which divides the childhood from the maturity of science. (Frazer 1909:153)

Following "Freud's suggestion that mythology is psychology projected upon the external world," Alan Dundes (1962:1037–38) claims that one "'endo-psychic' perception which could have served as the model" for myths of "cosmogonic creation from mud," including earth-diver ones, is "the existence of a cloacal theory of birth." He contrasts the interpretation of earth-diver myths with that of world-parent (Earth Mother, Sky Father) myths. Below, presentations of these two myth types precede a more general discussion of notions about conception in both biological ("earthly") and symbolic ("enlightened") terms, especially the ways men have defined them so as to appropriate for themselves sole creative and procreative power. The question of virginity figures in such cultural constructs, and Christian beliefs about the Virgin Mary as colorful (earthly) Dark Madonna and blue-and-white (enlightened) Immaculate Conception are explored more fully in the final section, "Earth Mother, Virgin Mother."

Earth-Diver

> In North American Indian myths of the origin of the world, the culture hero has a succession of animals dive into the primeval waters, or flood waters, to secure bits of mud or sand from which the earth is to be formed. Various animals, birds, and aquatic creatures are sent down into the waters that cover the earth. One after another animal fails; the last one succeeds, however, and floats to the surface, half dead, with a little dirt or sand in his claws. . . . [It] is then put on the surface of the water and magically expands to become the world of the present time. (Erminie Wheeler-Voegelin in Leach 1972:334)

Earth-diver creation myths are widely distributed in the Northern Hemisphere. After surveying some 230 versions, Earl W. Count (1952:55; also Rooth 1957:498–500; Köngäs 1960:166) reports:

> It appears that, setting aside the latter-day spread of Christianity, the cosmogonic notion of a primal sea out of which a diver fetches material for making dry land, is easily among the most widespread single concepts held by man. It stretches from Finland across Eurasia— roughly, over the USSR, the Balkans, Mongolia and Turkestan; it even appears in India and southeastern Asia; and it covers most of North America, excepting the Eskimo, the Northwest Pacific coast, the Southwest and most of the Southeast.

Some Eurasian earth-diver myths are dualistic, and Mircea Eliade (1972:106) claims that "it is only in Eurasia that the cosmogonic dive involves a hostile protagonist, an adversary of God." In her comparative study, Köngäs maintains that some of these may express the belief in reflection-souls. She includes a Finnish manuscript version (1906:161), of which Eliade (1972:82) summarizes a published variant:

> Before the Creation of the World God stood on a golden pillar in the middle of the sea. Seeing his image in the water, he cried: "Get up!" The image was the Devil. God asked him how the World could be made. The Devil answered: "By diving to the bottom of the sea three times!" God ordered the Devil to dive. The third time, he managed to bring back some mud. But he had a little of it in his mouth, and it swelled and hurt him. God took the mud from the Devil's mouth and threw it toward the north, and so the stones and rocks came into existence.

Psychoanalyst Géza Róheim, who asserts that the "*core*" of any myth is "*a dream actually dreamed once upon a time by one person*" and then "told and retold," interprets a similar Lett devil-as-earth-diver myth: "If we substitute the rectum for the mouth the myth makes sense as an awakening dream conditioned by excremental pressure" (1952:428, 429).

In nondualistic earth-diver cosmogonies from both Eurasia and North America, the diver is frequently an ornithomorphic deity (Eliade 1972:106), as in the following Pohonichi Miwok cosmogony told by a half-Miwok, half-Yokuts man living among the Chukchansi Yokuts in Madera County, California:

> Before there were people there was only water everywhere. Coyote looked among the ducks and sent a certain species (Chukchansi: yimeit) to dive. At first it said it was unable to. Then it went down. It reached the bottom, bit the earth, and came up again. Coyote took the earth from it and sent it for chanit (Yokuts name) seeds. When the duck brought these he mixed them with the earth and water. Then the mixture swelled until the water had disappeared. The earth was there. (Kroeber 1906–1907:202)

Köngäs (1960:167–69) interprets these as myths reflecting beliefs in a *Seelenvogel,* or bird soul, a widespread concept which "is especially prevalent in the Arctic area where shamanistic practice presupposes [it]—where the shaman sends his soul away to fulfill difficult tasks."

The bird soul, for example, can move independently of the owner's body, fulfil tasks which are not possible for the person himself, wander over seas, and visit the other world. Could we not think that the helpful animal in the Earth-Diver is the bird soul of the creator? In shamanistic terms, the soul is the *helping-spirit*. In the Earth-Diver myth the creator needs earth: he sends his spirit helper to fulfill the difficult task.

She also suggests a nongenetic identity between such myths and Genesis 1, when "the spirit of God moved upon the primeval water." In this myth, "the helper of the creator . . . was not any occasional animal, but a very definite kind of animal—'the spirit of the god,' the soul of the creator."[2]

To Géza Róheim (1952:428), the bird's flight is symbolically straight-forward: "The higher they fly or the deeper they dive the greater the penis becomes—since flying in dreams or diving is an erection." He identifies a "*basic* dream," in which "the dreamer falls into something, frequently a lake or a hole," and interprets it as "characterized by a *double vector* regression to the uterus, and the body as penis entering the vagina."[3] These terms suggest imagery related to the "alchemical reduction to the *prima materia*," as surveyed by Eliade (1962:154-56; also 1978b):

> Notably it may be equated with a regression to the pre-natal state, a *regressus ad uterum*. There is support for this seminal symbolism in a codex studied by Carbonelli [1925], in which it is written that before using gold in the *opus* "it is necessary to reduce it to a sperm." . . . "The vase is akin to the work of God in the vase of divine germination," writes Dorn [1602]. According to Paracelsus [1493–1541], "he who would enter the Kingdom of God must first enter with his body into his mother and there die." The whole world, according to the same writer, must "enter into its mother", which is the *prima materia*, the *massa confusa*, the *abyssus,* in order to achieve eternity. . . . The re-gressus ad uterum is sometimes presented in the form of incest with the mother. . . . The dissolution to the *prima materia* is also sym-bolized by a sexual union which is completed by disappearance into the uterus. In the *Rosarium Philosophorum* [in *Artis Auriferae,* 1593] we read: "Beya mounted Gabricus and enclosed him in her womb in such a fashion that nothing of him remained visible. She embraced him with so much love that she absorbed him entirely into her own na-ture."

Not surprisingly, perhaps, Henry Miller (in Ghiselin 1952:185) uses similar terms to describe his craft in "Reflections on Writing" (1941).

> Writing was not an "escape," a means of evading the every day reality: on the contrary, it meant a still deeper plunge into the brackish pool— a plunge to the source where the waters were being constantly renewed. . . . I had to throw myself into the current, knowing that I would probably sink. . . . Nobody can drown in the ocean of reality who voluntarily gives himself up to the experience. Whatever there be of progress in life comes not through adaptation but through daring, through obeying the blind urge.

A similar, though involuntary, "plunge" is described in J. N. B. Hewitt's Iroquoian creation myth (1903), which includes an earth-diver segment.[4] Heavenly beings called Ongwe exist above primordial waters teeming with water birds and a tortoise whose back eventually serves as foundation for the earth that is dived for. An Ongwe Chief pushes his wife and their baby daughter out of a hole in the heavens. Marie-Louise von Franz (1972:31) summarizes the narrative:

> The woman who has been pushed through the hole in heaven sinks down through deep darkness. Everything around her is a dark blue color; she can see nothing and does not know what will happen to her as she sinks further and further down. Sometimes she sees something but does not know what it is. It is the surface of a great water with a lot of water birds swimming about on it. One of the birds suddenly calls out and says that a human being, a woman, is coming up out of the water—he is looking into the water and sees the mirage—but another bird says that she is not coming up out of the water but falling down from above.

Jungian analyst von Franz (1972:38) remarks on the birds' simultaneous vision of the falling woman "in a mirrored image, as though she came from above and below." Both domains are equally "creative" in being unbidden and unexpected sources of the new.

> Creation is a sudden autonomous event which, from a psychological angle, we could say takes place in the collective unconscious for no outer reason. . . . In the Freudian view the unconscious is only—put

rather crudely—a dustbin into which the cast away facts of consciousness and personal experience are repressed or suppressed. . . . Jung, however, by watching his cases, came more and more to the conclusion that the unconscious is not only a response system, a reactive system which reacts to outer situations, e.g., conscious thoughts, conscious representations, but that it can, of itself, and for no outer or biographical reason, produce something new. In other words, it is creative in the essential sense of the term. . . . I am personally inclined to believe that we do not always have to look for outer reasons, but that actually the human unconscious psyche is capable of a *creatio ex nihilo;* the unconscious can suddenly produce a new impulse, and we cannot explain it as a reaction to anything—except perhaps to boredom! (von Franz 1972:36–37)

Viewed in this way, conception can be parthenogenetic in the fullest sense of the word. And it is a parthenogenesis originally inherent in the Earth Mother and only later ascribed to the Sky Father.

Earth Mother, Sky Father

The cosmic dualism of agrarian tribes places the powers of heaven and atmosphere in more or less clear opposition to the chthonic powers, especially to the deities of earth and water. . . . This confrontation is expressed in a power struggle between the thunderbird and the water snake. It is also expressed, perhaps more fundamentally, in the sexual distance between the celestial male and the chthonic female elements. Attention is then focused on the sky god and the earth goddess. According to the myth, the universe and mankind arose from the union of the heavenly father with Mother Earth. (Hultkrantz 1979:53)

K. Numazawa classifies Polynesian, Yuma, Zuni, Yoruba, Egyptian, Greek, and Gypsy myths as " 'Welternmythen' (Universal-parent myths)" in his 1953 study, "The Cultural-Historical Background of Myths on the Separation of Sky and Earth" (in Dundes 1984:186–87).[5] Anna Birgitta Rooth (1957:500–502) reports that "the World-Parents type [of creation myth] (i.e., the Sky-Father and the Earth-Mother) is limited in North America to southern California, Arizona, and New Mexico" and "in Eurasia to southeastern and southern Asia, as far west as the eastern Mediterranean area." She concludes: "Because of the relationship of the tradition of this area with the Pacific Islands, . . . the World-Parents type came by way of the Pacific Islands to southern California—or rather to the Meso-American tradition-area, whose northern part includes southern North America."

Myths of cosmic hierogamy are frequently related to agricultural societies. According to Eliade, hierogamy precedes and ensures fertility, and "it is probable that this sacred marriage between heaven and earth was the primeval model both of the fertility of the land and of human marriage" (1958:257). In many agricultural societies, public ritual intercourse as well as orgies in the plowed fields or elsewhere symbolize and stimulate this cosmic hierogamy, "arousing" the fertilizing rain from the sky. During periods of drought, women might also run naked through the fields to stir the heavens' desire (Eliade 1958:356–61). Parthenogenesis seems to be an older notion, stemming from a time when the man's role in conception was either unknown or minimized and when agriculture was more a woman's province. When the "true" causes of conception are understood and agriculture considered more a male than a female activity, the plow is often identified with the phallus, the furrow with the woman, and tilling the soil with the sexual act (Eliade 1978a:40–41; 1958:259–60).

Åke Hultkrantz (1979:55) observes in *The Religions of the American Indians,*

> From a mythological point of view it is true that agrarian peoples see the mother goddess as only one of the two primordial procreative beings. This idea of the emanation of life and the world through a sacred union seems to fade in practical faith, where the performance of the goddess is often enough emphasized at the expense of the sky god. She is mentioned . . . as the one who alone brings forth the earth and the plants, giving birth to them from herself. . . . For some peoples the procreative characteristics of the mother goddess have been transferred to the male god who has thus fully assumed her role as agrarian deity.[6]

Symbolically, then, "procreative" deities run the gamut from parthenogenetic Earth Mothers to their male equivalent, the gods who masturbate the cosmos into being.[7]

Gerda Lerner has traced evidence of major economic and social changes in second millennium B.C. myths of the ancient Near East, among them the change in "leading metaphors" or symbols "from the vulva of the goddess to the seed of man" (1986:146).

The supremacy of the Goddess is also expressed in the earliest myths of origin, which celebrate the life-giving creativity of the female. In Egyptian mythology the primeval ocean, the goddess Nun, gives birth to the sun-god Atum, who then creates the rest of the universe. The Sumerian goddess Nammu creates parthenogenetically the male sky-god An and the female earth-goddess Ki. In Babylonian myth the goddess Tiamat, the primeval sea, and her consort give birth to gods and goddesses. In Greek mythology, the earth-goddess Gaia, in a virgin birth, creates the sky, Uranos. . . . In the Assyrian version of an older Sumerian myth the wise Mami (also known as Nintu), "the mother-womb, the one who creates mankind," fashions humans out of clay, but it is the male god Ea "who opened the navel" of the figures, thus completing the life-giving process. In another version of the same story, Mami, at the urging of Ea, herself finished the creative process: "The Mother-Womb, the creatress of destiny/in pairs she completed them. . . . The forms of the people Mami forms."

Lerner (1986:149) calls such texts myths expressing "concepts deriving from earlier modes of the worship of female fertility," in which appear "snake-goddess, sea-goddess, virgin-goddess, and goddess molding humans out of clay—it is the female who holds the key to the mystery."

When the male holds the key, any number of myths are maintained, among them cosmogonies about masturbation and anthropogonies about the sperm's creative supremacy. In Egyptian mythology of the fourth millennium B.C., the creator god Atum or the sun-god Re masturbates the world into existence. A papyrus manuscript dating from around 310 B.C., "The book of knowing the creations of Re and of overthrowing Apophis," preserves language and material from some two thousand or more years earlier. In it, the "All-Lord" calls himself "he who came into being as Kephri," or the morning sun-god, "conceived as a scarab beetle," a notion that involves onomastic and mythic "play on the name Kephri and the word *kheper* 'come into being.'" The creator-god proclaims:

I planned in my own heart, and there came into being a multitude of forms of beings, the forms of children and the forms of their children. I was the one who copulated with my fist, I masturbated . . . with my hand. Then I spewed with my own mouth. I spat out what was Shu [god of air], and I sputtered out what was Tefnut [goddess of moisture]. (trans. John A. Wilson in Pritchard 1969:6)

S. G. F. Brandon (1963:23) claims, "Atum's act of masturbation . . . not only shows that the male factor in generation was already understood: it indicates that the male factor was regarded as decisive."

Wilson points out that the text is "a fusion of two myths, creation by self-pollution [*sic*] and creation by ejection from the mouth," and refers to the Memphite theology of the same period. In Memphis, the god Ptah was "proclaimed to have been the First Principle, taking precedence over other recognized creator-gods," among them Atum.

His [Ptah's] Ennead is before him in (the form of) teeth and lips. That is (the equivalent of) the semen and hands of Atum. Whereas the Ennead of Atum came into being by his semen and his fingers, the Ennead (of Ptah), however, is the teeth and lips in this mouth, which pronounced the name of everything, from which Shu and Tefnut came forth, and which was the fashioner of the Ennead. (trans. John A. Wilson in Pritchard 1969:5)

In the note to this text Wilson refers to Atum's "act of creation . . . through onanism" and Ptah's creation "through command speech with teeth and lips. Pronouncing a name was creative."

Both fornication and masturbation were considered cosmogonic and creative by members of the Gnostic sect of the Phibionites, whose fourth-century A.D. Alexandrian rites were described and decried by the Church Father St. Epiphanius in his *Panarion* (26.17.1ff.):

After they have intercourse in the passion of fornication they raise their blasphemy toward heaven. The woman and the man take the fluid of the emission of the man into their hands, they stand, turn toward heaven, their hands besmeared with the uncleanness, and pray . . . , bringing to the Father of the Nature of All, that which they have on their hands, and they say: "We offer to thee this gift, the body of Christ." And then they eat it, their own ignominy, and say: "This is the body of Christ." (trans. Stephen Benko 1967, as quoted in Eliade 1976:110)[8]

The Phibionite cosmology and theology includes the Primordial Spirit or Father, who brings forth the female Barbelo or Prounikos, who in turn gives birth to the male Ialdabaoth or Sabaoth, who in turn creates the lower world beginning with its rulers the Archons. When Ialdabaoth proclaims himself sole creator, Barbelo has a change of heart about her creation, and "she appeared to the Archons in a beautiful form, seduced them, and when they had an emission she took their sperm, which contained the power originally belonging to her" (*Panarion* 25.2.2ff., trans. Benko 1967, as in Eliade 1976:111).

Mircea Eliade (1976:111–12) calls this ritual an "approach to God through a progressive 'spermatization.'"

As Leisegang has pointed out, theological justification could be found in the First Epistle of John (3:9): "No one born of God commits sin; for the sperm of God abides in him, and he cannot sin because he is born of God." Moreover, according to the Stoic doctrine of *logos spermatikos,* understood as a fiery *pneuma,* the human seed contains a *pneuma,* thanks to which the soul is formed in the embryo.[9] The Stoic theory was the logical consequence of Alcmaeon of Crotona's locating the seed in the brain, that is, in the same organ in which the soul, *psyche,* was supposed to reside. As Onians [1951:119–20] points out, for Plato the *psyche* is "seed," *sperma* (*Timaeus* 73c), "or rather it is in the 'seed' (91a), and this 'seed' is enclosed in the skull and spine (73ff.). . . . It breathes through the genital organ (91b). . . . That the seed was itself breath or had breath (*pneuma*) and that procreation itself was such a breathing or blowing is very explicit in Aristotle."

In *Generation of Animals,* believed to have been written between 347 and 322 B.C., Aristotle acknowledges the necessity for both sexes' contributions to procreation but exalts the male "secretion" (semen) over the female "secretion" (menstrual blood).

(1) The male and the female are distinguished by a certain ability and inability. Male is that which is able to concoct, to cause to take shape, and to discharge, semen possessing the "principle" of the "form"; and by "principle" I do not mean that sort of principle out of which, as out of matter, an offspring is formed belonging to the same kind as its parent, but I mean the *proximate motive principle,* whether it is able to act thus in itself or in something else. Female is that which receives the

semen, but is unable to cause semen to take shape or to discharge it. And (2) all concoction works by means of heat. Assuming the truth of these two statements, it follows of necessity that (3) male animals are hotter than female ones, since it is on account of coldness and inability that the female is more abundant in blood in certain regions of the body. (*Generation* 4, 1, trans. A. L. Peck 1963:385, 387)

A similar Aristotelian "mythology" informs the anti-feminist diatribe by journalist-historian Ferdinand Lundberg and psychiatrist Marynia F. Farnham (1947:245):

Here, we should again like to point out to female egalitarians, is a good place to ponder this fact: for the male, sex involves an objective act of his doing but for the female it does not. . . . Any failure to carry through the act is *his* failure, not the woman's. Her role is passive. It is not as easy as rolling off a log for her. It is easier. It is as easy as being the log itself. She cannot fail to deliver a masterly performance, by doing nothing whatever except being only appreciative and allowing nature to take its course.

Aristotle's final "Cause 'for the sake of which'" is a superior "principle . . . derived from the upper cosmos," something eternal and divine," by which "Soul is better than body."

And as the proximate motive cause, to which belong the *logos* and the Form, is *better* and more divine in its nature than the Matter, it is *better* also that the superior one should be separate from the inferior one. That is why whenever possible and so far as possible the male is separate from the female, since it is something *better* and more divine in that it is the principle of movement for generated things, while the female serves as their matter. The male, however, comes together with the female and mingles with it for the business of generation, because this is something that concerns both of them. (*Generation* 2, 2, trans. Peck 1963: 129, 131, 133)

Aristotelian "logic" pervades the mythology of world-parents narrated by Manly Palmer Hall in his occult anatomy, *Man: The Grand Symbol of the Mysteries* (1947:132–34):

From the occult standpoint, then, the spermatozoon is the carrier of the archetype. It is a little *ark* in which the seeds of life are carried upon the surface of the waters that at the appointed time they may replenish the earth. A triad of forces—spiritual, psychical, and material—are contained within the head of the sperm. This triad originated from the three great centers of man referred to exoterically as the heart, the head, and the navel. The sperm also contains the Logoi, or generating gods—the Builders—those who are to establish their foundations in the deep and upbuild their thrones in the midst of the waters. With them come also the hierarchies of celestial powers—the star spirits— pioneer gods going forth to build new worlds. In the ovum is the plastic stuff which is to be molded by the heavenly powers. In the ovum lies the sleeping world, awaiting the dawn of manvantaric day. In it lurk the Chhaya forms of time and place. Suddenly above the dark horizon of the ovum appears the blazing spermatic sun. Its ray shoots into the deep. The mother ocean thrills. The sperm follows the ray and vanishes into the mother. The germ achieves immortality by ceasing of itself and continuing in its progeny. The mother ovum is fertile.

Earthly Versus Enlightened Conception

The Buddha descended from heaven to his mother's womb in the shape of a milk-white elephant. The Aztec Coatlicue, "She of the Serpent-woven Skirt," was approached by a god in the form of a ball of feathers. The chapters of Ovid's *Metamorphoses* swarm with nymphs beset by gods in sundry masquerades: Jove as a bull, a swan, a shower of gold. Any leaf accidentally swallowed, any nut, or even the breath of a breeze, may be enough to fertilize the ready womb. The procreating power is everywhere. (Campbell 1972:311–12)

In the revised and enlarged edition of the *Motif-Index of Folk-Litera-ture: A Classification of Narrative Elements in Folktales, Ballads, Myths, Fables, Mediaeval Romances, Exempla, Fabliaux, Jest-Books, and Local Legends,* Stith Thompson (1955–58:5, 390–96) lists a number of motifs of "Miraculous conception" (T510–539). The main categories of these motifs are:

T511   Conception from eating

T512   Conception from drinking

T513   Conception through another's wish

T514   Conception after reciprocal desire for each other

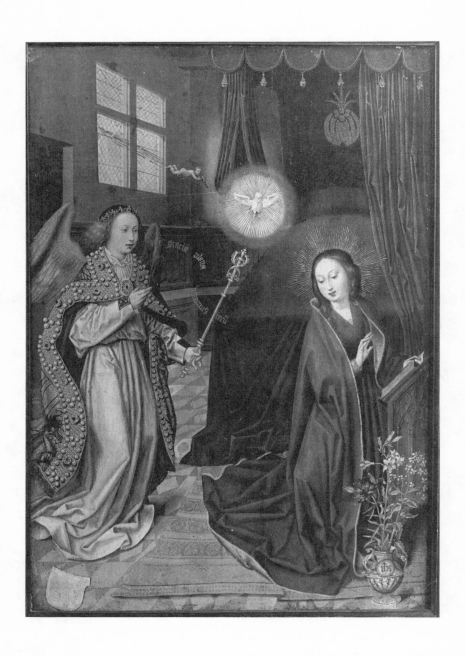

Earth-diver and Aristotelian imagery is evident in "Annunciation" ("Verkun-digung an Maria"), a sixteenth-century painting by Bartel Bruyn, Cologne.[10] Courtesy, Rheinisches Landesmuseum, Bonn.

According to Marina Warner (1976:38), "The influence of pagan bird meta-morphoses on ideas about Christ's birth appears to have been stronger in the western, Latin world, where it endures into the late Renaissance, than in eastern Christianity, where the Holy Spirit's gender was unclear. The Apostles' Creed, developed at the end of the fourth century and finally drawn up in the eighth, ex-presses the idea that the Holy Spirit carried the whole child into Mary's womb to be nourished there, rather than quickening it to life. Jesus Christ, it affirms, was 'conceived by the Holy Ghost, born of the Virgin Mary' (*conceptus est de Spirito Sancto, ex Maria Virgine*). The Holy Ghost, like a mother, conceived the child and then took possession of Mary until the day of the child's birth."[11]

Robert Graves (1966:157), whom Warner cites, relates this idea in the Apos-tles' Creed to the cosmogony in Genesis: "In Gnostic theory . . . Jesus was con-ceived in the mind of God's Holy Spirit, who was female in Hebrew [*shekinah*] and, according to Genesis I, 2, 'moved on the face of the waters.' The Virgin Mary was the physical vessel in which this concept was incarnate and 'Mary' to the Gnostics meant 'Of the Sea.' The male Holy Ghost is a product of Latin grammar—*spiritus* is masculine—and of early Christian mistrust of female deities or quasi-deities. Conception by a male principle is illogical and this is the only in-stance of its occurrence in all Latin literature."

Warner (1976:39) notes: "Later in the west, the dove's feminine aspect re-ceded and its action at the Annunciation came to be seen as more and more virile, while in iconography the scene of the Annunciation resembles more and more a restrained theogamy. The Virgin's first systematic theologian, Francisco Suarez (d. 1617), even felt bound to deny that the encounter was sexual: 'The Blessed Virgin in conceiving a son neither lost her virginity nor experienced any venereal pleasure . . . it did not befit the Holy Spirit without any cause or utility to pro-duce such an effect, or to excite any unbecoming movement of passion. . . . On the contrary the effect of his overshadowing is to quench the fire of original sin.'"

T515   Impregnation through glance

T516   Conception through dream

T517   Conception from extraordinary intercourse

T518   Conception from divine impregnation

T521   Conception from sunlight

T522   Conception from falling rain

T523   Conception from bathing

T524   Conception from wind

T525   Conception from falling star

T526   Conception because of prayer

T527   Magic impregnation by use of charm (amulet)

T528   Impregnation by thunder (lightning)

T531   Conception from casual contact with man

T532   Conception from other contacts (including flowers, magic trees, lettuce, smells, touching another's garment, shadows)

T533   Conception from spittle

T534   Conception from blood

T535   Conception from fire

T536   Conception from feathers falling on woman

T537   Conception from scarification

T538   Unusual conception in old age

The miscellaneous motifs (T539) include conception by a cry, from intercourse with a demon, and by a faraway husband.

Such notions of "animistic" pan-fecundity cannot be attributed to simple ignorance of the physiological "facts" of reproduction but must be viewed in cultural terms, as part of complex symbolic constructs about creation and procreation. Mircea Eliade (1960:164–65), for example, describes systems that assign primacy to the feminine, earthly powers:

> According to innumerable beliefs, women became pregnant whenever they approached certain places; rocks, caves, trees or rivers. The souls of the children then entered their bodies and the women con-

ceived. Whatever was the condition of these child-souls—whether they were or were not the souls of ancestors—one thing was certain: in order to become incarnate, they had been waiting hidden somewhere, in crevasses or hollows, in pools or woods. Already, then, they were leading some sort of embryonic life in the womb of their real Mother, the Earth. That was where children came from. And thence it was, according to other beliefs still surviving among Europeans of the nineteenth century, that they were brought by certain aquatic animals—fish, or frogs, and especially by storks.

By contrast, Carol Delaney (1986:502) discusses the "folk monogenetic theory of procreation" that characterizes monotheism in the vastly different systems of Judaism, Christianity, and Islam: "The male role in procreation reflects on the finite level God's power in creating the world. . . . Not only is there only one God, but divinity *is* creativity and potency—a principle animating the universe—and in these systems it is implicitly and explicitly masculine."

The Maori supreme creator deity is Io, of whom "it is interesting to note that no form of offering or sacrifice was made . . . , that no image of him was ever made, and that he had no *aria*, or form of incarnation, such as inferior gods had" (Best 1922:20). The Maori cosmogony tells how, in the beginning, Io exists in immense darkness, "with water everywhere." His first creation is to speak, saying, "Darkness become a light-possessing darkness," and his cosmogonic speech is now paradigmatic.

> The words by which Io fashioned the Universe—that is to say, by which it was implanted and caused to produce a world of light—the same words are used in the ritual for implanting a child in a barren womb. The words by which Io caused light to shine in the darkness are used in the rituals for cheering a gloomy and despondent hearth, the feeble aged, the decrepit; for shedding light into secret places and matters, for inspiration in song-composing, and in many other affairs, affecting man to despair in times of adverse war. For all such the ritual to enlighten and cheer includes the words (used by Io) to overcome and dispel darkness. Thirdly, there is the preparatory ritual which treats of successive formations within the universe, and the genealogical history of man himself. (Hongi 1907:113–14)[12]

Gerda Lerner (1986:150) has studied Near Eastern myths from the third and second millennia B.C., and found "evidence that a new concept of creation enters religious thinking: Nothing exists unless it has a name. The name means existence." Lerner (1986:151–52) claims that this "symbolification of the capacity to create . . . simplifies the move away from the Mother-Goddess as the sole principle of creativity."

> It is, so to speak, a higher level of thinking to move away from the common-sense observable facts of female fertility and conceptualize a symbolic creativity, which can be expressed in "the name," "the concept." It is not a very big step from that to the concept of "the creative spririt" of the universe. . . . Until people could imagine an abstract, unseen, unknowable power which embodied such a "creative spirit," they could not reduce their numerous, anthropomorphic, contentious gods and goddesses to the One God. The transitional stage is expressed in those creation myths, which describe the "creative spirit" as the god of the air, the god of the winds, the god of thunder, who creates by bringing to life mechanically fashioned beings through his "breath of life."

The symbolic or "conceptual" creativity of the Zuni deity Awonawilona, as presented by Frank Hamilton Cushing in his "Outlines of Zuñi Creation Myths," is a mist or breath.

> In the beginning of the new-made, Áwonawílona conceived within himself and thought outward in space, whereby mists of increase, streams of potent growth, were evolved and uplighted. Thus, by means of his innate knowledge, the All-container made himself in person and form of the Sun whom we hold to be our father and who thus came to exist and appear. With his appearance came the brightening of the spaces with light, and with the brightening of the spaces the great mist-clouds were thickened together and fell, whereby was evolved water in water: yea, and the world-holding sea. (Cushing 1896:379)[13]

Matilda Coxe Stevenson, one of Cushing's anthropologist contemporaries at Zuni, has erroneously portrayed A'wonawil'ona as a bisexual deity ("He-She is the blue vault of the firmament"),[14] who "with the ['tinted'] breath from his heart . . . created clouds and the great waters of the world." She also claims that "the Zuñi conception of A'wonawil'ona is similar to that of the Greeks of Athena" (1904:23, 24). Although it is not clear exactly what

Stevenson means, the common view of Athena as a primarily masculine goddess of wisdom (cf. Weigle 1982:77–79) suggests a similarity between Awonawilona and the Judeo-Christian tradition of Wisdom as a creator goddess.[15]

In the Old Testament, Wisdom (Hebrew *Hokhmah*, Greek *Sophia*) is said to proclaim: "The Lord created me at the beginning of his work, the first of his acts of old" (Proverbs 8:22). She announces to the assembly: "I came forth from the mouth of the Most High, and covered the earth like a mist" (Ecclesiasticus [Sirach] 24:3). Like Awonawilona's conceiving mists, Wisdom's creative blanketing contrasts with the conventional image of the "word of God" as "sharper than any two-edged sword, piercing to the division of soul and spirit, of joints and marrow" (Hebrews 4:12).

New Testament sources elaborate the male sword and not the female blanketing imagery. The apocalyptic "Revelation" of John begins on a Sunday, when

> I heard behind me a loud voice like a trumpet saying, "Write what you see in a book and send it to the seven churches. . . ."
>
> Then I turned to see the voice that was speaking to me, and on turning I saw seven golden lampstands, and in the midst of the lampstands one like a son of man, clothed with a long robe and with a golden girdle round his breast; his head and his hair were white as white wool, white as snow; his eyes were like a flame of fire, his feet were like burnished bronze, refined as in a furnace, and his voice was like the sound of many waters; in his right hand he held seven stars, from his mouth issued a sharp two-edged sword, and his face was like the sun shining in full strength. (Revelation 1:11–16)

Alan W. Watts (1968:29) sees the stars in the vision's hand as "his sevenfold spirit," and "the sword which comes out of his mouth is his Word," the Son, in the cosmogonic sense of John 1:1–3: "In the beginning was the Word, and the Word was with God, and the Word was God. He was in the beginning with God; all things were made through him, and without him was not anything made that was made."

Joan Chamberlain Engelsman traces the historical development of Wisdom from "a personified hypostasis [attribute] of God" in the fourth century B.C.E. to a first-century B.C.E. figure who had grown "in stature and importance for the Jews . . . until her power was virtually equivalent to that of any Hellenistic goddess." Jews at the beginning of the Christian era portrayed a Sophia "acting in history and assuming the roles of judge and savior," one who unquestionably "rivaled the power of Yahweh himself" (1979:119; also Patai 1978:255–56).

> Within a hundred years Sophia's power was broken and she was superseded by a masculine figure who took over her roles. In Hellenistic Judaism the personified Logos of Philo's philosophy became the firstborn image of God who was with God at creation, the principle of mind and rational order, and the intermediary between God and men. However, in deference to Jewish scripture, Sophia was not totally discarded, but was elevated to heaven, where she was relegated to a minor part in the divine/human drama. At the same time, the early Christians replaced her with Jesus and within a few decades of his crucifixion, all her powers and attributes had been ascribed to Christ. This was either done directly, as in Paul's letters and Matthew's Gospel, or indirectly, as in John which identified Christ with the Logos, a masculine figure similar to the one developed by Philo. Ultimately, Sophia's powers were so totally preempted by Christ that she herself completely disappeared from the Christian religion of that time. (Engelsman 1979:119–20; also Bruns 1973:35–59; Ruether 1974; Cady et al. 1986)

Sophia's elevation and extinction as a female co-creative power parallel evolving Christian notions of the Virgin Mary.

Earth Mother, Virgin Mother

> Hail Mary, full of grace, the Lord is with thee. Blessed art thou among women and blessed is the fruit of thy womb Jesus. (Roman Catholic prayer)

Carol Delaney criticizes the ethnocentrism and sexism in anthropological debates on parthenogenesis and "the meaning of paternity."[16] She (1986:511) notes:

> To say that the male has a role in the production of a child is to say nothing more than that; how that role is interpreted is what is important. Sexual intercourse may be considered irrelevant to the produc-

tion of a child but even when it is relevant there can be several interpretations: 1) the male opens the path for a foetus that may come by other means, 2) intercourse stops menstruation which allows for (1), 3) the product of ejaculation may feed the foetus, 4) the product of ejaculation may contribute to the formation of the foetus. As a corollary to these one must also ask whether one act or several are necessary to accomplish the purpose. None of these, however, is the same as "paternity" which has meant the formative, primary and creative role.

Those who debate concepts of paternity and virginity often themselves express folk traditions about monogenesis, which can be related to monotheistic doctrine.

> In cultures influenced by monotheism a whole world is symbolically constructed and systematically integrated between notions of conception and the conception of deity. Abraham, the person through whom the concept of monotheism allegedly enters history, means something like "the father is exalted" and the glorification of the father is, to me, what patriarchy is all about. These systems, spanned between monogenesis and monotheism, are systems not merely of male dominance, but of the dominance, objectification and institutionalisation of the idea that the male as father is creator of human life, as God is thought to be of life in general.

This is particularly evident in Christian tradition, for, "by means of the Virgin Birth, Christianity makes explicit the 'monogenetic theory' of procreation that is, I believe, consistent with the theological concept of monotheism" (Delaney 1986:502).

In *Alone of All Her Sex: The Myth and the Cult of the Virgin Mary,* Marina Warner (1976:47) claims that "there is no more matriarchal image than the Christian mother of God who bore a child without male assistance." And yet,

> It is highly paradoxical that this parthenogenetic goddess fitted into the Aristotelian biological scheme, and that it was a deeply misogynist and contemptuous view of women's role in reproduction that made the idea of conception by the power of the Spirit more acceptable. For many matrifocal societies also entertain erroneously exaggerated ideas about the material contribution of women in parturition and belittle

the biological role of the man. But in their case the imbalance leaves mothers in the ascendant, while in Christianity identification of the womb with the lower, carnal order, gives fathers precedence. Thus the self-same ideogram of the mother and child can be worshipped by both societies that respect and despise women for their maternity.

The Christian devaluation and disregard of women's procreative powers are evident in the shift from the traditional and ancient notion of virgin birth as a ritually renewable, symbolic sign of strength and purity to the recent sense of it as a literal "fact" of physical intactness and a moral imperative toward sexual chastity. Christianity "broadened the concept of virginity to embrace a fully developed ascetic philosophy," according to Marina Warner (1976:48, 49), "and it was this shift, from virgin birth to virginity, from religious sign to moral doctrine, that transformed a mother goddess like the Virgin Mary into an effective instrument of ascetism and female subjection." Furthermore, by the mid-nineteenth century, official church doctrine promulgated a remarkable redefinition of the Virgin's own conception.

The Dogma of Immaculate Conception, whereby Mary was declared exempt from original sin, was proclaimed by Pope Pius IX on December 8, 1854. This ushered in what church leaders call the Marian Age, from 1850 to 1950, when the Dogma of the Assumption was proclaimed. During this time there were numerous apparitions of the Virgin in western and southern Europe, including Paris (1830), LaSalette (1846), Lourdes (1858), and Pontmain (1871) in France; Fátima in Portugal (1917); and Beauraing (1932) and Banneaux (1933) in Belgium. In her study of the nineteenth-century Marian revival, Barbara Corrado Pope (1985:176) notes that the uneducated Sister of Charity (a country nun then living in Paris) Catherine Labouré's vision of the Virgin of the Miraculous Medal was of a woman "dressed in white with a blue mantle (the colors of innocence and purity, and of royalist France)," and that "the coloration of blue and white (or simply white in some reproductions) reappeared at Lourdes, Fátima, Beauraing, and Banneaux. This is in contrast to earlier depictions of the Virgin, which were often multicolored and followed local cults."

At Lourdes, Bernadette Soubirous, "the asthmatic fourteen-year-old daughter of a pitifully poor family, first saw her vision in February 1858 while gathering wood with her sister and a friend." She then saw it "seventeen times during the next five months, often in front of thousands of witnesses." Bernadette's Virgin was dressed in "a white robe and veil and a blue sash, and had two gold roses resting on her bare feet." The older motifs in this apparition include obedience to commands like that of building a church and "the identification of a supernatural being with a miraculous fountain." According to Pope (1985:179, 180, 189), "What was startlingly new was the apparition's identity. 'I am,' she replied to Bernadette's repeated question, 'the Immaculate Conception.'" French Catholics thus came to believe that they had been singled out, in effect chosen, for the epiphany of this "new" power.

In *Pure Lust: Elemental Feminist Philosophy,* Mary Daly (1984:110) explains how the doctrine of Immaculate Conception, or Immaculate Deception, is a strategy of tokenism, specifically, "the employment of the *delusion of exceptionalism.* The immaculate conception worked a symbolic transformation, rendering Mary an exception, free of 'original sin.' . . . The token woman believes herself to be an exception to the alleged incompetency and array of weaknesses ascribed to women in general, that is, to the 'original sin' of being a woman." The promulgated doctrine coincides with the crest of the so-called first wave of feminism in the mid-nineteenth century:

> In comparison with the immaculate conception, the virgin-birth-of-Jesus is but a pale perversion. The greater deception, the deeper mythic undermining of the Originally Parthenogenetic Goddess required the erasure of her own Self, prior to her role as mother-of-god.
>
> Such mythic erasure of Mary's Self was attempted through the immaculate conception doctrine. According to this inconceivable doctrine, Mary was "preserved" from original sin by the grace of her son immediately at the moment of her conception—not only in advance of *his* birth, but also in advance of her own. Nor was she merely "purified" as an embryo in the womb of her mother. Indeed, according to this astonishing doctrine, Mary never had a moment of life, even of embryonic life, without being "full" of the "grace" merited by her son through his death on the cross. Thus she was purified of autonomous be-ing before ever experiencing even an instant of this. (Daly 1984: 103–4)

As Rosemary Radford Ruether (1975:50) observes, this official Mary resembles

> the Mary of the monks, who venerate her primarily as virgin and shape her doctrine in an antisexual mold. But there is the Mary of the people

who is still the earth mother and who is venerated for her power over the secrets of natural fecundity. It is she who helps the woman through her birthpangs, who assures the farmer of his new crops, new rains, and new lambs. She is the maternal image of the divine who understands ordinary people in their wretchedness.

The so-called black madonnas preserve elements of these folk beliefs. However,

> Catholic sources, for the most part, have denied the possible connection between the black madonnas and earlier earth goddesses. Nevertheless, Saint Augustine noted that the Virgin Mary represents the earth and that Jesus is of the earth born. . . .
>
> At this point our hypothesis begins to emerge: the black madonnas are Christian borrowings from earlier pagan art forms that depicted Ceres, Demeter Melaina, Diana, Isis, Cybele, Artemis, or Rhea as black, the color characteristic of goddesses of the earth's fertility. (Moss and Cappannari 1982:65; also Begg 1985)

Barbara Corrado Pope (1985:194) contrasts the black madonnas with the blue-and-white virgins of the nineteenth-century Marian revival:

> This Virgin had no connection with fertility and sexuality, the two most obvious attributes of any symbol of female divinity. This connection could only belong to the underground interpretation of the Good Mother's role. Although the connection was recognized and utilized in village rituals and local cults, it went unrecognized (officially at least) in the cults of the famous Black Virgins, some of whom may have gotten their coloration from their connection with the earth and with pre-Christian goddesses. From the perspective of these earlier images, the blue and white Virgin seems not only immaculate but also bloodless and disconnected from the earth and from the experiences of most women.

The Mexican Virgin of Guadalupe, known as Moreneta (Little Dark One) or Virgin Morena due to her brown coloring, is a powerful New World image of "earthly" virginity. In 1531, on the Hill of Tepeyac, the Virgin of Guadalupe "appeared to Juan Diego, a Christianized Indian of commoner status, and addressed him Nahuatl." A shrine was built as directed by the Virgin, and it, "rebuilt several times in centuries to follow, is today a basilica, the third highest kind of church in Western Christendom."

> The shrine of Guadalupe was, however, not the first religious structure built on Tepeyac; nor was Guadalupe the first female supernatural associated with the hill. In pre-Hispanic times, Tepeyac had housed a temple to the earth and fertility goddess Tonantzin, Our Lady Mother, who—like Guadalupe—was associated with the moon. Temple, like basilica, was the center of large scale pilgrimages. That the veneration accorded Guadalupe drew inspiration from the earlier worship of Tonantzin is attested by several Spanish friars. (Wolf 1972:150; also Turner and Turner 1978:40–103)

The cult of Guadalupe grew in popularity during the sixteenth century and came into its own in the seventeenth century, when the first pictures, poems, and sermons were recorded.

Paula Gunn Allen claims Our Lady of Guadalupe is an apparition of the Aztec goddess Tinotzin (Tonantzin), "Our Mother," a synonym for the fertility goddess Cihuacoatl, Serpent Woman, Earth-Goddess, who rules childbirth and death. Tinotzin, she claims, resembles the Pueblo goddess Iyatiku or Ic'city, a later name for Uretsete, one of the twin sisters whom Thought-Woman gave birth to ritually. Iyatiku authorizes and counsels the cacique or hotchin, "Chief Remembering Prayer Sticks, to keep the people ever in peace and harmony and to remember that they are all her children and thus are all entitled to the harvest of her body/thought" (Allen 1986:20).

Iyatiku is depicted on the Keres Fire Society altar with imagery that produces medicine power related to the heart, which is the source of creative strength. Commenting on a drawing made in 1928 (Stirling 1942: plate 10), Allen (1986:26) notes that "Iatiku appears as a bird woman, with the body of a bird and the head of a woman."

> One of the interesting features of this depiction of Earth Woman is her resemblance of Tinotzin . . . who is known as Our Lady of Guadalupe today. The Virgin Morena (the dark virgin), as she is also called, wears a salmon-colored gown that is spotted yellow to represent the stars. She wears a cloak of blue, and her image is surrounded by fiery tongues—lightning or flames, presumably.

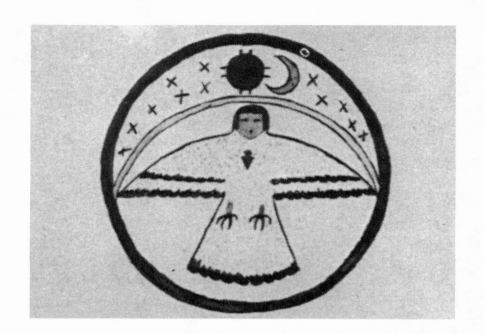

Acoma Pueblo altar sandpainting. "Fire society altar: The rim (blue) is the sky; the upper crescent contains the symbols for the sun (red), moon (yellow), and stars; the arc (pale gray) is the Milky Way; the face (yellow with black hair) below, Iatiku; and the spots (yellow) represent the earth; the triangular object (red) on breast is the heart, the center of the earth and the center of the picture" (Stirling 1942:121, and plate 10; also Appendix 10). Note that the figure is oriented to the east, from the top, above the sun and moon.

In Western tradition, however, enlightening power does not reside in the Earth Mother, as Simone de Beauvoir (1961:135) contends:

> But more often man is in revolt against his carnal state; he sees himself as a fallen god: his curse is to be fallen from a bright and ordered heaven into the chaotic shadows of his mother's womb. This fire, this pure and active exhalation in which he likes to recognize himself, is imprisoned by woman in the mud of the earth. . . .
> She also dooms him to death. This quivering jelly which is elaborated in the womb (the womb, secret and sealed like the tomb) evokes too clearly the soft viscosity of carrion for him not to turn shuddering away.

The Virgin Mary does not attain power until she is assumed bodily into heaven, a long-standing folk belief thought perhaps to have originated in Egypt. This popular belief had a firm hold in Europe by the fourteenth century, and, as Marina Warner (1976:89–90) maintains, it "inspired some of Christianity's masterpieces, including that ringing fanfare of the Renaissance, Titian's *Assumption,* painted in 1518, in which the apostles reach out in awe and ecstasy towards Mary's soaring form." Only in leaving the earth and shedding its dark, dank carnality (bodily odors were a sure sign of lacking sanctity) can a woman, and only this woman, gain true power.

In Native American cultures, on the other hand, all humans' ritual, spiritual, and social empowerment comes within, upon, and in reciprocal relationship with the Earth Mother. Her conception, gestation, and parturition is *not* a "one-time," physiological process, as demonstrated in Santa Clara Pueblo natives Rina Swentzell and Tito Naranjo's explication (1986: 36–37) of the complex Tewa word *gia,* or "mother." Biological *gias* are family mothers, some of whom become core *gias* with "special roles in counseling and healing." Community *gias* are both females and males who

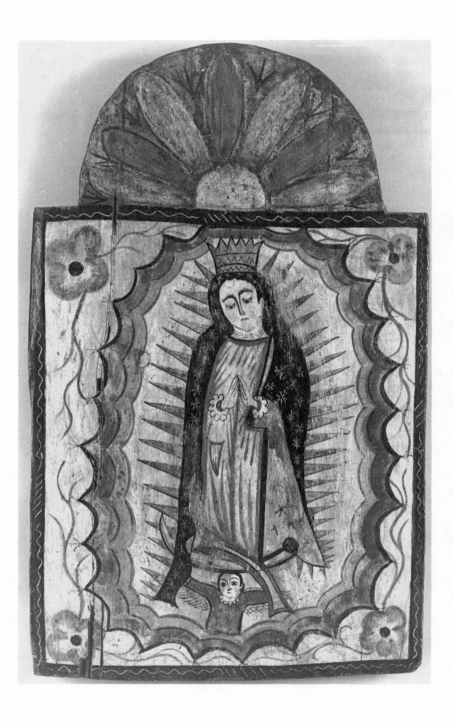

Our Lady of Guadalupe, by the Truchas Master, New Mexico, 1780–1840 (tree-ring range: 1700–1751). (Collection of the Taylor Museum, TM 852; William Wroth 1982:plate 159; 175. Courtesy, Taylor Museum of the Colorado Springs Fine Arts Center, Colorado Springs, Colorado.)

"serve the community and assure harmony in the social/political/religious realms. Almost any older woman is called a gia but so is a respected male leader, or cacique. . . . Possession of desirable qualities is shown, at this level, to be more important than the discrimination or distinction of sex roles." Some female and male deities—"the ones closest to the people [with] gia aspects of strength, courage, love of the people, and giving"—are also *gias*. Indeed, ideally, "To be alive is to be a nurturer," and the traditional paradigm for this life is Earth herself: "The Earth is the ultimate nurturer. She is our mother or *nung be gia*. We humans move in and out of her womb as is told in the emergence myths of the Pueblos. She is constant, reliable, and always giving and forgiving. She protects and heals."

5

Construction and Gestation

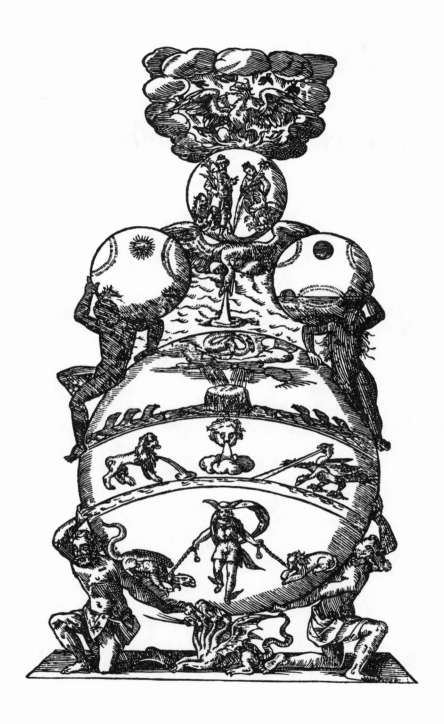

"Ichnographia operis Philosophia alia," from Libavius, *Alchymia*, 1606 (Lehner 1969:68, fig. 291). Libavius's explanation of this depiction of the stages in the alchemical process is translated in Carl G. Jung's *Psychology and Alchemy* (1968:285–87). Abstracting from that text, then: Base = earth; two giants (Atlases) support the sphere with a four-headed dragon (breathing four kinds of fire) beneath. *Bottom,* large sphere: Mercurius holds one-headed dragon (*left*) and green lion (*right*)—both = *prima materia*—with silver chain. *Middle:* Red lion (*left*) with blood, wind (*middle*) with spirit, three-headed silver eagle (*right*) with white Mercurial fluid—all flowing, mingling in the sea. *Top:* black waters of chaos (= *putrefactio*) with black ravens on both sides of a mountain with silver rain (= first dissolution and coagulation); dragon (ouroborus) at top is vision of heaven (= second coagulation). Ethiopian man (*left*) and woman (*right*), who = *nigredo* (second putrefaction), support spheres containing sun (*left*) and Mercurial sea and moon (*right*) and dark sea (= white fermentation). Between them, a swan (= white elixir or chalk, the philosopher's arsenic, common to both ferments) swims in pure silver sea of Mercurial fluid which unites the tinctures. *Top sphere:* King (*left*), clad in purple with golden crown, carrying a red lily, flanked by golden lion; Queen (*right*) with silver crown and white lily, stroking a white or silver eagle. *Atop:* "The phoenix on the sphere, cremating itself; many gold and silver birds fly out of the ashes" (= multiplication and increase).

While I am making a jar, I think all the time I am working with the clay about what kind of a design I am going to paint on it. When I am ready, I just sit and think about what I shall paint. I do not look at anything but just think what I shall draw and then when the pot is dry, I draw it. . . . I think about designs all the time. . . . I always know just how it will look before I start to paint. (woman potter from Zuni Pueblo [Bunzel 1972:49])[1]

This is what the sculptor must do. He must strive continually to think of, and use form in its full spatial completeness. He gets the solid shape, as it were, inside his head—he thinks of it, whatever its size, as if he were holding it completely enclosed in the hollow of his hand. He mentally visualizes a complex form *from all round itself;* he knows while he looks at one side what the other side is like; he identifies himself with its centre of gravity, its mass, its weight; he realizes its volume, as the space that the shape displaces in the air. (Henry Moore, "Notes on Sculpture" [from Evans 1937, as in Ghiselin 1952:74])

Western popular beliefs about conception bias interpretations of gestation mythologies. The woman is considered the passive nurturer of life actively engendered by the man. By herself she cannot beget a living being. Neither is that which she procreates a creative work. She only serves as material incubator for the male creator, whether inspiritor or craftsman. Aristotle elaborates these distinctions in *Generation of Animals*.

> The action of the semen of the male in "setting" the female's secretion in the uterus is similar to that of rennet upon milk. Rennet is milk which contains vital heat, as semen does, and this integrates the homogeneous substance and makes it "set." As the nature of milk and the menstrual fluid is one and the same, the action of the semen upon the substance of the menstrual fluid is the same as that of rennet upon milk. Thus when the "setting" is effected, *i.e.*, when the bulky portion "sets," the fluid portion comes off; and as the earthy portion solidifies membranes form all round its outer surface.

He maintains that "once the fetation has 'set,' it behaves like seeds sown in the ground," and its "growth is supplied through the umbilicus in the same way that a plant's growth is supplied through its roots" (*Generation* 2, 4, trans. A. L. Peck 1963: 191, 193).

Since "it is the female which provides the matter, and the male which provides the principle of movement," the latter is the sole creator: "Now the products which are formed by human art are formed by means of instruments, or rather it would be truer to say they are formed by the movement of the instruments, and this movement is the activity, the actualization, of the art, for by 'art' we mean the shape of the products which are formed, though it is resident elsewhere than in the products themselves" (*Generation* 2, 4, trans. Peck 1963: 193, 199, 201). In Aristotle's view, and in Western popular belief, then,

> the female is in the fullest sense of the word a "laborer." She passively takes on her task, laboring with her body to fulfill another's design and plan. The product of her labor is not hers. The man, on the other hand, does not labor but works. . . . Aristotle implied that the male is *homo faber*, the maker, who works upon inert matter according to a design, bringing forth a lasting work of art. His soul contributes the form and model of creation. (Horowitz 1976:197)

Microscopic investigations in the seventeenth and eighteenth centuries did little to alter the basic Aristotelian notions by then encoded in popular beliefs and mythology. Using "'perspectives,' or simple lenses of very low power," William Harvey substantially furthered embryology while not breaking entirely from Aristotelianism, according to Joseph Needham (1934:128–29):

> There can be no doubt that the doctrine *omne vivum ex ovo* was an advance on all preceding thought. Harvey's scepticism about spontaneous generation antedated by nearly a century the experiments of [Francesco] Redi [pub. 1684, 1688]. It is important to note that he was led to his idea of the mammalian ovum by observations on small embryos surrounded by their chorion and no bigger than eggs, for the follicle was not discovered until the time of [Nicholas] Stenson [Bishop of Titopolis, pub. 1664, 1667] and [Rene] de Graf [pub. 1672, 1677], and the true ovum not till the time of [Karl Ernst] von Baer [pub. 1828, 1837, posthumously 1888].

In his 1628 *De Motu Cordis et Sanguinis in Animalibus* and his 1651 *Exercitationes de Generatione Animalium,* Harvey also "settled for good the controversy which had lasted for 2200 years as to which part of the egg was nutritive and which was formative, by demonstrating the unreality of the distinction."

Seventeenth-century preformationists began to theorize about "the existence of visible miniatures" in either egg (ovism) or sperm (animalculism) and to dispute whether the fetus originates in egg or spermatozoon.[2] Pioneer microscopist Anton von Leeuwenhoek discovered animalcules in male semen in 1677 and wrote of his opposition to ovism in 1678.

> In a letter of 1685 he allowed himself to speculate on the possibility that the animalcule contains a miniature, but immediately contradicted this and insisted that anyone who had interpreted his reports to mean that the animalcules contained children was mistaken. The kernel of an apple is not a tree, and it is "no less improper to say, that the worms in mens' seed are children, tho' children come from them." Leeuwenhoek was certainly convinced that the spermatozoon could produce a child and was obviously tempted by the possibility that it might actually contain a miniature, but his own inability to discern such a structure seems to have prevented him from openly supporting such a claim. (Bowler 1971:232–33)

Karl Ernst von Baer's nineteenth-century discovery of the ovum was not well received, and it still has not revolutionized popular beliefs and mythology, Carol Delaney (1986:508) contends:

> The nature of [the ovum's] contents and function was hotly debated in
> medical and scientific circles throughout the century, partly, I suspect
> because of the implications of its meaning. In general, it was still held
> to be primarily nurturant material. With the re-discovery of Mendel's
> genetics in the twentieth century, the knowledge of what it contained
> (half the genetic constitution of a child) could be established, and thus
> also the knowledge that both men and women contribute essentially
> and creatively to a child. This theory was not widely assimilated in the
> West until the mid-twentieth century.

In contemporary society, she claims, "some women, at least, have been
learning that they are not merely vessels for the male seed, not merely
nurturers and supporters of life, but co-creators and (perhaps more than)
equal partners in this endeavour." Nevertheless, the traditional popular
belief in one male genitor or creator "persists not only in the 'soft' explanations to children about procreation, not only in theological language, but
also in the language of academia and in everyday speech."

Such language commonly portrays the egg as an inert and chaotic
material acted upon by a militant homunculus. It echoes the imagery in
animalculist Nicholas Andry's *De la generation des vers dans le corps de
l'homme* (1700). Andry

> pictured each egg as being like the Cavorite sphere in which H. G.
> Wells' explorers made their way to the moon, i.e. with one trap-door.
> The spermatazoa, like so many minute men, all tried to occupy an egg,
> but as there were far fewer eggs than spermatazoa, there were, when all
> was over, only a few happy animalcules who had been lucky enough to
> find an empty egg, climb in, and lock the door behind them. (Need-
> ham 1934:184)

William Harvey offered a remarkable feminine metaphor for the egg in
his 1651 *Generatione Animalium:* "An egge is, as it were, an exposed womb;
wherein there is a substance concluded, as the Representative and Substitute or Vicar of the breasts" (Needham 1934:130). Martin Llewellyn
prefaced his 1653 translation of Harvey's *Anatomical Exercitations Concerning the Generation of Living Creatures* with a poem (Needham 1934:131)
comparing the controversy sparked by Harvey's 1628 *De Motu Cordis* and
the hoped-for reception of his *Generatione Animalium:*

> A Calmer Welcome this choice Peice befall,
> Which from fresh Extract hath deduced all,

And for Belief, bids it no longer begg
That Castor once and Pollux were an Egge:
That both the Hen and Housewife are so matcht,
That her Son born, is only her Son hatcht;
That when her Teeming hopes have prosp'rous bin,
Yet to conceive, is but to lay, within.
Experiment, and Truth both take thy part:
If thou canst 'scape the Women! there's the Art.

Live Modern Wonder, and be read alone,
Thy Brain hath Issue, though thy Loins have none.
Let fraile Succession be the Vulgar Care;
Great Generation's Selfe is now thy Heire.

These "issues"—the construction and gestation of the egg, the brain, and the womb—are explored below in sections entitled "Cosmogonic Egg," "Cosmogonic Brain," and "Cosmogonic Womb."

Cosmogonic Egg

"Ta'aroa was the ancestor of all the gods; he made everything. From time immemorial was the great Ta'aroa, Tahi-tumu (The-origin). Ta'aroa developed himself in solitude; he was his own parent, having no father or mother. . . .

"Ta'aroa sat in his shell in darkness from eternity. The shell was like an egg revolving in endless space, with no sky, no land, no sea, no moon, no sun, no stars. All was darkness, it was continuous thick darkness . . ."

The record then proceeds to describe Ta'aroa's breaking his shell, which became the sky, his swimming in empty space and retirement into a new shell which, after he had again emerged, . . .

"he took . . . for the great foundation of the world, for stratum rock and for soil for the world.

"And the shell Rumia that he opened first, became his house, the dome of the gods' sky, which was a confined sky, enclosing the world then forming." (Polynesian cosmogony [Handy 1927:11–12])[3]

In her preliminary survey of "creation egg" myths worldwide, Anna-Britta Hellbom designates one group as "The *Cosmic Egg* or *World Egg*, i.e.

such stories as describe the creation of the universe, the world or the heavenly bodies out of an egg or egg-like object." She reviews texts from the Near East (Egypt, Israel, Phoenicia, Greece, Persia, India), Far East (Tibet, China, Japan, Assam; Indonesia: Sumatra, Java, Borneo), Polynesia (Hawaii, Raiatea, Tahiti, Tuamoto Islands), West Africa, Europe (Finland, Estonia), and Greenland. Hellbom concludes that "the *Cosmic Egg* occurs all over the Old World except North-Asia," and that "the rare occurrence of the egg theme within America is puzzling while especially its total lack in virtually all of North America seems incomprehensible" (Hellbom 1963:64, 65–73, 99; also Needham 1934:9–10; Gimbutas 1982:101–7).

Venetia Newall distinguishes various themes in creation egg myths, including: "The Primeval Waters," in which an egg comes into being; "The Egg of the Sun," as source of life; "The Cosmic Mountain," from or in which the egg evolves; "The Creation Struggle" within the egg; "Timelessness," associated with the broken or unbroken egg; and "The Universe Egg." Of the latter Newall (1971:35) notes: "In the beginning, according to many creation myths, the universe was a formless void, but containing a cosmic mass which resembled an egg."

The *Nihongi*, or "Chronicles of Japan," written in 720 (Saunders 1961:415), includes a universe egg myth.

> Of old, Heaven and Earth were not yet separated, and the In and Yo not yet divided. They formed a chaotic mass like an egg, which was of obscurely defined limits, and contained germs. The purer and clearer part was thinly diffused and formed Heaven, while the heavier and grosser element settled down and became Earth. The finer element easily became a united body, but the consolidation of the heavy and gross element was accomplished with difficulty. Heaven was therefore formed first, and Earth established subsequently. Thereafter divine beings were produced between them. (trans. W. G. Aston 1956:1–2; also Saunders 1961:417)

The Japanese cosmogony suggests European alchemical texts. Venetia Newall (1971:16) summarizes their creation egg elements as follows:

> In Europe as late as the Middle Ages an idea persisted that the earth was an egg itself, and metals grew like an embryo within its yolk. Man, wishing to imitate nature and prepare his own precious metal—the philosopher's stone, which would possess unbelievable magic pow-

ers—tried to reproduce what he took to be natural conditions. Hence the vessel used, the *aludel* or retort, was egg-shaped. This was also in imitation of the universe, so that the stars would be sure to influence the operation. The miraculous substance that was supposed to emerge was often called the "philosopher's egg", and is depicted as such in early woodcuts. Occasionally, with richer invention, it was shown as an infant. This creative aspect is emphasized by the word *Mutterschoss,* mother's womb, a common metallurgical term for a smelting kiln. Alchemists worked on two levels. Some only wanted to manufacture gold. Others, more mystically inclined, saw gold as representing spiritual rebirth. From the heat of the symbolic egg-shaped vessel, the phoenix or new soul would finally arise. An old woodcut shows the traditional alchemist cleaving an egg with a fiery sword, not to destroy it, but to release the new life within.

In a chapter entitled "Terra Mater. Petra Genetrix," Mircea Eliade (1962:43) abstracts "from the immense mass of lithic mythology" myths and beliefs "concerning men born from stone and . . . regarding the generation and ripening of stones and ores in the bowels of the earth. Both beliefs have implicit in them the notion that stone is the source of life and fertility, that it lives and procreates human creatures just as it has itself been engendered by the earth." Metallurgy is thus like agriculture, and man assists nature's procreation by properly cultivating and harvesting her children.[4]

The alchemist occupies "the same spiritual category"; he "takes up and perfects the work of Nature, while at the same time working to 'make' himself."

Like the metallurgist who transforms embryos (i.e. ores) into metals by accelerating the growth already begun inside the Earth-Mother, the alchemist dreams of prolonging this acceleration and crowning it by the final transmutation of all "base" metals into the "noble" metal which is gold.

In the *Summa Perfectionis,* a work on alchemy of the fourteenth century, we read that "what Nature cannot perfect in a vast space of time we can achieve in a short space of time by our art." The same idea is clearly expounded by Ben Jonson in his play, *The Alchemist* (Act II, Sc. 2). One of the characters, Surly, hesitates to share the alchemistic opinion which compares the growth of metals to the processes of animal embryology, whereby, like the chicken hatching out from the egg, any metal would ultimately become gold as a result of the slow maturation which goes on in the bowels of the earth. For, says Surly, "The egg's ordained by Nature to that end, and is a chicken in potentia." And Subtle replies: "The same we say of lead and other metals, which would be gold if they had time." Another character, Mammon, adds: "And that our art doth further." (Eliade 1962:47, 51)

Carl G. Jung concerns himself with the "soul-making" crucial to the alchemical discipline. He (1968:202) claims:

> In alchemy the egg stands for the chaos apprehended by the artifex, the *prima materia* containing the captive world-soul. Out of the egg— symbolized by the round cooking-vessel—will rise the eagle or phoenix, the liberated soul, which is ultimately identical with the Anthropos who was imprisoned in the embrace of [feminine] Physis [Nature].

Besides a fifteenth-century codex picture showing "the philosophical egg, whence the double eagle is hatched, wearing the spiritual and temporal crowns" (1968:201, fig. 98), Jung includes three images of Mercurius in the philosopher's egg or alchemical vessel (1968:66, fig. 22; 237, fig. 120; 238, fig. 121). In one from 1702 (p. 66): "As *filius* he stands [inside the egg] on the sun and moon, tokens of his dual nature. The birds [outside the egg] betoken spiritualization, while the scorching rays of the sun ripen the homunculus in the vessel."

Sally G. Allen and Joanna Hubbs (1980:220–21) explore similar imagery in their study of the iconography in *Atalanta fugiens* (Atalanta in flight), a seventeenth-century alchemical text by hermetic adept Michael Maier. They cite Jung's *Psychology and Alchemy,* wherein he observes,

> the equality of masculine and feminine in the alchemical opus is created in order to produce a masculine being, to right a masculine imbalance in masculine terms. The hermaphroditic nature of the *filius philosophorum* is a concession to the maternal by the dominant Father who thus encompasses the feminine (primordial animality) within the purer spiritual realm of the mind, the masculine "womb." The goal of the alchemical opus is to make conscious that which is hidden and to unite consciousness to the unconscious in such a manner as to contain the unconscious within the spiritual realm, that is, to masculinize it, by symbolically giving birth to the *filius,* not the *filia.*

The alchemical work anticipates contemporary reproductive technologies, and, "Today, the triumph of the test-tube baby seems to replicate the alchemical attempt to dominate the natural world by a 'self-inseminating, masturbatory' creation . . . and to demonstrate the strong obsession of patriarchy to control the creative aspects of nature."

Jung (1968:236–38) too emphasizes that the alchemical vessel "is no mere piece of apparatus."

> For the alchemists the vessel is something truly marvellous: a *vas mirabile*. Maria Prophetissa . . . says that the whole secret lies in knowing about the Hermetic vessel. "Unum est vas" (the vessel is one) is emphasized again and again. It must be completely round, in imitation of the spherical cosmos, so that the influence of the stars may contribute to the success of the operation. It is a kind of matrix or uterus from which the *filius philosophorum*, the miraculous stone, is to be born. . . . Hence it is required that the vessel be not only round but egg-shaped. . . . One naturally thinks of this vessel as a sort of retort or flask; but one soon learns that this is an inadequate conception since the vessel is more a mystical idea, a true symbol like all the central ideas of alchemy.

Marie-Louise von Franz (1972:226) summarizes the Jungian approach:

> The vessel represented something like the possibility of a unitary psychic concept of reality acquired, or built. . . . It is really a symbol of the human psyche as a whole, a microcosm, a vessel within which all the macrocosmic processes are caught and at the same time grasped and conceived. In the whole of alchemy, since the mental process is completely projected into the material operations, there is no difference between the actual retort and what we would call the psyche.

Both Greek and Roman philosophers located the psyche or soul in the head, which was thought to survive and enter the afterworld (Onians 1951:131–38).[5] In this sense, perhaps, the skull becomes the alchemical retort for the transmutable *prima materia* of the brain. The whole is cosmogonic, suggesting the cosmogonic egg in the Kashmir poet Somadeva's *Kathasaritsagara,* or "Ocean of the Streams of Story" (written between 1063 and 1081). One of Somadeva's poetically retold Sanskrit narratives

> tells how Shiva created the world from a drop of blood which he let fall into the primeval water. Of this became an egg and from it came

Portavit eum ventus in ventre suo.

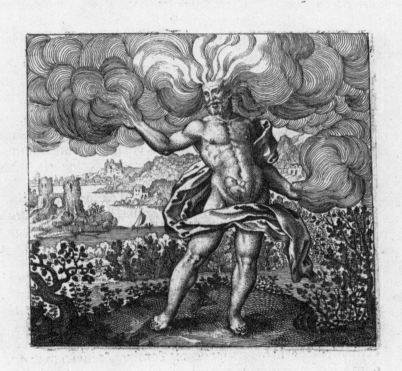

EPIGRAMMA I.

EMbryo ventosâ BOREÆ qui clauditur alvo,
  Vivus in hanc lucem si semel ortus erit;
Unus is Heroum cunctos superare labores
  Arte, manu, forti corpore, mente, potest.
Ne tibi sit Cæso, nec abortus inutilis ille,
  Non Agrippa, bono sydere sed genitus.

B 3   HER-

From Hermetic adept Michael Maier, *Atalanta fugiens* [Atalanta in flight] (Oppenheim, 1618): "The first image—and stage—shows us the muscular and bearded figure of the phallic god Hermes Trismegistus, the mythical founder of alchemy. His powerful body is drawn in a manner which suggests that he is not simply a messenger of the gods from heaven to earth but, rather, that in him earth and heaven are united. The caption, 'Portavit eum ventus in vetre sui' [The wind carried him in his womb],[6] refers to the lightly etched outline of an infant in fetal position placed at the base of his belly, indicating the inseminating role of the male and, even more explicitly, the desire to appropriate the function of maternity.[7] This remarkable image is followed by that of a woman suckling a child; it is entitled: 'Nutrix eius terra est' [His nurse is the earth]. In these two introductory engravings, then, we see the birth of a child from the male; the female's function is reduced to that of nurse, a notion consistent with the Aristotelian view of woman as the passive 'nurse' or carrier of the active male seed, the *form* of the foetus" (Allen and Hubbs 1980:211). Facsimile reproduction courtesy Beinecke Rare Book and Manuscript Library, Yale University.

Purusha, the Supreme Soul. Of the egg halves heaven and earth were fashioned. But as to shape the world resembles a skull. Shiva ends his story with these words: "Moreover, this world, resembling a skull, rests in my hand; for the two skull-shaped halves of the egg before-mentioned are called heaven and earth." (Hellbom 1963:68; citing N. H. Penzer's 1923–28 ed.)

Orphic and cabalistic traditions about cosmogonic egg/skulls are somewhat similar. In some of the former cosmogonies, Chronus (Time) is the first principle with Adrasteia (Necessity). Aether, Chaos, and Erebus come from Chronus, who "in Aether . . . fashioned an egg that split in two and from this appeared the first-born of all gods, Phanes, the creator of everything, called by many names, among them Eros" (Morford and Lenardon 1985:290; also Alderink 1981:36–41). According to Manly Palmer Hall (1947:121), " 'When the skull-like, wide-yawning egg did break' is a statement attributed to Orpheus which links the Greek and Jewish systems." In the Cabala, "the egg . . . is identical with the great cranium of *The Zohar,* the spherical envelope surrounding the world."

Cosmogonic Brain

At the beginning all things were in the mind of Wako[n]'da. All creatures, including man, were spirits. They moved about in space between the earth and the stars (the heavens). They were seeking a place where they could come into a bodily existence. They ascended to the sun, but the sun was not fitted for their abode. They moved to the moon and found that it also was not good for their home. Then they descended to the earth. They saw it was covered with water. They floated through the air to the north, the east, the south, and the west, and found no dry land. They were sorely grieved. Suddenly from the midst of the water uprose a great rock. It burst into flames and the waters floated into the air in clouds. Dry land appeared; the grasses and the trees grew. The hosts of spirits descended and became flesh and blood. They fed on the seeds of the grasses and the fruits of the trees, and the land vibrated with their expressions of joy and gratitude to Wako^{n}'da, the maker of all things. (Omaha creation myth [Fletcher and La Flesche 1911:570–71])[8]

Roland Barthes (1972:68–69) analyzes Einstein's brain as "a mythical object." This genius "is commonly signified by his brain, which is like an object for anthologies, a true museum exhibit." The mythic Einstein is virtually a "robot" who has "no diffuse power in him, no mystery other than mechanical: he is a superior, a prodigious organ, but a real, even a physiological one." His brain is "so lacking in magic that one speaks about his thought as of a functional labour analogous to the mechanical making of sausages, the grinding of corn or the crushing of ore: he used to produce thought, continuously, as a mill makes flour, and death was above all, for him, the cessation of a localized function: *the most powerful brain of all has stopped thinking.*'"

Einstein's brain thus becomes a magic object like the magic mill, a motif (D1263) identified by Stith Thompson (1955–58:2, 158) and related to motifs "D1318.15. Mill will not grind stolen wheat. D1338.6. Rejuvenation in magic mill. D1601.21. Self-grinding mill. Grinds whatever owner wishes. D1601.21.1. Self-grinding salt mill. D1601.27. Automatic mill. D1676. Mill refuses to work on Sunday. D1677. Mill refuses to work when saint is mistreated." An Indian folktale contains the "absurdity" motif "J1531.1.1. Mill has given birth to horse" (Thompson 1955–58:4, 121). Among the most familiar is mythological motif A1115.2.: "*Why the sea is salt: magic salt mill.* Stolen by sea-captain, who takes it aboard and orders it to grind. It will stop only for its master; ship sinks and mill keeps grinding salt" (Thompson 1955–58:1, 195).[9]

What Einstein's magic-mill brain "was supposed to produce was equations." In doing this, electricity was generated:

A photograph shows him lying down, his head bristling with electric wires: the waves of his brain are being recorded, while he is requested to "think of relativity." (But for that matter, what does "to think of" mean, exactly?) What this is meant to convey is probably that the seismograms will be all the more violent since "relativity" is an arduous subject. Thought itself is thus represented as an energetic material, the measurable product of a complex (quasi-electrical) apparatus which transforms cerebral substance into power. (Barthes 1972:69, 68)

Einstein's electroencephalogram is a contemporary manifestation of angels, the first, *ex nihilo* creations of the Holy Trinity according to Christian mythology of the late thirteenth century:

The angels of every order are winged to designate their spiritual nature, as well as the instantaneous manner in which they discharge all their activities. For an angel is where it thinks, and thus any number of angels can stand on the point of a pin because any number of angels can think of the point of that pin. As thought can move faster than light, jumping instantaneously from earth to the utmost nebulae, so likewise the angels can move from heaven to earth, and from end to end of the universe in almost no time at all. Furthermore, angelic thought is said to be many times faster than human thought because it does not require the cumbersome instrumentality of material images, which take time and effort to form within the mind. (Watts 1968:39–40)

Einstein's angelic glory is a single, key formula to unlock the cosmogonic egg or "safe":

There is a single secret to the world, and this secret is held in one word; the universe is a safe of which humanity seeks the combination: Einstein almost found it, this is the myth of Einstein. In it, we find all the Gnostic themes: the unity of nature, the ideal possibility of a fundamental reduction of the world, the unfastening power of the word, the age-old struggle between a secret and an utterance, the idea that total knowledge can only be discovered all at once, like a lock which suddenly opens after a thousand unsuccessful attempts. The historic equation $E = mc^2$, by its unexpected simplicity, almost embodies the pure idea of the key, bare, linear, made of one metal, opening with a wholly magical ease a door which had resisted the desperate efforts of centuries.

Although Einstein is often photographed "standing next to a blackboard covered with mathematical signs of obvious complexity," cartoons portray him as a mythic creator *ex nihilo,* showing "him chalk still in hand, and having just written on an empty blackboard, as if without preparation, the magic formula of the world." Barthes compares such insight to alchemy, in that "it is simple like a basic element, a principal substance, like the philosopher's stone of hermetists, tar-water for Berkeley, or oxygen for Schelling" (Barthes 1972:69).

In photographs and cartoons, Einstein usually appears with hair in wild disarray (cf. Leach 1958; Firth 1973), significant of the structures and processes within. This suggests the derivation of *cerebrum,* "the Roman name for the contents of the head, the brain," as traced by Richard Broxton Onians (1951:125–26):

> It has been vaguely connected with *kapa,* etc., with a suggested basic meaning, "the topmost part of the body"; but . . . the obvious Latin cognate is the old verb *cereo,* more familiar as *creo,* "I beget, I engender." . . . Cf. . . . for *cerebellum: flo, flabrum, flabellum,* etc. We may compare also *Ceres,* the name of the goddess of fertility identified particularly with the seed in the "head" of the corn-stalk, and the masculine *Cerus* (with various Italic by-forms) meaning "engenderer." . . . A garland for the head, formed of corn-ears or "heads", was the distinctive offering to Ceres.

The generative brain of the disheveled Einstein is a convoluted one, "a wholly material organ which is monstrous only by its cybernetic complication." This is a "prodigious organ" of mythic proportion, and "Einstein himself has to some extent been a party to the legend by bequeathing his brain, for the possession of which two hospitals are still fighting as if it were an unusual piece of machinery which it will at last be possible to dismantle" (Barthes 1972:69, 68).

Jill Purce (1980:97, 98) calls the convoluted brain "the labyrinth of the mind." She compares the "mystic spiral" of "the first vibrations of the egg of the world, which unfold to the confines of the universe," to images of the head as "the inner sanctuary of the temple of man's body, both created and protected by the windings of the labyrinth. With each turn man completes a stage in his evolution. In the centre of the spiral he meets himself . . . ; this is his higher or complete Self." Purce notes that "the number of *gyri* (windings) or folds of the cerebral cortex . . . is greater in man than in any other creature, since an increased surface area is necessary for higher mental processes." Those processes apparently transpire in a brain whose "overall form" she compares to "the vaginating embryo, . . . the kidney or the archetypal growth form of the mushroom," claiming it "resembles the natural form of flow." The labyrinth of the mind thus becomes the symbolic equivalent of the labyrinth of the earth, and Einstein's brain rivals Earth's womb.

Cosmogonic Womb

Anon in the nethermost of the four cave-wombs of the world, the seed of men and the creatures took form and increased; even as within eggs in warm places worms speedily appear, which growing, presently burst their shells and become as may happen, birds, tadpoles or serpents, so did men and all creatures grow manifoldly and multiply in many kinds. Thus the lowermost womb or cave-world, which was Anosin tehuli (the womb of sooty depth or of growth-generation, because it was the place of first formation and black as a chimney at night time, foul too, as the internals of the belly), thus did it become overfilled with being. Everywhere were unfinished creatures, crawling like reptiles one over another in filth and black darkness, crowding thickly together and treading each other, one spitting on another or doing other indecency, insomuch that loud became their murmurings and lamentations, until many among them sought to escape, growing wiser and more manlike. (Zuni creation myth outline, "The Gestation of Men and the Creatures" [Cushing 1896:381])[10]

In *The Second Sex,* Simone de Beauvoir (1961:467) characterizes the pregnant woman as an uncreative, noncosmogonic egg.

The transcendence of the artisan, of the man of action, contains the element of subjectivity; but in the mother-to-be the antithesis of subject and object ceases to exist; she and the child with which she is swollen make up together an equivocal pair overwhelmed by life. Ensnared by nature, the pregnant woman is plant and animal, a stockpile of colloids, an incubator, an egg. . . .

Ordinarily life is but a condition of existence; in gestation it appears as creative; but that is a strange kind of creation which is accomplished in a contingent and passive manner.

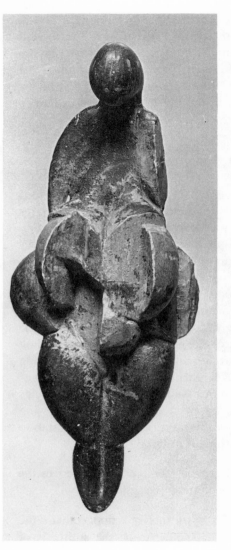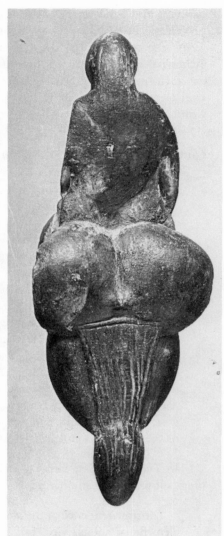

Venus of Lespugue, St. Germaine en Laye, ivory, Haute Garonne, France, Aurignacian period, ca. 24,000 B.C., now in Musée de l'Homme, Paris. (Photographie Giraudon 34604, 1935, courtesy Art Resource, New York.)

According to Jungian analyst Erich Neumann (1963:95–96), "With their emphasis on the impersonal and transpersonal, these figures of the Great Mother Goddess are primordial types of the feminine elementary character. In all of them the symbolism of the rounded vessel predominates. The belly and breasts, the latter often gigantic, are like the central regions of this feminine vessel, the 'sole reality.' In these figures the fertility of the Feminine has found an expression both prehuman and superhuman. The head is sightless, inclined towards the middle of the body; the arms are only suggested, and they too stress the middle of the body. The gigantic thighs and loins taper off into thin legs; the feet have broken off, but there is no doubt that they were frail and by no means conceived as supports of the giant body-vessel. In the magnificent Lespugue figure, whose breasts, belly, thighs, and triangular genital zone form a single cluster, this symbolic fullness of the elementary character is still more evident than in the naturalistic and therefore less symbolic Venus of Willendorf."

Feminist artists Monica Sjöö and Barbara Mor (1987:46) see these "first human images known to us" (35,000–10,000 B.C.) as "cult images—to Mother Guardians of the daily life, death, and rebirth of the people." The carved images "are very fleshy, more or less stylized to represent pregnancy and abundance." Archeologists no longer view the Venuses "as Cro-Magnon 'bunnies' . . . [or] sex objects. They are magic images of the mysterious power of the female to create life out of herself, and to sustain it."

This "contingent and passive" gestation suggests spontaneous generation and even the popular belief in generation from mud or excrement.

De Beauvoir voices what Erica Jong (1979:27) calls "the unexamined lie" of "creativity vs. generativity." Creation "demands conscious, active will," while pregnancy requires "only the absence of ill-will" toward the growing fetus.

> Most often, literary creativity is sheer hard labor, quite different from the growing of a baby in the womb, which goes on despite one's conscious will and as, properly speaking, God's miracle, or nature's, and does not belong to the individual woman who provides it with a place to happen. On the contrary, the growing of the fetus in the womb is DNA's triumph, the triumph of the genes, the triumph of the species. The woman whose body is the site of this miracle is, in a sense, only being used by the species temporarily in its communal passion to survive. (Jong 1979:27)

The pregnant woman's service to the species brings a false sense of creativity. De Beauvoir (1961:474) disparages the women during gestation who

> muse endlessly on their new importance. With the slightest encouragement they revive in their own cases the masculine myths: against the light of the mind they oppose the fecund darkness of Life; against the clarity of consciousness, the mysteries of inwardness; against productive liberty, the weight of this belly growing there enormously without human will. The mother-to-be feels herself one with soil and sod, stock and root; when she drowses off, her sleep is like that of brooding chaos with worlds in ferment.

De Beauvoir's "brooding chaos" suggests that of the Roman poet Ovid, whose "Chaos (*Metamorphoses* 1.1–75) is not a gaping void but rather a crude and unformed mass of elements in strife from which a god [*sic*] (not named) or some higher nature formed the order of the universe" (Morford and Lenardon 1985:32). It also resembles the unsavory mess of the "sooty" womb in Cushing's Zuni creation myth outline.

The "filthy," reptilian, "unfinished" Zuni "creatures" are like the *daimones* of ancient Greek belief. They are characterized by Jane Ellen Harrison (1980:6–7; also Nilsson 1961:18–21, 71–72) in a chapter of her *Prolegomena to the Study of Greek Religion* (1903) entitled "Olympian and Chthonic Ritual." Harrison takes issue with "lofty" views of Greek religion, among them Plutarch's "instructive treatise on 'the fear of the supernatural,'" *de Superstitio.*

> Plutarch deprecates the attitude of the superstitious man who enters the presence of his gods as though he were approaching the hole of a snake, and forgets that the hole of a snake had been to his ancestors, and indeed was still to many of his contemporaries, literally and actually the sanctuary of a god. . . . It can, I think, be shown that what Plutarch regards as superstition was in the sixth and even the fifth century before the Christian era the *real* religion of the main bulk of the people. . . . The beings worshipped were not rational, human, law-abiding *gods,* but vague, irrational, mainly malevolent *daimones,* spirit-things, ghosts and bogeys and the like, not yet formulated and enclosed into god-head.

The confused chaos of the subterranean, "feminine" womb in Cushing's Zuni myth outline and Greek folk belief may be contrasted with the apparently orderly, paired population aboard Noah's mythic boat. Alan Dundes (1962:1039) suggests: "If one were inclined to see the Noah story as a gestation myth, it would be noteworthy that it is the man who builds the womb-ark. It would also be interesting that the flood waters abate only after a period roughly corresponding to the length of human pregnancy." Noah's counterparts in contemporary, androcentric myths of gestation are found in popular culture, visual images like *The Silent Scream* and *2001: A Space Odyssey*. Rosalind Pollack Petchesky (1987:271) claims:

> The dominant view of the fetus that appears in still and moving pictures across the mass-cultural landscape . . . is one where the fetus is not only "already a baby," but more—a "baby man," an autonomous, atomized mini-space hero. This image has not supplanted the one of the fetus as a tiny, helpless, suffering creature but rather merged with it. . . . We should not be surprised, then, to find the social relations of obstetrics—the site where ultrasound imaging of fetuses goes on daily—infiltrated by such widely diffused images.

Among the scientific examples Petchesky (1987:276) quotes is the following by obstetrician Dr. Michael Harrison and his colleagues, who write about " 'fetal management' through ultrasound" in the *Journal of the American Medical Association* (1981):

> The fetus could not be taken seriously as long as he [*sic*] remained a medical recluse in an opaque womb; and it was not until the last half of this century that the prying eye of the ultrasonogram . . . rendered the once opaque womb transparent, stripping the veil of mystery from the dark inner sanctum and letting the light of scientific observation fall on the shy and secretive fetus. . . . The sonographic voyeur, spying on the unwary fetus, finds him or her a surprisingly active little creature, and not at all the passive parasite we had imagined.

Such voyeurism eclipses the mother's participation, with important consequences for the politics of reproduction:

> What we have here, from the children's standpoint, is a kind of *panoptics of the womb*, whose aim is "to establish normative behavior for the fetus at various gestational stages" and to maximize medical control over pregnancy. Feminist critics emphasize the degrading impact fetal-imaging techniques have on the pregnant woman. She now becomes

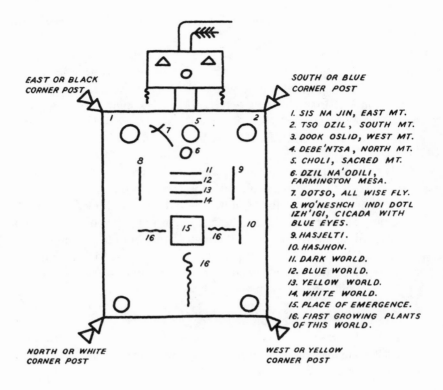

EAST OR BLACK
CORNER POST

SOUTH OR BLUE
CORNER POST

1. SIS NA JIN, EAST MT.
2. TSO DZIL, SOUTH MT.
3. DOOK OSLID, WEST MT.
4. DEBE'NTSA, NORTH MT.
5. CHOLI, SACRED MT.
6. DZIL NA'ODILI,
   FARMINGTON MESA.
7. DOTSO, ALL WISE FLY.
8. WO'NESHCH INDI DOTL
   IZH'IGI, CICADA WITH
   BLUE EYES.
9. HASJELTI.
10. HASJHON.
11. DARK WORLD.
12. BLUE WORLD.
13. YELLOW WORLD.
14. WHITE WORLD.
15. PLACE OF EMERGENCE.
16. FIRST GROWING PLANTS
    OF THIS WORLD.

NORTH OR WHITE
CORNER POST

WEST OR YELLOW
CORNER POST

Navajo sandpainting of the female earth, showing the underworlds (nos. 11–14) through which the first people emerged. Aileen O'Bryan (1956:22) provides this caption: "Sand Painting of the Earth. (The plan of the earth.) From the top of the mask projects a breath feather, tied with a white cotton string, the spider's gift. Coral and turquoise ear pendants are indicated. The body is dark gray. Borders, mask, neck, etc. The two arms and two legs as kos ischin, triangles set upon one another and symbolizing forming clouds or cloud terraces. (Sam Ahkeah and Gerald Nailor got this from medicine men at Shiprock.)"

According to this version of the Navajo emergence myth (see Appendix 11), after raising the sky, the Holy Ones "planned just how the earth should be. They made the face of the earth white, with eyes and nose and mouth. They made earrings of turquoise for the ears; and for a border they placed a black ring, a blue ring, a yellow ring, and a white ring, which is the earth's edge. These rings are for the earth's protection; no power shall harm her." Numbers 1–6 (3 and 4 are not marked) are the sacred mountains that bound the Navajo cosmos, guarding it from the chaos outside. Dotso (no. 7) often acts as a messenger for the gods in mythology, while the cicada (no. 8) or locust is usually thought to have emerged first from the fourth underworld into this fifth world. In O'Bryan's version, Hasjelti (no. 9) and Hasjohon (not Hasjhon, no. 10) are powerful supernatural figures associated with healing ceremonies known as mountain chants (O'Bryan 1956:23; also Wyman 1970:65–102).

---

the "maternal environment," the "site" of the fetus, a passive spectator in her own pregnancy. (Petchesky 1987:277)

In effect, the obstetricians' mythic pregnant woman ceases to act as co-generator and becomes instead a passive, material nurturer. J. A. Barnes (1973:68) finds little of note in the co-optation: "The denial of physical maternity usually means merely that the mother is thought to contribute nothing of importance to the foetus during pregnancy, as for example was believed in ancient Egypt . . . and is stated by Apollo in Aeschylus' *Eumenides* (lines 657–61), when defending Orestes against the charge of matricide." Barnes cites Needham, who (1934:25) quotes Diodorus of Sicily: "The Egyptians hold the father alone to be the author of generation, and the mother only to provide a nidus and nourishment for the foetus"; and Aeschylus's Apollo: "The mother of what is called her child is no parent of it, but nurse only of the young life that is sown in her. The parent is the male, and she but a stranger, a friend, who, if fate spares his plant, preserves it till it puts forth."

In Zuni mythology, however, *both* the Earth-mother and the Sky-father undertake an active gestational role. Cushing's second myth outline

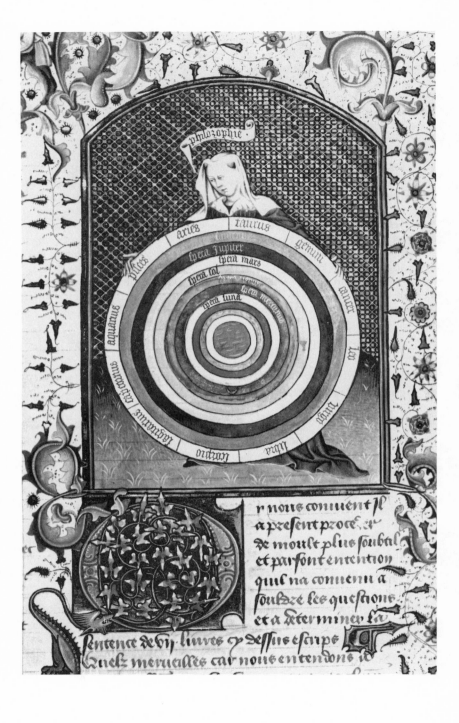

Philosophia with the World Disk. Miniature from a manuscript of St. Augustine's *De civitae Dei*, Flanders, ca. 1420. Ms. 9005, fol. 287 verso. (Copyright Bibliothèque Royale Albert Ier, Bruxelles.)

Erich Neumann includes this among the plates showing "Spiritual Transformation." Analyzing some of these images, Neumann (1963:326) asserts: "In the patriarchal Christian sphere Sophia is reduced to an inferior position by the male god, but here too the female archetype of spiritual transformation makes itself felt. Thus in Dante's poem the sacred white rose belonging to the Madonna is the ultimate flower of light, which is revealed above the starry night sky as the supreme spiritual unfolding of the earthly. In the Crescent Madonna the Feminine stands again at the center of the earthly and heavenly spheres. And the same is true of the medieval painting of Philosophia, one of the medieval forms of Sophia, gathering the arts around her, teaching the philosophers, and inspiring the poets. . . . She remains the Great Mother even when as Philosophia [reproduced here] she bears within her the world disk, zodiac, planets, sun, and moon. . . . And the queen sitting with her child in her lap, enthroned in the center of paradise, surrounded by the Evangelists and the virtues, is again the feminine self as the creative center of the mandala."

(1896:379–80; see Appendix 9.2) tells how Earth-mother consults with "All-covering Sky-father" about the way their progeny are to be nurtured when she does facilitate their growth and emergence: "As a woman forebodes evil for her first-born ere born, even so did the Earth-mother forebode, long withholding from birth her myriad progeny and meantime seeking counsel with the Sky-father." She prepares a terraced bowl and, like the Zuni women potters interviewed by Ruth Bunzel, "paints" it with foam.

The gestational Zuni Earth-mother's concerned, consultive crafting is far from the passive, "brooding chaos" envisioned by de Beauvoir and Western embryologists and obstetricians.[11] Cushing's Zuni myth, like most emergence accounts, suggests an active gestation within and upon the Earth-mother. Paula Gunn Allen (1986:27–28) calls this a ritual process of vitalization, not mere submission to biology:

> Pre-Conquest American Indian women valued their role as vitalizers. Through their own bodies they could bring vital beings into the world—a miraculous power whose potency does not diminish with industrial sophistication or time. They were mothers, and that word did not imply slaves, drudges, drones who are required to live only for others rather than for themselves as it does so tragically for many modern women. The ancient ones were empowered by their certain

knowledge that the power to make life is the source of all power and that no other power can gainsay it. Nor is that power simply of biology, as modernists tendentiously believe. When Thought Woman brought to life the twin sisters, she did not give birth to them in the biological sense. She sang over the medicine bundles that contained their potentials. With her singing and shaking she infused them with vitality. She gathered the power that she controlled and focused it on those bundles, and thus they were "born."

6

Couvade and Parturition

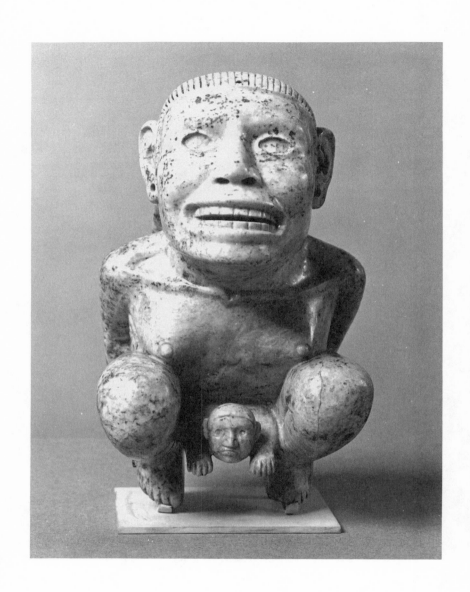

Aztec goddess Tlazolteotl in the act of childbirth. Aplite with inclusions of garnets, 20.2 cm. h. × 12.0 cm. w. × 14.9 cm. d., object D.O. B–71.AS. Courtesy, Dumbarton Oaks Research Library and Collections, Washington, D.C.

Known as Eater of Filth, Goddess of Dirt, Earth Mother, and various other names, Tlazolteotl "was extensively worshipped and was also synonymously known as the 'Mother of the Gods.' Primarily an earth-goddess, she, alone of the goddesses, had a moral significance, since in eating refuse she consumed the sins of mankind, leaving them pure." She is also identified as a goddess of childbirth (Vaillant 1966:187, 185, plate 55). As Eater of Filth, she is associated with witch-craft, the third phase of the moon, and a once-a-lifetime rite of confession to her priests which, properly performed, assured forgiveness for all previous sins. In this aspect too she blesses married life and the home with fertility and peace (Burland 1980:36–37, 106).[1]

That was the time people lived in darkness, in the very first begin-ning, when there were only men and no women. . . .

Woman was made by man. It is an old, old story, difficult to under-stand. They say that the world collapsed, the earth was destroyed, that great showers of rain flooded the land. All the animals died, and there were only two men left. They lived together. They married, as there was nobody else, and at last one of them became with child. They were great shamans, and when the one was going to bear a child they made his penis over again so that he became a woman, and she had a child. They say it is from that shaman that woman came.

That is all I know about people. I have also heard that the earth was here before the people, and that the very first people came out of the ground from tussocks. But these are hard things to understand, diffi-cult things to talk about, all this about where something began, where the first people came from. It is sufficient for us to see that they are here and that we ourselves are here.

And there are those who say that the children of the earth were not the first people, and that they only came to make people many. Women who happened to be out wandering found them sprawling in the tussocks and took them and nursed them; in that way people became numerous. (Nâlungiaq, a Netsilik Eskimo woman [Rasmussen 1931: 208–9])[2]

S. G. F. Brandon, a scholar of comparative religion, begins his study of ancient Egyptian, Mesopotamian, Israelite, Greek, and Iranian creation myths with a chapter titled "The Dawning Concept of Creativity" and claims that the idea "that the world had a beginning [is] a strange one for human beings to entertain." Its "very conception" requires "a high order of detachment from one's physical environment, as well as the power to contemplate that environment as an integrated whole in terms of its duration backward in time beyond the range of personal memory, indeed to its imagined far-off beginning." Once this detachment was achieved, Brandon asks, "what happenings or objects within the world of their experience were likely to have given the earliest peoples the idea of 'beginning'?" (Brandon 1963:1, 3–4). He proposes a double stimulus: biological birth and artistic creation.

The observation of biological birth, whether animal (especially from an egg) or human, is insufficient to conceptualize a true cosmogony.

> Such a biological pattern would mean, in ignorance of the cause of generation, that "beginning" would essentially connote the emergence of a pre-existing but immature individual being from the womb of a mature individual of the species concerned. The process of parturition would be seen as initiating a separate individual existence. As a conceptual image of beginning, biological birth would, accordingly, have been applicable only to animals; whether it was imaginatively extended by early man to explain the origin of other forms of organic life such as trees we cannot know. It would certainly seem, at least to our minds, that experience of biological "beginning" was unlikely to have prompted speculation about the beginning of the world or to have supplied the imagery for its conception. (Brandon 1963:5)

The stimulus for that all-important imagery "might reasonably be assumed to have come from Palaeolithic man's technical and artistic ability."

> The Palaeolithic artist who drew upon the blank wall of a cave the figure of an animal instinct with life, or carved from shapeless stone the figure of a woman, was a creator. He must have felt, and his fellow tribesmen must have recognised, that he was possessed of a marvellous power to bring into being a new and significant form—moreover, in terms of intent, these artistic creations were not mere depiction but were believed to be endowed with magical efficacy. (Brandon 1963:7)

Attitudes like Brandon's help explain the devaluation of procreation myths and the paucity of descriptions and interpretations of women's parturition. Most mythographers and ethnographers eagerly undertake the task of gathering and interpreting creation myths and rituals but do not similarly attend to the beliefs, myths, rites, and practices surrounding pregnancy, labor, delivery, and postpartum care, unless, of course, couvade is involved. Childbearing, however, is not a simple, dumb, physiological, biomedical circumstance but a complex, interactional, biosocial, cultural event, easily the equivalent of elaborate all-male rituals of couvade and initiation.

Helen Callaway begins her discussion of "'The Most Essentially Female Function of All': Giving Birth" with a reference to two essays by Robert Hertz—"The Representation of Death" (1907) and "The Pre-eminence of the Right Hand" (1909)—in which he "selected salient facts of nature and showed how these have been transformed by culture, how various societies have taken these biological facts as focal points in their collective systems of ideas and actions which invest their everyday world with meaning."

> Birth is another salient fact of nature. As a biological event it is "universal" among human groups, yet its practices in different societies show considerable diversity. . . . While birth might be considered as a focal event of the same order as death and marriage, compared to these widely investigated categories it has been relatively neglected in anthropology. Like these categories, birth is a focus of social rules and strategies which define and reinforce the classifications of male and female, and thus its study holds particular interest today. (Callaway 1978:163–64)

Such study would serve to counterbalance the voluminous literature on couvade and other forms of male parthenogenesis.

By the same token, in mythology, emergence myths have been overlooked, deemed cosmogonies unworthy the kinds of analysis to which *ex nihilo,* earth-diver, and other more "male" creation myths have been subjected. Emergence myths recount how

> men, animals, and vegetation live in a cave in the earth. When the earth is ready for people they are instructed in all ceremonies, customs, and crafts; they can now emerge to the surface and begin their wanderings to their present sites. The corn-mother, the sun twins, or a hero is sent to lead them out into the sun from the dark, narrow cave where they

have lived in misery. Sometimes the wandering is pictured as a climbing of a tree or vine which, reaching up to the roof of the cave, pierces a
crevice in the stone. . . . Sometimes animals are sent to dig a hole into
"heaven" or the roof. (Rooth 1957:503)

Anna Birgitta Rooth maps instances throughout the American Southwest,
"with offshoots in the Plains area," and suggests that they are related to
Meso-American tradition and possibly to certain insular Pacific, notably
Trobriand Island, and East Asian traditions.

Washington Matthews (1902:739) calls these "myths of gestation and
parturition." He points out various features—including subterranean
worlds or wombs, ascent by a vine or reed (a *funis,* he claims), and emergence in a lake or accompanied by a flood of water—which "must be
suggestive to the tocologist." Erminie Wheeler-Voegelin and Remedios W.
Moore (1957:73–74) make a similar observation in their comparative study
of 120 versions of emergence from Native North American tribes: "The
'Earth-mother' concept of creation enters into the story as a motif; we have
not gone into the study of it as a type, although certain of the versions do
reflect the psychological attitude toward the emergence as childbirth in an
extended sense, after a period of gestation." This association between
emergence and childbearing has contributed to its being overlooked, as in
Wheeler-Voegelin and Moore's study, or devalued, as in the usual ethnocentric and androcentric creation mythologies.

As Susan Stanford Friedman (1987:51) asserts for literary discourse, this
devaluation results from cultural and not textual considerations. "The
context of the childbirth metaphor is the institution of motherhood at
large. Consequently the meaning of the childbirth metaphor is overdeter-
mined by psychological and ideological resonances evoked by, but independent of, the text." That context supports what Friedman calls "the [child-
birth] metaphor's dangerous biologism" with its "fundamental binary
oppositions of patriarchal ideology between word and flesh, creativity and
procreativity, mind and body." In the final section below, validating readings of emergence—in the allegories of Plato's *Republic* and myths from
Sioux and Southwest Indian cultures—are suggested.

Defecation and Parturition

A Chukchee myth from northeastern Siberia tells how Raven protests to his
wife that he cannot do as she wishes and create the earth. She counters that

"I, at least, shall try to create a 'spleen-companion,'" and goes to sleep while Raven intermittently watches her transformation from bird to pregnant human.

> Again he looks at his wife. Her abdomen has enlarged. In her sleep she creates without any effort. He is frightened, and turns his face away. . . . Then he looked again, and, lo! there are already three of them. His wife was delivered in a moment. She brought forth male twins. Then only did she awake from her sleep. . . . Raven said, "There, you have created men! Now I shall go and try to create the earth."

Raven, who does not change during his creation, consults various "benevolent Beings" and finally finds a group of naked men "created from the dust resulting from the friction of the sky meeting the ground." They implore him to create the earth, and one man accompanies Raven as he "flies and defecates," and "every piece of excrement falls upon water, grows quickly, and becomes land." Raven's companion tells him it is not sufficient, so Raven "began to pass water. When one drop falls, it becomes a lake; where a jet falls it becomes a river. After that he began to defecate a very hard substance. Large pieces of excrement became mountains, smaller pieces became hills. The whole earth became as it is now" (Bogoras 1910:151–53).[3]

It is Freud's contention in "The Sexual Life of Man" that "children are all united from the outset in the belief that the birth of a child takes place by the bowel: that is to say, that the baby is produced like a piece of feces" (1952:328). In "On the Sexual Theories of Children," Freud (1959:219) claims that "in later childhood" the unacceptable "anal sexual components" must be repressed, and so, "when . . . the same question is the subject of solitary reflection or of a discussion between two children, the explanations probably arrived at are that the baby emerges from the navel, which comes open, or that the abdomen is slit up and the baby taken out—which was what happened to the wolf in the story of Little Red Riding-Hood." Initially though, young children's

> ignorance of the vagina also makes it possible for [them] to believe [that] . . . if the baby grows in the mother's body and is then removed from it, this can only happen along the one possible pathway—the anal aperture. *The baby must be evacuated like a piece of excrement, like a stool.* . . . At that time [of childhood] a motion was something which could be talked about in the nursery without shame. The child was still

not so distant from his constitutional coprophilic inclinations. There was nothing degraded about coming into the world like a heap of faeces, which had not yet been condemned by feelings of disgust. The cloacal theory, which, after all, is valid for so many animals, was the most natural theory, and it alone could obtrude upon the child as being a probable one.

Neither the "primitive" Chukchee's mythic Raven nor Doctor Freud's hypothetical Viennese children are alone in their metaphors of parturition. Many ethnographic accounts of childbirth imply that it is a strictly "natural" act and somehow not a "cultural" performance. This common notion of "primitive" (or "peasant" or "poor") women simply "dropping the child" like feces is implied in Knud Rasmussen's brief description of Netsilik Eskimo childbirth: "She brings her child into the world while on her knees and alone, without help. If it is winter, she allows the child to glide down into a small hollow in the snow on the platform itself. No skin lining is placed in the hollow for the child, which falls straight into the snow" (Rasmussen 1931:258).[4] The literary counterpart is perhaps "Tennessee Williams's description of 'trying to shit a watermelon'" (Poston 1978:28).

Sheila Kitzinger notes that "the squatting position is the one spontaneously adopted by human beings for defecation, and childbirth entails release of the same pelvic floor muscles that are used in emptying the bowels." She suggests cultural and class variables for the variety of postures "which women are expected to adopt during advanced labor . . . , from the sitting posture used in European medieval labour chairs or stools (changed only in the reign of Louis XIV when obstetricians delivered his mistress on a flat table so that he could hide behind a curtain to see everything), to swinging from the rafters of a hut."

> When I was doing research in a big Jamaican maternity hospital there was a constant battle between labouring women and midwives, the women wanting to get up and crouch down or rock their pelvises back and forward with knees bent, and the midwives trying to get them on the bed, where they were expected to lie still and be good patients.
>
> One middle-class labour ward sister, who was embarrassed that I, an outsider [white], should witness this, said, "I don't know why you want to see them do this. They are just like animals!" (Kitzinger 1980:93, 92, 91)

Both defecation and parturition are partly "involuntary" processes and are so described in the gynecological texts reviewed by Emily Martin (1987:58–59). The technological accounts easily match the coprological ones.

Since the uterus is seen as an involuntary muscle, it, rather than the women, is seen as doing most of the labor. What the uterus does is expressed in terms that would be familiar to any student of time and motion studies used in industry to analyze and control workers' movements: "Labor is work; mechanically, work is the generation of motion against resistance. The forces involved in labor are those of the uterus and the abdomen that act to expel the fetus and that must overcome the resistance offered by the cervix to dilation and the friction created by the birth canal during passage of the presenting part." Note that the kind of "work" meant is mechanical work, as defined in physics, a narrow conception of force working against resistance.

This work is often evaluated using the "time and motion studies" more appropriately applied to production than reproduction.

Uteruses produce "efficient or inefficient contractions," good or poor labor is judged by the amount of "progress made in certain periods of time." In the obstetrician Emanuel Friedman's well-known representations of average dilation curves, the amount of time it takes a woman's cervix to open from 4 to 8 cm is described as a "good measure of the overall efficiency of the machine." Presumably the "machine" referred to is the uterus.[5]

The mechanical imagery with its time and motion evaluation contrasts starkly with the sense of parturition in emergence myths, wherein each underworld or womb has its own sacred characteristics and expected social behaviors. The Navajo first beings journey through perilous black, blue, yellow, and white worlds before emerging into this fifth, "changeable" one, according to the Hastin Tlo'tsi hee version (Appendix 11). Gill (1983:502) identifies Navajo texts characterizing the environment and populations of from two to fourteen such "worlds described as either platters or hemispheres." Frank Hamilton Cushing's Zuni myth outlines (1896; see Appendix 9) designate the "cave-wombs" of the "Four-fold Containing Mother-earth" as: Womb of Sooty Depth or Growth-Generation; Umbilical-womb or Place of Gestation; Vaginal-womb or Place of Sex-generation or Gestation; and Ultimate-uncoverable or Womb of Parturition.

The questions posed by literary critic Carol H. Poston (1978:20) apply as well to gynecology, ethnography, and most mythology:

> Given that birth is such an overwhelming experience, why do we find it so rarely described in literature? Babies might indeed be found under cabbages, so magically and without travail do they usually appear on the written page. Furthermore, when we do find examples of birth, why is the experience so rarely that of the birthing woman; in other words, where is the authentic voice?
>
> Because female experiences, from menstruation to menopause, have been consistently slighted in our literature, childbirth is a virtually unexplored literary topic. "Childbed," says Hortense Calisher [1971: 225–26], "is not a place or an event; it is merely what women do." . . . Women's experiences are not regarded as fully human experiences, so they do not have literary currency—though it need hardly be said that men's experiences not shared by women have been taken as universal.

Poston (1978:21) identifies two literary metaphors of birth, both initially in the language of men, "and so great has the tyranny of language been that women began experiencing birth from the male point of view."

> It was, first of all, men who began to write about birth in literature; and most of them saw (and see) it as an activity which is savage, barbaric, primitive, or loathsome in some other way. This attitude produces what I would call the "savage" tradition of childbirth and its practitioners have been men and women. The other side of this is the "heroine" tradition, which reaches its apogee in the view that birth is a woman's highest moment, that adulation of childbirth as the crown of the mature woman, what J. W. De Forest in *Miss Ravenel's Conversion* calls "the apotheosis of womanhood." Women have refined this "heroine" stance by using a kind of understatement, a withdrawal from the details of birth as a way of implicitly assuming the experience is so wrenching that all women recognize what one has got through. The "savage" tradition also seems to have a female refinement as well, especially interesting in the context of the audience point of view; and

that is the schizoid split, wherein the woman feels the agony of birth as an event which tears her into two selves, one watching the other.

When women cease to view themselves as schizoid savages, crowned heroines, or forced labor, Emily Martin (1987:157–58) demonstrates, they create a range of "new key metaphors, core symbols of birth." Some

> stress a process that develops from within and the continuity of this process with the past and future. *A river:* "the continuous flow of labor narrows into an intense stream of life-filled birth"; *a ripening fruit:* "like fruit ripening on a tree, birth takes time. If we start too soon or try to rush, it will be like picking unripe fruit: harder work, longer hours, and possible damage to the crop."
>
> Other writers focus more explicitly on the energy people feel to be present during birth: "At birth, you, the laboring woman, are the channel for the Life Force, the energy of creation and transformation." They choose metaphors that capture how the woman seems to "ride" this energy, actively adapting to it: "It is not possible to control your labor, but it is both possible and necessary to control yourself, in the way that a surfer controls himself in riding the big waves by maintaining equilibrium at the same time that he surrenders to them." Dwelling on heightened energy leads these writers to stress the similarities between the experience of birthing and the experience of sexual union: "Birth is fundamentally a creative act, as is the act of sexual union."[6]

Other key metaphors focus on the pregnant and parturient mother as an initiate, undertaking a transformative rite of passage equivalent to that of the baby itself or of male heroes and initiates. Martin (1987:158) quotes Gayle Peterson's *Birthing Normally* (1984:52): "Birth is a journey. . . . The view of pregnancy and birth as a journey inward has begun at the end of the first trimester. Birth becomes an opportunity for psychological growth and an event to which a laboring woman relates intimately and uniquely, weaving a learning experience all her own." It becomes a parthenogenesis like that described by Anne G. Dellenbaugh (1982:44):

> Within a phallocentric semantic context, parthenogenesis is a method of reproduction.[7] But wrenched from this context and heard with a radical feminist consciousness, *Parthenogenesis* names a wholly different phenomenon. Hearing it in this new way requires a qualitative

leap into Self-consciousness, for Parthenogenesis names nothing less than the process of a woman creating her Self.

Couvade and Parthenogenesis

But a mist went up from the earth and watered the whole face of the ground—then the Lord God formed man of dust from the ground, and breathed into his nostrils the breath of life; and man became a living being. . . . So the Lord God caused a deep sleep to fall upon the man, and while he slept took one of his ribs and closed up its place with flesh; and the rib which the Lord God had taken from the man he made into a woman and brought her to the man. (Genesis 2:6–7, 21–22)

She [Rheia] wrapped a great stone in baby-clothes,
   and this she presented
to the high lord [Kronos], son of Ouranos,
   who once ruled the immortals,
and he took it then in his hands
   and crammed it down in his belly. . . .
     —Hesiod, *Theogony*, 485–87 (trans. R. Lattimore, in Lattimore 1959:152)

As part of his study of "Couvade in Genesis," Alan Dundes (1983:35, 36) presents a valuable survey of the vast couvade literature. The first mention is from the early second century B.C., in *The Argonautica* by Apollonius of Rhodes: "Soon after leaving them [the Chalybes] behind, the Argonauts rounded the headland of Genetaean Zeus and sailed in safety past the country of Tibareni. Here, when a woman is in childbirth, it is the husband who takes to his bed. He lies there groaning with his head wrapped up and his wife feeds him with loving care" (trans. E. V. Rieu, in Rieu 1959:101). The term first appeared in print in Charles de Rochefort's 1665 description of the Carib Indians, *Histoire naturelle et morale des Iles Antilles de l'Amérique*. Two hundred years later, in his *Researches into the Early History of Mankind* (1865), E. B. Tylor used the anthropological term, "derived from the French *couver*, to brood or hatch, . . . to refer to a widespread custom whereby fathers or men about to become fathers ritually went through the motions of confinement and childbirth." Psychological perspectives owe much to Bruno Bettelheim's 1954 study, *Symbolic*

Wounds: Puberty Rites and the Envious Male, in which he (1962:111) asserts: "Women, emotionally satisfied by having given birth and secure in their ability to produce life, can agree to the couvade; men need it to fill the emotional vacuum created by their inability to bear children."

Dundes argues that three key elements of couvade appear in the male creation myth of Genesis 1–3: rest following the six days of creation, creation from dirt and from flesh, and the injunction about painful childbirth. The seventh-day rest in Genesis 2:2 is "the very essence of couvade."

> In theory, an omnipotent God, capable of creating the heaven and earth and all else, would not need to rest. Of course, it is possible that the sanctification of a seventh day may have been merely a device to offer a sacred charter for a religious system which demanded that individuals devote one day a week to that system. Still, in the context of couvade, it makes perfect sense for a male creator to rest after his creative act. (Dundes 1983:46)

The woman's "curse" ("I will greatly multiply your pain in childbearing; / in pain you shall bring forth children" [Genesis 3:16]) is essentially the end of this practice, "a myth providing a sociological charter for non-couvade" by men (Dundes 1983:52).

The male *Deus faber*'s earthen and flesh creations are more problematic, especially the latter. Dundes cites William E. Phipps's review essay on "Adam's Rib: Bone of Contention," where the latter traces "the beginning of the clash between biology and religion" to Andreas Vesalius's 1543 *De Humani Corporis Fabrica Libri Septem:* "The ribs are twelve in number on each side in man and woman. . . . The popular belief that man is lacking a rib on one side and that woman has one more rib than man is clearly ridiculous, even though Moses, in the second chapter of Genesis, said that Eve was created by God from one of Adam's ribs" (Phipps 1976–1977:263). Dundes (1983:50, 52) adds to this discussion observations from folklore showing "that the [human] phallus has been commonly perceived as 'the boneless one,'" and concludes:

> I believe that the initial act of creation by God (which ends in a day of rest) and the creation of a female from a male body genital— remember that females give birth from their genital parts—and the specific details of God's curse upon women (referring to labor pains) all support the idea that the first two chapters of Genesis consist in part

of a form of literary couvade. The critical importance of this psychological constellation is indicated by the widespread distribution of
couvade among peoples in many areas of the world, e.g., Asia, Europe,
South America, and by its manifestations among individual males in
most, if not all, modern urban societies (under the couvade syndrome
label).[8]

According to such interpretations, male creativity simulates female
procreativity. In the study "The Special Position of the Artist in Biogra-
phy," for example, Ernst Kris and Otto Kurz (1979:115–16) identify clusters
of motifs, including "the tradition—one that extends from classical antiquity into modern times—which regards the work of art as the 'child' of the
artist and attempts to view the process of artistic creation according to the
model of sexual life."

> A painter is asked how it is that his own children are so hideous,
> when those that he paints are quite the opposite. The reason, he
> replies, is that he engenders the latter by daylight, but the former at
> night. This quip derives from a classical source, the *Saturnalia* (2:2.10)
> of Macrobius, where it is attributed to the Roman painter Lucius
> Mallius. It is cited by Petrarch in one of his letters, when he comes to
> speak of the unappealing exterior of great artists. In the fourteenth
> century this ancient anecdote is still told, this time of Giotto, with
> Dante as the questioner. . . . Another remark of Michelangelo's shows
> us this anecdote in a different interpretation. When he was asked why
> he had never married, Michelangelo indicated that his works were his
> children.

Dundes (1983:45) affirms this view when he claims that "Athena, Zeus's
literal brainchild, is male creativity (without female assistance) par excellence."
   On the other hand, female procreativity par excellence may be Rhea's
presentation of the artfully swaddled stone to an oblivious Cronos, no less
an act of craft than Yahweh's transformed rib presented to the oblivious
Adam. Hesiod's poem resembles the Old Testament scripture.

> The fundamental struggle of the *Theogony* is over the power of
> reproduction. In the three generations that culminate in the rule of
> Zeus, the male moves progressively closer to appropriating the re-

productive process. Ouranus tries to block the birth of his children by keeping them within the body of Gaia; Cronus moves closer to the female role by swallowing his children so that they are kept within his own body. But even this measure is not wholly successful, since Rhea, when she is about to give birth to Zeus, asks Gaia and Ouranus for a *mētis* by which to elude Cronus (468–478). The trick they devise is to substitute a stone wrapped in swaddling clothes for the real infant. Here is the primary *mētis,* the first imitation, one that seems to symbolize a supposititious child. For Cronus is baffled by the disguise, as any man would be, when his wife presents him with what she says is his child, for who except his wife can vouch for his true child, the legitimate heir to his property and his proper name. Only the female has the knowledge necessary to tell the true from the false heir, but it is this very knowledge that also makes her able to substitute for the truth, a false thing that resembles it.

The appropriation is complete when Zeus "improves upon Cronus' attempt to control reproduction by swallowing not the children alone, but the mother Metis as well, thus ensuring that he alone will now possess the knowledge and power she represents" (Bergren 1983:74).

The next step symbolically is to claim either that women simulate male creativity in projects or erections (so-called penis envy) or that they have absolutely no need to create since they "naturally" reproduce. James Joyce (in Jong 1979:27), for example, wrote to his wife: "Men have the feeling that women can create life in their bodies, therefore, how dare they create art?" This sort of sexism is overt in articles like G. W. B. James, "Psychology and Gynaecology," from a 1963 textbook edited by A. Claye and A. Bourne, *British Obstetric and Gynaecological Practice.* "Femininity tends to be passive and receptive, masculinity to be more active, restless, anxious for repeated demonstrations of potency, requiring worldly [*sic*] success and its external signs. Childbirth should be the crowning fulfilment of a woman's sexual development; her physical and psychological destiny have been achieved" (Callaway 1978:169).

In a psychological and political study of womb envy, Eva Feder Kittay (1983:99–100, 98) argues "that just as 'penis envy' derives its force not from mere biological difference—although that difference is a potential source of envy—but from the context of cultural male supremacy, so 'womb envy' assumes its strength and fury within this same context." Some of this "fury" comes because "within the context of patriarchal male dominance, where

Aurum plůit, dum naſcitur Pallas Rhodi, & Sol concumbit Veneri.

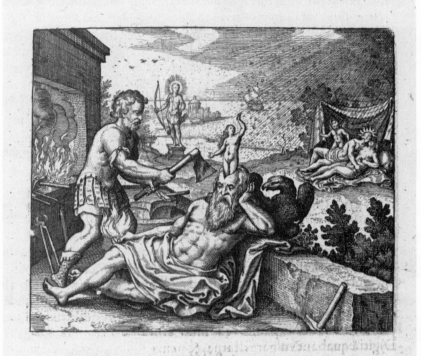

EPIGRAMMA XXIII.

R Es eſt mira, fidem fecit ſed Græcia nobis
    Ejus, apud Rhodios quæ celebrata fuit.
Nubibus Aureolus, referunt, quòd decidit imber,
    Sol ubi erat Cypriæ junctus amore Deæ:
Tum quoque, cum Pallas cerebro Jovis excidit, aurum
    Vaſe ſuo pluviæ ſic cadat inſtar aquæ.

N 3   AURUM

Emblem XXIII of alchemist Michael Maier's *Atalanta fugiens* [Atalanta in flight] (Oppenheim, 1618). Facsimile reproduction courtesy Beinecke Rare Book and Manuscript Library, Yale University.

According to Kurt Seligmann (1971:108–9), it shows an alchemical allegory, the golden rain. In it, Maier (1568–1622) "depicts in breathless simultaneity several events of mythology associated with the alchemist's work. The adept (or is it the god Vulcan?) splits sleeping Jupiter's head. In his right hand, the maltreated god holds the sign of his power: the flame of lightning. He is leaning against his bird, the eagle. From the wounded head arises naked Pallas Athene. A shower of gold falls upon her. Like the sun, the head of Apollo's statue in the background rises above the horizon. The god Apollo himself embraces Venus in an improvised tent. They are observed by Eros. The explanation of the representation is given as follows: 'It rained gold when Pallas was born in Rhodes, and the sun mated with Venus. This is a marvel, and its truthfulness is affirmed by Greece. The happening was celebrated in Rhodes where they say that the clouds yielded a golden rain. And the sun was joined to Cypria, the goddess of love. At the time when Pallas emerged from Jupiter's brain, from the vessel fell gold as if it were rain-water.'"

In their feminist interpretation, Sally G. Allen and Joanna Hubbs (1980:218) note: "Emblem XXIII represents the birth of Athena from the head of Zeus, a birth aided by the alchemist who brandishes an axe with which he has to split the head of the Greek Father God. Athena is greeted by a golden shower from the sky, the heavenly source of life and seed, and the motto reads: 'Gold rains down from the sky while Pallas was born in Rhodes, and Sol [Apollo] cohabits with Venus.' The sexual act empowered from above (Apollo and the golden shower) generates the birth of woman out of man, that is, reverses the natural relationship of male child emerging out of the body of the female."

". . . There can / be a father without any mother. There she stands, / the living witness, daughter of Olympian Zeus, / she who was never fostered in the dark of the womb, / yet such a child as no goddess could bring to birth" (Aeschylus, *The Eumenides,* lines 662–66, trans. Richmond Lattimore [in Lattimore 1953:158]).

Man is the Essential and Woman the Other, sexual differences cannot be simply differences . . . [and] take on symbolic significance as hierarchical differentia so that features of men are positively marked and those of women are lacks, defects, or excesses"—except, of course, when properly appropriated by men.

Writer H. D. expresses elements of this "fury" in her *roman a clef, Asphodel,* according to Susan Stanford Friedman (1987:70–71):

> H. D. expresses the fear she felt during her first pregnancy that the attempt to combine speech and childbirth was a form of madness: when her flaming mind beat up and she found she was caught, her mind not taking her as usual like a wild bird but her mind-wings beating, beating and her feet caught, her feet caught, glued like a wildbird in bird lime. . . . No one had known this. No one would ever know it for there were no words to tell it in. . . . Women can't speak and clever women don't have children. So if a clever woman does speak, she must be mad. She wouldn't have had a baby, if she hadn't been.

H. D.'s "image of a wild bird caught in bird lime [as] a metaphor for the tie between creation and procreation" (Friedman 1987:71), which is also a parthenogenesis metaphor, may be contrasted with the joyous parthenogenesis of the mythic Sioux ancestor as recounted by Chief Luther Standing Bear (1933, in Turner 1974:125–26):

> Our legends tell us that it was hundreds and perhaps thousands of years ago since the first man sprang from the soil in the midst of the great plains. The story says that one morning long ago a lone man awoke, face to the sun, emerging from the soil. Only his head was visible, the rest of his body not yet being fashioned. The man looked about, but saw no mountains, no rivers, no forests. There was nothing but soft and quaking mud, for the earth itself was still young. Up and up the man drew himself until he freed his body from the clinging soil. At last he stood upon the earth, but it was not solid, and his first steps were slow and halting. But the sun shone and ever the man kept his face turned toward it. In time the rays of the sun hardened the face of the earth and strengthened the man and he bounded and leaped about, a free and joyous creature. From this man sprang the Lakota nation.

Women's equivalent mythic ancestor of emergent parthenogenesis is Tiamat, according to Anne G. Dellenbaugh (1982:56):

Tiamat is an image of She Who Is and Is Not Yet, she who has always been, will always be, and yet is never the same. She Who will not be held back. It is impossible to stop her movement. Like the "unconscious," which, in dreams for instance, breaks through the barrier into consciousness, this wild sea monster will sooner or later burst through the patriarchally constructed pseudo-cosmos to real-ize herself. When a woman dares to know and be conscious of her Self, the earth moves, the "cosmos" erupts, and she is plunged into the depths of chaos.

In reappropriating Tiamat, the Babylonian/Assyrian primeval salt-water ocean who is portrayed as mother of the gods and later their chaotic adversary whom Marduk slays (cf. Heidel 1951:83–101),[9] the parthenogenetic parturients symbolically invert the supposed Other and create new images for cosmogonic chaos and emergence.

> Many women have described their first "moment of insight" . . . as "a volcano erupting," or "a dam breaking loose." They later spoke of "touching the bottom of a pit," or "the *very center of one's being*." . . . The abyss in which they were plunged was not the void of nothingness, but primordial chaos itself. Even the metaphors they used to describe the experience are ones of a tremendous life force breaking loose, erupting. Both a volcano and a flood can be acts of creation. The one may cause the birth of an island, the other fertilize a plain. "It is one of the paradoxes in the ways of earth and sea," writes Rachel Carson [1961:84], "that a process seemingly so destructive, so catastrophic in nature, can result in an act of creation." (Dellenbaugh 1982:57)

Emergence

> They came out of the earth, from Iatik'u, the mother. They came out through a hole in the north called Shipap. They crawled out like grasshoppers; their bodies were naked and soft. It was all dark; the sun had not yet risen. All of the little people had their eyes closed; they hadn't opened them yet. Iatik*u* lined them all up in a row facing east. Then she had the sun come up. When it came up and shone on the babies' eyes they opened. They crawled around. In eight days they were bigger and stronger. They walk around now. (White 1932:142)[10]

In the *Republic*, his famous dialogue constructing the ideal state, Plato uses two allegories of emergence to speak about politics and philosophy. The former is called "a sort of Phoenician tale"; the latter is an explicit comparison between the process of education and being led out (*educere,* "to lead out") from a "subterranean cavern."

Early in the dialogue (Book II) Socrates banishes from education the "composed false stories" of Hesiod, Homer, and "other poets." He proposes "a censorship over our storymakers," lest "our children . . . listen to any chance stories fashioned by any chance teachers and so . . . take into their minds opinions for the most part contrary to those that we shall think it desirable for them to hold when they are grown up." Acceptable stories "we will induce nurses and mothers to tell to the children and so shape their souls by these stories far rather than their bodies by their hands" (377b–d, trans. Paul Shorey, 1930, in Hamilton and Cairns 1961:624).

Socrates refers to this part of the dialogue in Book III, after a discussion of the ideal city's proper guardians, "watchers against foemen without and friends within, so that the latter shall not wish and the former shall not be able to work harm." He proposes to "contrive one of those opportune falsehoods of which we were just now speaking, so as by one noble lie to persuade if possible the rulers themselves, but failing that the rest of the city." He claims his "fiction" is "nothing unprecedented, . . . but a sort of Phoenician tale, something that has happened ere now in many parts of the world, as the poets aver and have induced men to believe, but that has not happened and perhaps would not be likely to happen in our day and demanding no little persuasion to make it believable." Telling the tale requires "audacity" and "the words to speak" in order

> to persuade first the rulers themselves and the soldiers and then the rest of the city that in good sooth all our training and educating of them were things that they imagined and that happened to them as it were in a dream, but that in reality at that time they were down within the earth being molded and fostered themselves while their weapons and the rest of their equipment were being fashioned. And when they were quite finished the earth as being their mother delivered them, and now as if their land were their mother and their nurse they ought to take thought for her and defend her against any attack and regard the other citizens as their brothers and children of the selfsame earth. (414c–e, trans. Paul Shorey, 1930, in Hamilton and Cairns 1961:658–59)

Monique Canto calls "the drama of the *Republic,* the first certain entry of women's bodies into the city." They are envisioned as fully functional members of the political community whose only difference from men is that he "begets" while she "bears."

> But since the meaning of the community of men and women is in the first place political, only a political idea of procreation would be capable of neutralizing the effects of this difference. That procreation should be the city's first concern is actually what Socrates is proposing when he calls for child-rearing in common. . . . Children are turned over to nurses at birth to live in a special quarter of the city. Mothers will come to suckle offspring only so long as their breasts are full of milk, and children are to be presented to them in such a way that no mother will recognize her own. Hence there is nothing to distinguish the mother from the father of a child. A man "will call all male offspring born in the tenth and seventh month after he became a bridegroom his sons, and all female, daughters, and they will call him father." Similarly, every possible step is to be taken to prevent a woman from calling a child her own (V, 460b–461e). The living all belong to the city.

Women's former gynaeceum has thus been expanded to coincide with the city walls, its place now occupied by a communal nursery.

> Socrates suggests that it may be necessary to tell the men and women of the city "a sort of Phoenician tale," a myth of foundation, according to which all citizens believe that they are brothers (414c–417b)—even the women, because, as political bodies, they are the same as men, and because, like the men, they work to drive otherness to the periphery of politics. This shows that within the city woman is in no sense the representative of otherness. (Canto 1986:342, 343, 344)

What Socrates's "contrived fiction" does to motivate and govern the male and female citizens of his ideal city, emergence myths do for *all* (animals, plants, minerals, humans, etc.) living in the world outside the place of emergence from the underworld(s)/womb. Among the Lakota, for example, the Buffalo nation is "the metaphor for humans living in the subterranean world," and this "very name by which humans living [there] are designated in the creation myth—'Buffalo People'—means that the Lakotas are a people *born of woman,* really and spiritually." Women and buffalo are "frequently . . . interchangeable metaphors." During rites at menarche, the young woman was reminded that the buffalo was the most important of all animals. It provided food, clothing, shelter, and even fuel. It was a natural symbol of the universe, for it symbolically contained the totality of all manifest forms of life, including people. According to one story the buffalo originated under the earth like the Oglalas, who emerged from a subterranean place; this demonstrated that the buffalo and the Oglalas are one, the Buffalo Nation (Dorsey 1894). (M. N. Powers 1986:38, 69)

In emergence myths, those in the underworld(s) are shown as instructed and "enlightened" by those who, like the ritual specialists and storytellers, lead them out into the present world. This instruction is evident in the final paragraph of Cushing's Zuni myth outline, "The Birth and Delivery of Men and the Creatures," about the "Womb of Parturition."

Here it was light like the dawning, and men began to perceive and to learn variously according to their natures, wherefore the Twain taught them to seek first of all our Sun-father, who would, they said, reveal to them wisdom and knowledge of the ways of life—wherein also they were instructing them as we do little children. Yet like the other cave-worlds, this too became, after long time, filled with progeny; and finally, at periods, the Two led forth the nations of men and the kinds of being, into this great upper world, which is called Ték'ohaian úlahnane, or the World of Disseminated Light and Knowledge or Seeing. (Cushing 1896:383)[11]

Probably it is not coincidental that Cushing's reworked Zuni myths show a journey like the educational process depicted by Socrates at the beginning of Book VII of the *Republic:*

Picture men dwelling in a sort of subterranean cavern with a long entrance open to the light on its entire width. Conceive them as having their legs and necks fettered from childhood, so that they remain in the same spot, able to look forward only, and prevented by the fetters from turning their heads. Picture further the light from a fire burning higher up and at a distance behind them, and between the fire and the prisoners and above them a road along which a low wall has been built, as the exhibitors of puppet shows have partitions before the men themselves, above which they show the puppets. . . .

See also . . . men carrying past the wall implements of all kinds that rise above the wall, and human images and shapes of animals as well, wrought in stone and wood and every material, some of these bearers presumably speaking and others silent.

The educator unfetters the prisoner and "compels" him to behold the firelight and then proceeds to "drag him thence by force up the ascent which is rough and steep, and not let him go before he had drawn him out into the light of the sun," which is at first excruciating and blinding and in which he is only gradually able to discern shadows, reflections, and the heavens at night, until at last "he would be able to look upon the sun itself and see its true nature" (514–517, trans. Paul Shorey, 1930, in Hamilton and Cairns 1961:747, 748).

Gladys A. Reichard (1974:16) elucidates a similarly difficult process in Navajo emergence mythology.

Upon arriving in a new world the primordial ancestors of the Navaho made vows to co-operate with the natives; as they learned more and more they kept their promises longer and longer. At each pause in the upward migration they accepted more social curbs—some were learned from the old residents, some were commands of their own leaders. The leitmotiv of the earlier worlds—confusion, uncertainty, error—led to evil, witchcraft, and death. Each subsequent step in the emergence changed the emphasis until now, in this world, stability, knowledge, and cooperation are ideals, the chrysalis of ignorance having been shed in the lower worlds.

Plato's "Phoenician tale" and "cave" emergence allegories are ascribed to Socrates, who is presented in dialogue with two young men, Glaucon and his brother Adimantus. It takes place in the Piraeus on the day of a newly inaugurated festival to the goddess. The older Thrasymachus has discontinued his "case," and young Glaucon challenges Socrates, asking, "Is it your desire to seem to have persuaded us or really to persuade us that it is without exception better to be just than unjust?" (Book II, 357, trans. Paul Shorey, 1930, in Hamilton and Cairns 1961:605). Socrates's subsequent, lengthy dialogue with the young men is both a validation of himself and an education for them.

The performance dimension is crucial. Karl W. Luckert stresses the Navajo emergence myth's validation of ritual knowledge in his editor's introduction to Father Berard Haile's typescript, "Creation and Emergence Myth of the Navajo, According to the *haneelnéehee* Moving-up Rite":

> The interest of Westerners in cosmogonies notwithstanding, the *hane-elnéehee* myth was never told to enlighten curious listeners about human origins in general. It was narrated specifically to get into focus the process of which "downward illness" and the corresponding "upwardness of healing power" were brought into the proximity of humankind. This myth was told not to satisfy an intellectual curiosity about the origin of things, but rather to substantiate Navajo soteriology and medicinal knowledge. (Luckert in Haile 1981:ix)

An Oglala narrative apparently had a similar meaning. It

> tells us the Oglalas believed that a man who dreamed of buffalo and thus acted like one had a buffalo inside him, and that a chrysalis lay near his shoulder blade so that no matter how often he was wounded he would not die. The chrysalis means that the buffalo (man/woman) has the power to renew himself (procreate). There is constant metamorphosis, for there is a mechanism for revitalization within the organism. (M. N. Powers 1986:69)

Emergence, like the chrysalis, is a powerful symbol. Barre Toelken was made aware of an equally powerful Navajo symbol associated with emergence, the red ant.[12]

> When I lived with Yellowman's family in Montezuma Canyon, I once came down with what appears to have been pneumonia and was diagnosed by a Navajo practitioner as one in need of the Red Ant ceremony. A medicine man (in Navajo, literally, a "singer") was sent for who knew the ceremony, and I was later advised I was being treated for red ants in my system which I had no doubt picked up by urinating on an anthill. Some time after the ritual, which was quite successful I must point out, I had occasion to discuss the treatment with the singer: Had I really had ants in my system, did he think? His answer was a hesitant "no, not ants, but Ants" (my capitalization, to indicate the gist of his remark). Finally, he said, "We have to have a way of thinking strongly about disease." (Toelken and Scott 1981:90)

Just so, there is need for a way of thinking strongly about birth, whether actual, ritual, or imaginative. The mothers, midwives, and gossips who think and act strongly about childbirth must be counted among the enablers of powerful symbolic processes. Emergence myths must be included in mythology as paradigms of creation that empower in the same way as so-called true cosmogonies. All are expressions of pro/creation and renewal.

7

Midwifery and the Dialogue of
Mythos *and* Mundus

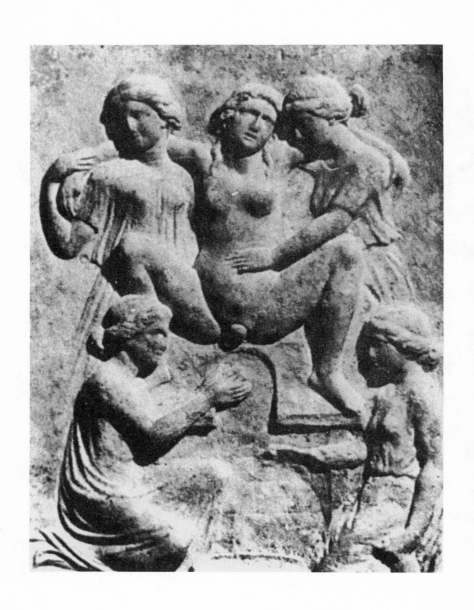

"Birth scene. Early Greek relief. The nude parturient is supported on either side by attendants, one of whom presses against her uterus; while the midwife and another assistant, kneeling before the birthstool, await the infant, whose head is presenting through the vulva" (Speert 1973:83).[1]

Myth tells how, through the deeds of Supernatural Beings, a reality came into existence, be it the whole of reality, the Cosmos, or only a fragment of reality—an island, a species of plant, a particular kind of human behavior, an institution. . . . In short, myths describe the various and sometimes dramatic breakthroughs of the sacred (or the "supernatural") into the World. It is this sudden breakthrough of the sacred that really *establishes* the World and makes it what it is today. Furthermore, it is as a result of the intervention of Supernatural Beings that man himself is what he is today, a mortal, sexed, and cultural being. (Mircea Eliade 1963:5–6)

As the [Maya] baby's head begins to show (sometimes still covered by the unbroken membranes), the excitement in the little house reaches a new pitch. Birth talk is continuous, punctuated only by the midwife's progress reports. She will tell the mother that the baby is "at the door" and ready to be born, she might make an estimate of how many more pushes will be required, and she might report that she can see the baby's beautiful hair. Finally, the head crowns, and with the next contraction or two the product of all this effort emerges in a splash of blood-tinged fluid. Sometimes the baby begins to cry as soon as the head is born, but in any case [midwife] Doña Juana is quick to suction the mucus from its nose and mouth to facilitate breathing. (Brigitte Jordan and Nancy Fuller [in Jordan 1980:28])[2]

Rudolf Otto's description of the religious experience in his 1917 study, *Das Heilige,* or "The Sacred," translated in 1923 as *The Idea of the Holy,* has influenced definitions and interpretations like Mircea Eliade's. Otto claims that the sacred "breaks through" into this world, confronting mortals as a phenomenon wholly other (*ganz andere*), totally different. The experience is a numinous one, derived from the Latin *numen,* meaning god and, significantly, nod. Faced with the numinous, man is as nothing and experiences "the *feeling of terror* before the sacred, before the awe-inspiring mystery (*mysterium tremendum*), the majesty (*majestas*) that emanates an overwhelming superiority of power . . . [and] *religious fear* before the fascinating mystery (*mysterium fascinans*) in which perfect fullness of being flowers" (Eliade 1961:9–10).[3] In Judeo-Christian tradition the paradigm is Moses and the burning bush:

> Now Moses was keeping the flock of his father-in-law . . . ; and he led his flock to the west side of the wilderness, and came to Horeb, the mountain of God. And the angel of the Lord appeared to him in a flame of fire out of the midst of a bush; and he looked, and lo, the bush was burning, yet it was not consumed. . . . God called to him out of the bush. "Moses, Moses! . . . Do not come near; put off your shoes from your feet, for the place on which you are standing is holy ground." And he said, "I am the God of your father. . . ." And Moses hid his face, for he was afraid to look at God. (Exodus 3:1–6)

Experiences of the holy as wholly other figure in Alan W. Watts's (1968:7–8) definition of myth "as a complex of stories—some no doubt fact, and some fantasy—which, for various reasons, human beings regard as demonstrations of the inner meaning of the universe and of human life." They recount events that "have a miraculous or 'numinous' quality which marks them as special, queer, out of the ordinary, and therefore representative of the powers or Power behind the world." These experiences must be proclaimed in richly symbolic expressions, in myth, which "is quite different from philosophy in the sense of abstract concepts, for the form of myth is always concrete—consisting of vivid, sensually intelligible narratives, images, rites, ceremonies, and symbols."

The contrast between the sacralizing and valorizing hierophany and parturition as usually considered is blatant, even ludicrous, if Moses is seen as a midwife or gossip who hides his face from the birth event. Childbirth is not *ganz andere* or extraordinary but an ordinary process *involving* all participants—mother, baby, midwife, gossips—in this world, *mundus*. It is *mundane* in the most important sense of physical, social, and cultural survival. And, although concrete, vivid, and sensually intelligible, it is rarely the subject of mythological study.

Androcentrism clearly plays an important role in this devaluation. David Meltzer (1981:2–3) begins his anthology, *Birth,* "with a quotation by an Abyssinian woman recorded by the anthropologist Leo Frobenius in the early twentieth century":

> How can a man know what a woman's life is? A woman's life is quite different from a man's. God has ordered it so. A man is the same from

the time of his circumcision to the time of his withering. He is the same before he has sought out a woman for the first time, and afterwards. But the day a woman enjoys her first love cuts her in two. She becomes another woman on that day. The man is the same after his first love as he was before. The man spends a night by a woman and goes away. His life and body are always the same. The woman conceives. As a mother she is another person than the woman without child. She carries the fruit of the night nine months long in her body. Something grows. Something grows into her life that never again departs from it. She is a mother. She is and remains a mother even though her child dies, though all her children die. For at one time she carried the child under her heart. And it does not go out of her heart ever again. Not even when it is dead. All this the man does not know; he knows nothing.[4]

"Birth," Meltzer claims, "is the art and mystery of woman and her powerful presence is infused throughout this collection."

By contrast, poet Padraic Colum associates his collection of "great" examples of "stories regarded as sacred that form an integral and active part of a culture," and "in which there is matter that can be 'sympathized' with—recognized as being of proper present interest—by readers of today," with male-dominated mysteries locating the heart of things in death and the underworld:

> I have called the collection "Orpheus," naming it after the minstrel who, according to the poet of the Argonautica, sang "how the earth, the heaven, and the sea once mingled together in one form, after deadly strife were separated each from the other; and how the stars and the moon and the paths of the sun ever keep their fixed place in the sky; and how the mountains rose, and how the resounding rivers with their nymphs came into being, and all creeping things." (Colum 1930:viii–ix, xxviii)

That Colum's collection of choice examples contains few myths that may be called gynocentric or "women's" is not unexpected, given the attitudes documented in the following ethnographic account of Ojibwa women by Ruth Landes (1971:9, 10–11), whose sarcasm could as easily apply to Western views of mythology:

> Women "dream" beadwork patterns, songs, decorations for a dress, complicated dance patterns; men dream traditional tales, or tales

about culture heroes, or have visions of the architecture of the after-world. . . .

Whenever men fulfill their duties creditably, they are lauded. In company they tell endless stories about their adventures, for their duties are always "adventures"; they hold stag feasts of religious importance after a successful hunt. Even the mythology occupies itself with the pursuits and rewards of men. The important visions, which men have been driven all their youth to pursue, bestow power for the masculine occupations. A successful hunter can parade this fact in ways licensed by his visions: songs that he sings publicly, amulets that are conspicuous and worn in public, charms that he can sell. . . . Women's work on the contrary "is spoken of neither for good nor for evil"—at least in a gathering of men. Conventionally it is not judged in any way, it is simply not given any thought. . . . The women themselves live in a world of values all their own, a world closed to the men. Mothers and daughters discuss the merits of their work just as men do the merits of theirs, and when the village quarter of the year comes about, the various families visit, and wider groups of women discuss their own interests. But these discussions and boasts are not formal, as the men's are; they belong to the level of gossip.[5]

Anthropologists Yolanda Murphy and Robert F. Murphy (1974:140–41, 133) have reported a similar attitude among the Mundurucú Indians of Amazonian Brazil.

Rituals are social affairs to both sexes, yet to the women they are mainly social affairs. They like to listen to myths, although they are far less absorbed in their content than are the men and usually keep up a subdued conversation among themselves during the narration. And they never tell myths themselves. . . .

The women are secular and pragmatic in their orientation to life. There is a matter-of-factness and straightforward earthiness in their manner and world view. . . . They believe the myths, they credit the efficacy of the ritual, they are sure that there are spirits—they believe all these things, but they do not think too much about them.

What the Mundurucú women *want* to tell, listen to, and participate in, what they do believe and enjoy, is gossiping together in work and dwelling-house groups apart from the men. Then, they collaboratively create an absorbing, ongoing narrative through the "exchange of valuable information about people" of this world.

The mundane specifics and intense evanescence of this talk makes it virtually impossible to anthologize, let alone conceptualize or mythologize. But that vivid ephemerality makes it no less significant.

Padraic Colum entitles his preface to *Orpheus* "The Significance of Mythology." The examples he uses initially are Greek and Roman, and he cites mythographers Vico and Goethe. The third scholar noted is Jeremiah Curtin, said to be "one who loved and studied the mythologies of diverse peoples." The beginning of the passage Colum quotes (from Curtin's 1890 *Myths and Folklore of Ireland*) suggests the present orientation to myth as midwifery, having to do with many different languages:

> There are two nouns in the Greek language which have a long and interesting history behind them; these are *mythos* and *logos*. Originally they had the same power in ordinary speech; for in Homer's time they were used indifferently, sometimes one being taken, and sometimes the other, with the same meaning that *Word* has in our language. . . . *Logos* grew to mean the inward constitution as well as the outward form of thought, and consequently became the expression of exact thought—which is exact because it corresponds to universal and unchanging principles—and reached its highest exaltation in becoming not only the reason in man, but the reason in the universe—the Divine Logos, the Son of God, God Himself. . . . *Mythos* meant, in the widest sense, anything uttered by the mouth of man—a word, an account of something, a story understood by the narrator. (Colum 1930:vii)

In "Earth-Diver: Creation of the Mythopoeic Male," Alan Dundes (1962) has elaborated the languages of two such "mouths"—the oral and anal. This chapter (and this book) is an attempt to consider a third—the vaginal/vulval. It is the *language* of birthing—the substantive speech of specialist midwives, of the participants known as gossips, and of the mother and emerging child during parturition—that is the pro/creation of the "mythopoeic female." And, in the dialogue between what has been known as myth and what has previously been ignored as *mundus,* there are many languages and mythologies.

Midwives—Birthing Specialists

> Cast away vngostly and olde wyves' fables. (1 Timothy 4:7 [Tindale, 1526; "Have nothing to do with godless and silly myths," 1971])

Folklore. . . . There is also, beside the juvenile, a strong feminine element in folklore, because its origin antedates the emergence of reason and belongs in the instinctive and intuitional areas. It is irrational and highly imaginative: much of it truly is termed "old wives' tales." Women have always been the savers and conservators of beliefs, rites, superstitions, rituals, and customs. (Charles Francis Potter [in Leach 1972:401])

The Shorter *Oxford English Dictionary* defines an old wife as 'an old woman, now usu. disparagingly'. 'Old wives' tales' it registers as 'trivial stories, such as are told by garrulous old women'. Indeed, the ultimate dismissal for a piece of advice is to term it 'an old wives' tale'. (Mary Chamberlain 1981:3)

In "The Structural Study of Myth," Claude Lévi-Strauss analyzes a deep structure of common concern with autochthony in the Oedipus myth and the Zuni emergence myth. Both cultures "understand the origin of human life on the model of vegetal life (emergence from the earth)" (1967:217; also Bahr 1977). Among Lévi-Strauss's data is Cushing's myth outline, which includes the following: "Therewith ['grasses and crawling vines'] the two [culture hero twin sons of the Sun-father and Foam-cap mother] formed a great ladder whereon men and the creatures might ascend to the second cave-floor, and thus not be violently ejected in aftertime by the throes of the Earth-mother, and thereby be made demoniac and deformed" (Cushing 1896:382).[6]

Washington Matthews (1902:741–42) compares this Native American metaphor of "vegetal life" to Norse myths about the World Tree Yggdrasill.

The Scandinavian Tree of Existence, it is said, sprung from three roots. This feature of the myth might be easily explained by saying that three was a sacred number with the northern myth-makers. . . . Yet it must occur to the anatomist that the funis consists of three obvious elements—two arteries and a vein—and that, before circulation ceases, it apparently arises from three roots.

. . . I believe a careful study of the Gothic myths will yet reveal that the wonderful Ygdrasil [*sic*], "a most sublime and finished myth," as Professor Anderson truly calls it, was, in the beginning, nothing more poetic than that which every midwife beholds when she performs her special functions.

Apparently, the female midwife is able only to make literal, naturalistic observations rather than "poetic" myths. Her "special functions" are not worthy of further scrutiny. Matthews hereby reduces the role of the midwife to nonpoetic, dumb functionary.

This is not inconsistent with the implications of a study such as Lévi-Strauss's, "The Effectiveness of Symbols" (1967:181–201). It is not until the Cuna shaman is called in by the confused midwife that poetry worthy of being analyzed by Lévi-Strauss is produced, when the shaman provides the sick woman with a language that the midwife cannot. Otherwise, there is simply no reason to pay attention to the language of childbirth and midwifery.

A similar deprecation is expressed by Socrates in Plato's dialogue *Theatetus* (149a, 150a–d, trans. Francis Macdonald Cornford, 1935, in Hamilton and Cairns 1961:853, 855):

> All this [drugs, incantations, techniques, matchmaking] lies within the midwife's province, but her performance falls short of mine. It is not the way of women sometimes to bring forth real children, sometimes mere phantoms, such that it is hard to tell the one from the other. If it were so, the highest and noblest task of the midwife would be to discern the real from the unreal. . . .
>
> My art of midwifery is in general like theirs; the only difference is that my patients are men, not women, and my concern is not with the body but with the soul that is in travail of birth. And the highest point of my art is the power to prove by every test whether the offspring of a young man's thought is a false phantom or instinct with life and truth. I am so far like the midwife that I cannot myself give birth to wisdom. . . . Heaven constrains me to serve as a midwife, but has debarred me from giving birth. So of myself I have no sort of wisdom, nor has any discovery ever been born to me as the child of my soul.

Eva Feder Kittay (1983:108; also Kittay and Lehrer 1981:49–57) notes this passage as evidence for "male direct devaluation of our corporality . . . [in] that childbirth is conceived to be split into a spiritual and a physical component, wherein men are responsible for the former and women for the latter." In this, one of the strategic "writings of such foundational figures of western civilization as Plato, Aristotle, and Aquinas," since "it is dependent on the higher value placed on what is ideational rather than sensible, the devaluation is largely implicit."

With the rise of the Western medical profession, the spiritual/physical split was reversed; the "superstitious" midwife was relegated the former, the "scientific" doctor the latter. The historical process has been well documented (e.g., Oakley 1976; Miller 1978; Chamberlain 1981; Leavitt 1984, 1986). Barbara Ehrenreich and Deirdre English's pamphlet, *Witches, Midwives, and Nurses: A History of Women Healers* (1973) is pivotal.[7] They outline the relationship between witchcraft (mostly female) and medicine (increasingly male) during the middle ages.

> The distinction between "female" superstition and "male" medicine was made final by the very roles of the doctor and the witch at the trial. The trial in one stroke established the male physician on a moral and intellectual plane vastly above the female healer he was called to judge. It placed him on the side of God and Law, a professional on par with lawyers and theologians, while it placed her on the side of darkness, evil and magic. He owed his new status not to medical or scientific achievements of his own, but to the Church and State he served so well. (Ehrenreich and English 1973:19)

Women healers continued to practice after the witch hunt craze, but were "branded . . . forever as superstitious and possibly malevolent."

> So thoroughly was she discredited among the emerging middle classes that in the 17th and 18th centuries it was possible for male practitioners to make serious inroads into that last preserve of female healing—midwifery. Nonprofessional male practitioners—"barber-surgeons"—led the assault in England, claiming technical superiority on the basis of their use of the obstetrical forceps. (The forceps were legally classified as a surgical instrument, and women were legally barred from surgical practice.) In the hands of the barber surgeons, obstetrical practice among the middle class was quickly transformed from a neighborly service into a lucrative business, which real physicians entered in force in the 18th century. Female midwives in England organized and charged the male intruders with commercialism and dangerous misuse of the forceps. But it was too late—the women were easily put down as ignorant "old wives" clinging to the superstitions of the past. (Ehrenreich and English 1973:19, 20)

Mary Chamberlain (1981:3–4) declares the result for the wisdom of old wives:[8]

Old wives' tales—the body of popular medical lore—have now almost died, killed off by the monopoly achieved by the medical profession and its intellectual hegemony over scientific ideas. They are now regarded largely as supersition—as ritual devoid of content. This view ignores . . . an approach to health care which sought as much comfort in explanation and participation (albeit often in a ritualistic way) as in a solution. Old wives' tales and the old wife represented communal healthcare—they were a neighbourhood resource with no barriers of class, education or money to separate them from the community.

The triumph of male instrumentation, physicalization, and commercialization is seen in the contemporary medical language of birth examined by Emily Martin (1987:64):

If the doctor is managing the uterus as machine and the woman as laborer, is the baby seen as a "product"? It seems beyond reproach for doctors to be concerned with the "fetal outcome" of a birth. What seems significant is that cesarean section, which requires the most "management" by the doctor and the least "labor" by the uterus and the woman, is seen as providing the best products. "Doctors have created the attitude that a cesarean delivery implies a perfect baby." Some accounts even celebrate the "dramatic increase" in cesarean rates. "Credit" should be given to earlier colleagues who advocated the increased rate (from 3 to 8 percent ten years ago to 15 to 23 percent today) and fostered a change in attitude (clearly one to be desired): "formerly focus was on the mother and delivery, and now it is centered on fetal outcome." It follows that the current rate may not be as high as it will go. The *New York Times* quotes Dr. Robert Sokol: "Doctors are not going to hesitate to do a Cesarean if there is any possibility it could improve the outcome." By this criterion alone, he said, "a 20 percent rate might not be too high." Others detect a "new principle": "The long-held concept of vaginal delivery is rapidly giving way. The new growing principle seems to be, *vaginal delivery only of selected patients.*"[9]

In this technological midwifery the surgeon's divisive metal is the *logos* of the two-edged sword (Hebrews 4:12; Revelation 1:16). Only vaguely reminiscent of the mythological helpers in the emergence—among them, badger (Acoma, Appendix 10), locust (Navajo, Appendix 11), and spider (Navajo, Chapter 2), it is a far cry from the relational massage, voice, and even purgatives of the traditional midwife and the gossips.

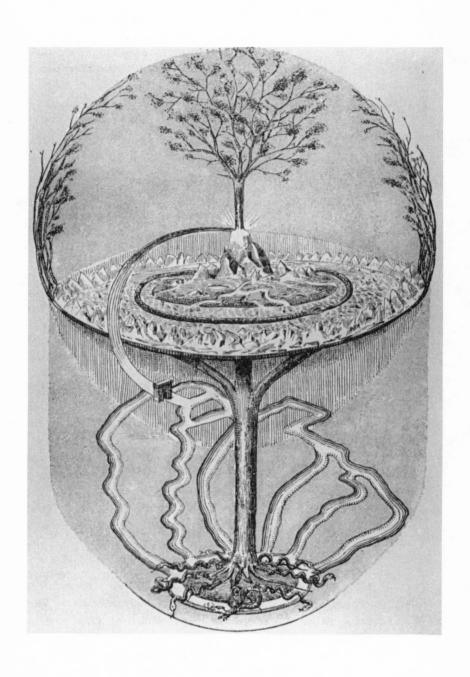

Yggdrasill, the world tree of the Edda. From *Finnur Magnusson's edition of the Elder Edda,* eighteenth century. (Drawing from Folkard 1884:facing p. 2 in Neumann 1963:249, fig. 55. For a similar version—in color—the frontispiece of Bishop Percy's *Northern Antiquities,* see Michell 1975:41, pl. 17.)

Neumann (1963:248, 250) discusses this as it appears in alchemy, where "the psychological significance of birth from tree or flowers is particularly evident. A birth of this sort is always the ultimate result of processes of development and transformation, which cannot be assigned to the sphere of animal instinct. It arises from psychic strata in which—as in the plant—the elements are synthesized and achieve a new unity and form through a transformation governed by the unconscious. They belong to the 'matriarchal consciousness' whose nature and symbolism are as intimately bound up with the plant world as with the world of the Feminine."

Neumann quotes Martin Ninck, *Wodan und germanischer Schicksalsglaube* (1935): "The tree is a symbol of destiny because it is rooted in the depths. . . . All-dominating stands Yggdrasill, the 'greatest and best of all trees' in the mythical world picture of the Edda, putting forth its crown aloft, so that 'its branches tower over the heavens,' reaching deep down into the depths with its tree roots, which embrace Niflheim, Asgard, and Jotunnheim, the realm of the frost giants.

". . . Fate grows slowly out of them like a tree rooted in the depths, like the tall and mighty ash that reaches back to a stone age and in the depths embraces nine realms of the world with its three mighty roots.

"Fate is the sacred center of life. From its womb flow wealth and want . . . , happiness and unhappiness, life and death. ON. *skop,* used in the plural, means 'fate' and also means genitals; it is related to Goth. *gaskapjan,* OE. *scyppan* . . . , 'to create, order, determine.' . . . Thus the working of fate is an eternal becoming . . . , a weaving and creating, and to everything that is, fate assigns its part in life and its peculiar character."[10]

Gossips—Birthing Participants

Thou shalt not go up and down as a talebearer among thy people. (Leviticus 19:16 [King James, 1611; "You shall not go up and down as a slanderer among your people," Revised Standard Version, 1952])

Etymologically, *gossip* means "god-related." As a noun, the word originally designated a godparent, of either sex; then its meaning enlarged to include any close friend—someone belonging to the group from which godparents would naturally be chosen. But the word undergoes a process of degradation. Dr. Johnson, in the middle of the eighteenth century, offered a second meaning of "tippling companion" and a third definition for the first time connecting gossip unambiguously and officially with women: "One who runs about tattling like women at a lying-in." Not until 1811, according to the *Oxford English Dictionary*, did the noun designate a mode of conversation rather than a kind of person: "idle talk, trifling or groundless rumour; tittle-tattle."

In the late twentieth century, *gossip,* as noun and as verb, appears to have lost all dignity in its dictionary definitions. . . . They convey no vestige of the emphasis on close human association that earlier definitions reveal. (Patricia Meyer Spacks [1985:25–26])

Gossip *n* ["A familiar acquaintance, friend, chum. Formerly applied to both sexes now only (somewhat *archaic*) to women. . . . *esp.* Applied to a woman's female friends invited to be present at a birth."—*O.E.D.*]: a Female Friend and/or Familiar, esp. applied to the Fates, Fairies, Familiars, and Friends who invite themselves to be Present at any Female Act of Creation. (conjured by Mary Daly in cahoots with Jane Caputi [1987:132])[11]

Gossips are expected at parturition. Sometimes, but not always, they are women, as in seventeenth-century rural England:

It was customary, when travail began, to send for all the neighbours who were responsible women, partly with the object of securing enough witnesses to the child's birth, partly because it was important to spread the understanding of midwifery as widely as possible because any woman might be called upon to render assistance in an emergency. (Clark 1968, in Oakley 1976:24)

The performance of godsiblingship is crucial, what Brigitte Jordan (1980:9) calls "the doing of birth by *participants,* [and] by 'participants' I mean all persons (professionals and nonprofessionals) (including myself) who are engaged in the common task of producing an event and making it visible as the business at hand, as doing a birth."

Godsiblingship is shared by all in the Navajo origin myth told to Aileen O'Bryan (1956:102–3) by Hastin Tlo'tsi hee in 1928:[12]

The Sun brought a turquoise man fetish and gave it to Yol gai esdzan, the White Bead Woman. She ground white beads into a powder and made a paste with which she molded a fetish like the one the Sun had given her, but it was a woman. When it was finished they laid the two side by side. Then they took the white corn which was brought up from the Dark World where the First Man was formed and they laid it beside the turquoise man fetish. And the yellow corn from the Dark World, which was formed with the First Woman, was laid by the side of the White Bead Woman fetish.

Here the chanting begins. It covers the two fetishes, the two ears of corn and the four clouds and the four vapors. There are many chants sung here. They were sung before the fetishes could move. Then the two fetishes, the Turquoise Man and the White Bead Woman, and also, the two ears of corn, white and yellow, moved.

When they began to move the Coyote came. He jumped on the bodies and put something first up one nostril and then up the other nostril. He said to the first nostril: "You shall be saved by this." To the second nostril he said: "This shall be your shield." The first turned out to be the trickery of man; the second, the lies that they tell. But once in a while they are saved by their own lies. That was what Coyote had in mind.

The fetishes and the ears of corn moved but they were not able to rise. So word was sent to all the Holy Beings and to the Upper World where the Five Chiefs of the Wind dwelt. Gifts were offered to the Winds and they accepted them. They sent the Little Breeze down, and it entered the bodies of the two fetishes and the two ears of corn. Little, fine hairs appeared over the bodies, for it is through these that air comes out of the body. It was after that, that the four, the two fetishes and the two ears of corn, became human beings.

Godsiblingship is shared but ultimately controlled by a male deity in the similar, but for the most part misogynist, classical myth of Pandora,[13] of whom Sarah Pomeroy (1975:2) writes: "Her name is ambiguous. It can mean 'giver of all gifts,' making her a benevolent fertility figure, or 'recipient of all gifts.' Hesiod chooses the latter interpretation in order to attribute to the first woman the woes of mankind." Mythologist Jane Ellen Harrison (1980:284, 285) calls Hesiod to task for the choice.

Pandora is in ritual and matriarchal theology the earth as Kore, but in the patriarchal mythology of Hesiod her great figure is strangely changed and minished. She is no longer Earth-born, but the creature, the handiwork of Olympian Zeus. On a late, red-figured krater in the British Museum, obviously inspired by Hesiod, we have the scene of her birth. She no longer rises halfway from the ground, but stands stiff and erect in the midst of the Olympians. Zeus is there seated with sceptre and thunderbolt, Poseidon is there, Iris and Hermes and Ares and Hera, and Athene about to crown the new-born maiden. Earth is all but forgotten, and yet so haunting is tradition that, in a lower row, beneath the Olympians, a chorus of men, disguised as goat-horned Phanes, still dance their welcome. It is a singular reminiscence, and, save as a survival, wholly irrelevant. . . .

Zeus the Father will have no great Earthgoddess, Mother and Maid in one, in his man-fashioned Olympus, but her figure *is* from the beginning, so he remakes it; woman, who was the inspirer, becomes the temptress; she who made all things, gods and mortals alike, is become their plaything, their slave, dowered only with physical beauty, and with a slave's tricks and blandishments. To Zeus, the archpatriarchal *bourgeois,* the birth of the first woman is but a huge Olympian jest: "He spake and the Sire of men and of gods immortal laughed."

Zeus's role as superordinate gossip is also seen in many modern medical delivery rooms, where obstetrical "teams" of suitably subordinated "females" are headed by a "male" doctor.

All-male godsiblingship is evident in most of the initiations analyzed by Bruno Bettelheim in *Symbolic Wounds: Puberty Rites and the Envious Male* (1962). In "A Psychoanalytic Study of the Bullroarer," used in many of these rites, Alan Dundes (1980:196) maintains: "It may now be more clear why the initiation rites must be kept secret from the women. Whether it is males attempting to emulate female procreativity by means of anal power, or homosexual intercourse in lieu of heterosexual intercourse, or ritual masturbation, the consistent element is that men seek to live without recourse to women." Life without recourse to men either, dispensing with godsiblingship altogether, is the male parthenogenesis enacted by the space man in Stanley Kubrick's movie *2001: A Space Odyssey,* according to Herbert W. Richardson.

Richardson (1969:104, 105) identifies what he calls "three myths of transcendence," or "story-images" that "form habitual modal feelings in the lives of [religious community] members." He claims: "Differences in religious images imply differences both in the feeling of wholeness and in the Wholes themselves." Because they give personal, psychic identity to those who experience them, these myths are exemplified by particular heroes (not heroines). The three are instructive:

1. Separation-and-return (dust-to-dust, womb-to-t/womb), a cycle of participation exemplified by Odysseus.

2. Conflict-and-vindication (good vs. evil, we vs. them), a polarizing of linear history as an "overagainstness" exemplified by Jesus.

3. Integrity-and-transformation, wherein "to be 'integral' . . . is not to need to complete ourselves through others (or from 'outside'), but to need to express and expand ourselves from within," exemplified by Kubrick's *2001: A Space Odyssey,* wherein the space man's journey "takes him . . . nowhere. The end of his seeking is neither a place nor (given the infinity of space itself) is it a 'conquest.' . . . It is, rather, his own self-transformation into a higher being, his spiritual rebirth, his divinization." (Richardson 1969:111–12)

The integral space man, whether *in utero* in the maternal amniotic chaos or in the classical abyss of *nihilo* chaos, is reborn without the help of gossips:

> This rebirth (with which *2001* ends) is not from the maternity of a mother. It is the result of man's integrity to his own creative vision, to his own project for himself. By his integrity to this vision, man gains for himself his own positive identity, his own aseity of being. He no longer lives by dependence or obedience. He no longer lives by being "a part of" or "overagainst." He no longer needs another to complete him or compensate for his negatives. He can now live by what he is.

The space man has no godsiblings; "conventionally speaking, the 'integral' man has no needs at all—that is, he needs nothing outside himself in order to establish an identity or be happy" (Richardson 1969:111).

The *2001* space man becomes the ultimate mythological solution to the dilemmas posed by procreation. His is an appropriated transcendence—reminiscent of the alchemical, and, in contemporary society, the technological (e.g., Corea 1985; Stanworth 1987). He should not be consulted as a godsib, for he is not engaged like those about whom Ralph Waldo Emerson lectured in 1845: "Our globe discovers its hidden virtues not only in heroes, and archangels, but in gossips and nurses."[14]

Mouths—Birthing Speech

> When the waters saw thee, O God,
>   when the waters saw thee, they
>   were afraid,
>   yea, the deep trembled.

The clouds poured out water;
   the skies gave forth thunder;
   thy arrows flashed on every side.
The crash of thy thunder was in the
      whirlwind;
   thy lightnings lighted up the world;
   the earth trembled and shook.

—Psalms 77:16–18

Then deep from the earth you shall
   speak,
   from low in the dust your words
   shall come;
your voice shall come from the
      ground like the voice of a ghost,
   and your speech shall whisper out
   of the dust.

—Isaiah 29:4

Gossip *v* ["To be a gossip or sponsor to; to give a name to. *Obs.* . . . To act as a gossip, or a familiar acquaintance; to take part (in a feast), be a boon-companion; to make oneself at home. . . . To tell like a gossip; to communicate. Also with *out*. 1650 'The secret lay not long in the Embers, being gossiped out by a woman.' . . . 1827 'And wisdom, gossip'd from the stars.'" —*O.E.D.*] 1: to exercise the Elemental Female Power of Naming, especially in the Presence of other Gossips 2: to take part in the festivity of wordplay among Boon-Companions 3: to tell like a Gossip; to divine and communicate the secrets of the Elements, the wisdom of the stars. (conjured by Mary Daly in cahoots with Jane Caputi [1987:132–33])

In "'Temple and Sewer': Childbirth, Prudery, and Victoria Regina," John Hawkins Miller (1978:27) documents the nineteenth-century medical men's assault against female gossips and their gossip or birth talk.

The presence of gossips at a confinement . . . was not encouraged by the emerging medical specialists, the "man-midwives," or obstetricians; and many Victorian medical guides condemned the practice. One guide advised the pregnant woman not to comply with the request of her female friends to be sent for at the onset of labour, for, the author wrote, "the patient will find quietness and composure, of far greater service than the noisy rallying round of friends, to awaken and cherish the idea of danger." Another medical handbook recommended that even the mother of the woman in labour should not be allowed into the room though she could be present in the house.[15]

By defining traditional birthing as noisy (gossipy), the medical specialists remove it from what R. Murray Schafer (1980:76) calls "Sacred Noise."

We have already noted how loud noises evoked fear and respect back to earliest times, and how they seemed to be the expression of divine power. We have also observed how this power was transferred from natural sounds (thunder, volcano, storm) to those of the church bell and pipe organ. I called this Sacred Noise to distinguish it from the other sort of noise (with a small letter), implying nuisance and requiring noise abatement legislation. This was always primarily the rowdy human voice. During the Industrial Revolution, Sacred Noise sprang across to the profane world. Now the industrialists held power and they were granted dispensation to make Noise by means of the steam engine and the blast furnace, just as previously the monks had been free to make Noise on the church bell or J. S. Bach to open out his preludes on the full organ.

The association of Noise and power has never really been broken in the human imagination. It descends from God, to the priest, to the industrialist, and more recently to the broadcaster and the aviator. The important thing to realize is this: to have the Sacred Noise is not merely to make the biggest noise; rather it is a matter of having the authority to make it without censure.

Alan Dundes analyzes the Sacred Noise of the whirring bullroarer as both an anal and a phallic component of many male initiation rites in which men give birth to boys. He (1980:184) lauds Ernest Jones as "the only writer to have discussed in painstaking detail the anal erotic elements of the bullroarer complex."

Jones, in a brilliant essay, "The Madonna's Conception through the Ear," first published in 1914, lucidly articulates the symbolic transformations of the expulsion of intestinal gas (1951:278). Males, he maintains, create by a blowing movement (breath, wind) or by sound.

Although Jones does tend to make such categorical statements as the following: "That the idea of thunder is exceedingly apt, in dreams and other products of unconscious fantasy, to symbolize flatus, particularly paternal flatus, is well known to all psycho-analysts" (1951:287 . . .), he supports his assertions with extensive documentary evidence.

Dundes (1980:197, 198) notes that "etymological antecedents of *bull* refer to testicle and penis, but several also refer to swelling and blowing as in a pair of bellows." He claims: "The roar of a bullroarer would be analogous to a 'bronx cheer' or a 'raspberry.' To razz somebody is to direct at him a derogatory flatulent sound (*razz,* from *raspberry tart* which in rhyming slang substitutes for *fart*)."

The "noise" of the vagina/vulva and its attendants is far subtler and more varied—surely no less worthy of substantial consideration as an equivalent Sacred Noise. Consider Brigitte Jordan's account of childbirth in the Yucatan, where there is constant talk of many sorts.

While the contractions are weak and far apart, the talk which fills the long hours of waiting has to do with everyday concerns, rambling perhaps from divorce to the high cost of living, or from community affairs . . . to building a new house for the growing family. . . .

When contractions become stronger and more frequent, talk begins to focus on the business at hand. Stories are told about such things as miscarriages, abortions, the horrors of hospital deliveries, and, especially, the birth experiences of the women present. . . .

The question of the nature of the topics which are admissible during the birth process deserves detailed investigation since such talk can be expected to convey not only pragmatic and instructional information but it is also likely to contain symbolic messages regarding the meaning of the event. It seems to be the case that one topic that needs to be dealt with in such situations is the topic of death. In our own culture, it is hardly ever permitted to be addressed directly. It nevertheless crops up regularly, in more or less disguised form. (Jordan 1980:23, 92)

The talk is also tangible, literally *touching*. The parturient Mayan woman's husband, her mother, and other women who have given birth act as "helpers" who "substantially contribute to a successful birth," as "jointly and by turns they give the woman the mental and physical support she needs."

When a woman needs encouragement to renew her flagging strength, helpers respond to her with what we came to call "birth talk." At the onset of a contraction, casual conversation stops. A rising chorus of helpers' voices pours out an insistent rhythmic stream of words whose intensity matches the strength and length of the contraction. *"Ence, ence, mama," "jala, jala, jala," "tuuchila," "ko'osh, ko'osh"* comes from all sides of the hammock. With the "head helper" behind her, not only holding her but physically matching every contraction, the laboring woman is surrounded by intense urging in the touch, sound and sight of those close to her. (Jordan 1980:24, 26)

Sometimes the helpers become irritated and scold the flagging mother.

Although the expectation is of a quick, fairly easy birth, at least some pain is recognized as a normal part of bearing a child. It figures in the birth stories which have been told all along, preparing the mother for what is to come. . . .

   As the baby's head begins to show . . . the excitement in the little house reaches a new pitch. Birth talk is continuous, punctuated only by the midwife's progress reports. (Jordan 1980:27, 28)

Talk does not return to normal until after the cord is cut, the afterbirth passed, the mother and baby bathed, and the latter swaddled and, if a girl, her ears pierced.

   Birth speech is substantive—verbally and bodily—involving mouth and vagina, words and blood. All must be attended; all are equally and crucially pro/creative. Yet Susan Griffin maintains in her 1976 essay, "Feminism and Motherhood," "I think men do not relate to children or infants but to the idea of children and the idea of motherhood. They do not want to touch the blood of birth or the body of the child" (1982:76). It is apparently preferable to talk about creation through flatus, excrement, and other effluvia as well as to enact elaborate male rites of couvade and initiation and not to attend childbirth.

   it is all blood and breaking,
   blood and breaking.the thing
   drops out of its box squalling
   into the light.they are both squalling,
   animal and cage.her bars lie wet, open

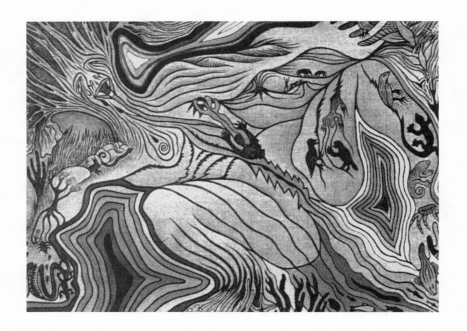

---

and empty and she has made herself again
out of flesh out of dictionaries,
she is aways emptying and it is all
the same wound the same blood the same breaking.
— Lucille Clifton, "She Understands Me," from *An Ordinary Woman*
(1974:50)

Pro/creation—The Dialogue of Mythos *and* Mundus

From the moment of their appearance these spirits—the angels—were startled out of everlasting sleep into the lightning-shock of a direct, unshielded vision of the Glory. . . . At the same instant, all the nine choirs or spheres into which they were divided, burst into the exultant hymn which they have never ceased singing to this day.

"Agios! Agios! Agios! Kyrie Sabaoth!
Holy! Holy! Holy! Lord of Hosts!
Heaven and earth are full of Thy Glory!
Hosanna in the Highest!"
— Alan W. Watts (1968:36), recording the *Divine Liturgy of St. John Chrysostom*

We did continuous tape recording during the birth from the time we arrived at each house until we left. . . .
At births we always did a playback of the baby's first cry for the family, and that re-experiencing was invariably an occasion for relief, laughter, and satisfied remarks about the successful outcome of the birth. (Brigitte Jordan and Nancy Fuller [Jordan 1980:15, 16])

An encompassing and enabling mythology of pro/creation such as is broached in this volume would anthologize not just nine kinds of "true" and not-so-"true," mythic cosmogonies but also the languages that create and sustain this world, *mundus*. In the case of the Papago it might include the following texts:

Of cosmogony:

In every Papago village there is an old man whose hereditary function is to recite this "bible" [of song and story]. The accepted time for the recitation is those four nights in winter "when the sun stands still" before turning back from that southern journey which, it seemed, might take its light away forever.

On those nights—four nights, for everything holy goes by fours— the Papago men gathered in the ceremonial house. One by one they puffed the ceremonial cigarette, native tobacco in a hollow cane tube. Tobacco smoking among the Papagos is like the burning of incense: a solemn function, not a recreation. Each man took four puffs, then passed the cigarette sunwise, calling his neighbor by the term of relationship. Of course they were all kin. "Kinsman" and "neighbor" are the same word in Papago.

The men sat cross-legged, their arms folded, their heads bowed. This was the position required by propriety, as sitting upright in a church pew was required by our Victorian ancestors. No one must interrupt the speaker by a question or even by a movement. No one must doze. If he did, some neighbor would poke the burning cigarette between his sandaled toes. If the speaker saw it, he stopped suddenly and there was no more storytelling that night. (Underhill 1973:10–11)

Of creation:

I knew all about Coyote and the things he can do, because my father told us the stories about how the world began and how Coyote helped our Creator, Elder Brother, to set things in order. Only some men know these stories, but my father was one of them. On winter nights, when we had finished our gruel or rabbit stew and lay back on our mats, my brothers would say to my father: "My father, tell us something."

My father would lie quietly upon his mat with my mother beside him and the baby between them. At last he would start slowly to tell us about how the world began. This is a story that can be told only in winter when there are no snakes about, for if the snakes heard they could crawl in and bite you. But in winter when snakes are asleep we tell these things. Our story about the world is full of songs, and when the neighbors heard my father singing they would open our door and step in over the high threshold. Family by family they came, and we

made a big fire and kept the door shut against the cold night. When my
father finished a sentence we would all say the last word after him. If
anyone went to sleep he would stop. He would not speak any more.
But we did not go to sleep. (Underhill 1979:50)[16]

Of gossip:

We women sat in the dark [in summertime], under the shelter, and
told about the strange things we had heard. We told how there is a root
which men carry to make the deer come to them and it makes women
come, too. It smells strong and sweet, and you can smell it on the
sweaty hands of a man beside you in the dance. If it is very strong and
has been used in many love matches, sometimes it turns into a man. It
walks up beside a woman while she is sleeping and makes her dream.
We told how, in our village, a girl was struck by lightning. Someone
must have been menstruating and not have confessed it, said the
medicine man. So he called all the girls, took out his crystals and
looked at them. "It was the girl herself," he said. "She has killed
herself."
We told how, when a woman does not seem to care for any man or a
man for any woman, that person is really married to a snake. There was
a man in our village who used to go out alone into the desert and
disappear in a wash. His parents followed him and found there a little
red snake with her baby snakes on her back. They said to their son,
"What! have you a family of snakes?" He said, "No, she is a beautiful
woman." That is how snakes fool you. The older women used to tell
us, too, that if we thought too much about any boy before we married,
that boy would seem to come to make love to us. But it would not be
he, it would only be a snake. So girls must not think too much about
boys. That was what the old women told us. We must not think about
boys and we must not talk to boys. When we were married it would be
time enough to speak to a man. Now it was better to work and be
industrious.
So I worked. But I used to think while I was sitting under the shelter
with my basketry, about whether I would get a good man and whether
I would like being married. (Underhill 1979:53–54)

Of parturition:

We were careful when the first baby was coming. Our men were not
going to war any more, so I did not have to keep my husband home.

That had always worried my mother, for if a man kills an enemy at such a time, his child will die a violent death. But probably a man will not kill an enemy, he will be killed himself, he is so weak from his wife's weakness. But my husband did not kill any rabbits so that the baby should not have a choking sickness, and he kept away from rattlesnakes so it should not have convulsions. I was kind to the people in our village who looked sick or ugly, and I never laughed at them, so that my baby should have a good body.

I did not know just when the time would be, but I knew that I felt pain when I stooped out of our little door. I said to my husband's aunt: "I think I will go to the Little House. I would not like such a dreadful thing to happen as for me to be caught inside the house in childbirth." "Well, go," she said. This was the first I had said to her or to my mother-in-law either, the whole thing being so new.

There was a gully behind our house and the Little House was on the other side of it. When I reached the near edge of that gully, I thought I had better run. I ran fast; I wanted to do the right thing. But I dropped my first baby in the middle of the gully. My aunt came and snipped the baby's navel string with her long finger nail. Then we went on to the Little House. My sisters-in-law said to me afterward, "Why didn't you tell us? We didn't know you were suffering in there. We heard you laughing." I said, "Well, it wasn't my mouth that hurt. It was my middle." (Underhill 1979:66)

The purpose of such a panoply of pro/creation would be to empower language from all "mouths"—to establish a dialogue, what Dennis Tedlock (1983:322, 323) calls "a 'speaking alternately'—or, to translate the Greek *dialogos* literally, a 'speaking across.'" It is a realm of "*betweenness*," and "the anthropological dialogue creates a world, or an understanding of the *differences between* two worlds, that exists between persons who were indeterminately far apart, in all sorts of different ways, when they started out on their conversation."

In the case of that most famous of Mesoamerican ethnohistorical documents, the Popol Vuh, the opening creation story, which contains allusions to the Bible, has been dismissed by a hundred years of scholarship as "an accommodation to Christian notions" or "a syncretistic paraphrase of Genesis" not to be compared with the rest of what is otherwise a perfect document—never mind that it was all written in the Roman alphabet.

From a dialogical point of view, such documents as these are interesting not in spite of the fact that some European got there first but precisely because of it. They show, from both sides and with moments of thunderbolt clarity, the dialogical frontier between European and Mesoamerican cultures during the colonial period. In some ways, the opening of the Popol Vuh tells us more about the sixteenth-century Quiché Maya than anything else in that document, precisely because it simultaneously shows us, with respect to the question of cosmogony, who those Quichés were and who our Spanish cousins were, how they met up and how they did not meet up. (Tedlock 1983:333–34)

The epilogue to Dennis Tedlock's work on "the emergence of a dialogical anthropology" can serve to conclude these "reflections" on a proper pro/creation mythology and lead to placing the murmuring waters and the midwives in complement and full equivalency with the thundering heavens and the *ex-nihil*-ators.

But [Franz] Boas did note that there are, in northern California, myths in which "creation by will" takes place. When we reread the Maidu and Kato versions of these myths,[17] it turns out that there are two creators, male and female, and that they are present in a world that already has physical existence at the very beginning of the story. The changes that then take place in the world come about when this man and woman engage in a dialogue—there is no solitary male nude saying, "Let there be this and that." A similar dialogue is at work in the Popol Vuh, and it constitutes the Popol Vuh's profound rejection of Genesis. To argue that "underneath the veneer" of myths such as these lie the workings of a single universal Logos is to cast a vote for the Western metaphysic and against dialogue. But the Popol Vuh asks to be approached dialogically, and the way to write about the Popol Vuh might be to set down the opening words, *Are uxe oher tzih uaral Quiche ubi,* and then go on from there, quoting and questioning all along the way. (Tedlock 1983:338)

This is the account, here it is:
    Now it still ripples, now it still murmurs, ripples, it still sighs, still hums, and it is empty under the sky.
    Here follow the first words, the first eloquence:

. . .

    Whatever might be is simply not there: only murmurs, ripples, in the dark, in the night. Only the Maker, Modeler alone, Sovereign

Plumed Serpent, the Bearers, Begetters are in the water, a glittering light. They are there, they are enclosed in quetzal feathers, in blue-green.

. . .

And of course there is the sky, and there is also the Heart of Sky. . . .

And then came his word, he came here to the Sovereign Plumed Serpent, here in the blackness, in the early dawn. He spoke with the Sovereign Plumed Serpent, and they talked, then they thought, then they worried. They agreed with each other, they joined their words, their thoughts. Then it was clear, then they reached accord in the light, and then humanity was clear, when they conceived the growth, the generation of trees, of bushes, and the growth of life, of humankind, in the blackness, in the early dawn. (*Popol Vuh*, "Council Book," of the Quiché Maya, or "The Mayan Book of the Dawn of Life," trans. Dennis Tedlock [1985:72–73])

By Way of Epilogos and Epimundus

Then the Lord answered Job
out of the whirlwind:

. . .

"Where were you when I laid the
foundations of the earth? . . .
"Or who shut in the sea with doors,
   when it burst forth from the womb;
when I made clouds its garment,
   and thick darkness its swaddling
      band,
and prescribed bounds for it,
   and set bars and doors,
and said, 'Thus far shall you come,
   and no farther,
   and here shall your proud waves
      be stayed'?"

—Job 38:1, 4, 8–11

The fiat of Genesis and the midwifery of the Popol Vuh are not only separated by geography, history, and sociocultural context but by a reason that does not equally empower the *mythos* of other worlds and the *mundus* of this one. In most mythology, this world is valued primarily as the product, expression, or epiphany of a creator, not as the midwifery of gossips and procreators. Cosmogony, the "very first" beginnings of the cosmos, claims hegemony over origins—the subsequent, mundane beginnings. Yet these myriad midwiferies, an unceasing process of engendering, are as much the gossip of life itself as are the specific rites of birthing.

As a rule, creation, not procreation, provides the valued mythological paradigm. Thus, an account like the following is highlighted by mythographer Mircea Eliade (1963:21) in declaring the "Magic and Prestige of 'Origins,'" in which "the creation of the World being *the* pre-eminent instance of creation, the cosmogony becomes the exemplary model for 'creation' of every kind."

> Among the Osage, on the birth of a child "a man who had talked with the gods" was sent for. On his arrival he recited to the infant the story of the Creation and of the animals that move on the earth. Then, after placing the tip of his finger on the mother's nipple, he pressed that finger on the lips of the child, after which he passed his hands over the body of the child. Then the infant was allowed to take nourishment. Later, when the child desired to drink the water the same or a like man was sent for. Again the ritual of the Creation was recited, and the beginning of water was told. The man then dipped the tip of his finger into water and laid it on the lips of the child and passed his hands over its body from head to foot. After this ceremony the child could be given water to drink. When the child reached the age when it needed or desired solid food, the same man or one of his class was again sent for. Once more the Creation story was recited and the gift of corn and other food was recounted. At the close the man placed the tip of his finger upon the food prepared for the child and then laid this finger on the lips of the child, after which he passed his hands over its body. This ceremony prepared the child to receive solid food. Fees were given to the man who performed these rites. (Fletcher and La Flesche 1911:116, note a)

But the narrative of procreation, the midwifery that enacts *mundus* may be no less pre-eminent and exemplary, as in the following myth text:

> So from the moment that a Manus baby is born, it is caught into a system which emphasizes the active rhythmic reciprocity with the

world around it, deemphasizes differences in size and strength and sex, and stresses its existence as an independent organism. Before the cord is cut, the old woman who takes care of the newborn starts to lull it in time to its own crying so that the sound it makes and the sound it hears are as nearly one as it is possible to make them. (Mead 1956:346)[18]

Mythologies of pro/creation will establish the dialogue—the dia-*mundus*—the full range of *mythos* as many mouths—between these and numerous other texts. Their anthologists and analysts will eschew the facile, sexist notions of compensation that authorize male rites of couvade, parthenogenesis, and initiation and ignore female rites and processes of conception, gestation, and parturition. In feminist terms, the fiat of Elohim, the "first labor" of Yahweh, cannot remain the sole empowering. Chaotic parturition is not the symbolic inversion of orderly cosmogony; rather, the watery (gossipy) chaos that the whirlwind Yahweh dam(n)s instead both heralds and constitutes the parturience that the mother/midwife exalts.

the labor of She Who carries and bears is the first
labor all over the world
the waters are breaking everywhere
everywhere the waters are breaking
the labor of She Who carries and bears
and raises and rears is the first labor,
there is no other first labor.
     —Judy Grahn, "She Who," from *The Work of a Common Woman* (1978:85)

Appendix: Selected Texts of Creation and Procreation

1. Ekoi Folktale, "How All Stories and All History Came Among Men"

This African etiology is a metanarrative account of how stories originate. All the protagonists are women—Mouse, who weaves multi-colored story-children to compensate for her lack of "real" children, Sheep, Leopard, Sheep's daughter, and the powerful Nimm woman.

According to collector Percy Amaury Talbot (1912:337), "Sheep and tortoise are credited with cunning above all other animals, and hold in this respect somewhat the position of Brer Rabbit and Reincke Fuchs in the Folk-lore of other continents." Among the Ekoi, "Nimm is the special object of devotion to . . . women, and her cult, founded, according to tradition, by a Divine woman who came down to earth for the purpose, seems to provide satisfactory expression for the religious feelings of her human sisters. . . . Each 'Nimm woman' has a little shrine built in the corner of her room. On this stands a pot, usually an ancient earthenware one, containing 'medicine', peculiar to the cult, together with some queerly shaped pieces of carved wood, corn cobs, a Juju knife, and the feathers of the white 'Ebekk'" (Talbot 1912:94–95).

Talbot had served with the Nigerian Political Service since 1907. He (1912:335) states: "Most of the tales recorded were taken down from sources never before brought into contact with white influence. . . . All have been taken down exactly as they were told, except the one given on p. 337, 'How all Stories and all History came on Earth [*sic*].' The introduction to this was related by one man, and the bulk of the tale by another, but the *finale* so obviously belongs to that of which the first otherwise disjointed fragment, forms the beginning, that it seemed better, in this one case, to combine the two." Thus, the portion of "How all Stories and all History came among Men" (Talbot 1912: 337–40) before the asterisks was told by Agra of Mbeban.

Mouse goes everywhere. Through rich men's houses she creeps, and visits even the poorest. At night, with her little bright eyes, she watches the doing of secret things, and no treasure-chamber is so safe but she can tunnel through and see what is hidden there.

In old days she wove a story-child from all that she saw, and to each of these she gave a gown of different colours—white, red, blue, or black. The stories became her children, and lived in her house and served her, because she had no children of her own.

* * * * *

Now in olden days a sheep and a leopard lived in the same town. In course of time Leopard became *enceinte* and Sheep also. Sheep bore a daughter and Leopard a son.

There was a famine in all the land, so Leopard went to Sheep and said, "Let us kill our children and eat them." Sheep thought, "If I do not agree, she may kill my child in spite of me," so she answered "Good."

Then Sheep went and hid her own babe, and took all that she had and sold for a little dried meat. This she cooked and set before Leopard, and they both ate together. Leopard killed her own child, and ate that also.

In another year they both became *enceinte* once more. This time again the townsfolk were hungry. Leopard came as before and said, "Let us kill these children also." Sheep agreed, but she took her second child and hid her in the little room where the first child was, then went out, and begged till someone gave her a few pieces of dried meat. These she cooked and set before Leopard as she had done before, in place of her babe. Leopard ate and said nothing.

Some years afterwards Leopard sent to Sheep and said, "Come; to-day you shall feast with me."

Sheep went, and found a great calabash on the table. She opened it, and found if full of food, and by it three spoons laid ready.

She was astonished and questioned Leopard. "Formerly we used two spoons, you and I. Why should there be three to-day?"

Leopard laughed, opened the door of the inner room, and called, "Come, daughter, let us eat." Her daughter came, and they all ate together. Then the mother said, "When my first child came, I killed and ate him because we were very hungry; but when I learned how you had saved your child, I thought, 'Next time I also will play such a trick on Sheep.' Therefore I saved my daughter alive."

After that Sheep went home, and tended her two children. Years passed by, and all the daughters began to grow up. Leopard put her child into the fatting-house. Then she went to Sheep and said, "Give me one of your daughters to stay with mine in the fatting-house. She is alone and cannot eat."

Now Sheep and both her daughters were quite black, but there were some young goats in the house which served them as slaves. These were white, so before Sheep sent her daughter to Leopard's house she rubbed her all over with white chalk, then dyed one of the young goats black, and sent them together.

When they both arrived at the house, Leopard thought that the goat was Sheep's daughter. All three of the young ones were placed in the fatting-house. During the night Leopard entered the room, took Goat and killed her, then cooked the meal and gave her own daughter to eat, thinking it was the daughter of Sheep whom she had slain.

Next day Leopard went to Sheep and said, "Give me your other child, that our three daughters may be in the fatting-house together."

Sheep consented, but before this child went she advised her what to do.

When therefore the second lamb reached the fatting-house she took out a bottle of rum and gave it to Leopard's daughter, saying "Drink this. It is a present which my mother has sent you." So Leopard's child drank and fell asleep. The two young sheep kept awake until their companion slept. They then got up, carried her from her own bed, and laid her on one of those prepared for themselves.

It was very dark in the room, and, when Leopard came in to kill one of the young sheep, she killed her own daughter instead. She was pleased and thought, "Now I have finished with the children whom Sheep hid from me." Next morning, very early, she went out to the bush to get palm wine that she might drink it with her daughter while they feasted on the young sheep.

No sooner had she left the house than the two sheep ran out. One of them went home to her mother's house, but the other followed after Leopard. The latter was at the top of a high palm tree, so Sheep's child stopped some way off and called in a loud voice:

"Last night you tried to kill me as you did the young goat, but you made a mistake, and killed your own child instead."

No sooner had Leopard heard this than she jumped from the tree and ran after the young sheep.

The latter ran to the cross-roads, and when Leopard reached the place she could not tell which way Sheep had gone. After thinking a while she took the wrong road and ran on.

Now when Sheep had run a long way she met the Nimm woman walking along with her Juju [knife] round her waist. The woman looked as if she had come a long way, and Sheep said, "Let me carry your Juju for you."

To this the Nimm woman agreed. When they came to her house she was very tired and her head hurt her.

Sheep said, "Let me fetch water and firewood while you rest."

The Nimm woman was very thankful, and went into her house to lie down.

When the young Sheep had done as she promised, she went into the other part of the house where the Nimm shrine was. On it she saw the "medicine." This she took and rubbed over herself.

Next day the Nimm woman said, "Will you go and fetch me my 'medicine' which stands on the shrine of Nimm?"

Sheep asked her, "Do you not know that I was 'born' into your medicine last night?"

At this the Nimm woman was very angry and sprang up. Sheep ran, and the Nimm woman followed her. In her hurry to escape, Sheep ran against the door of the house where Mouse lived. The door was old and it broke, and all the stories on earth, and all the histories ran out. After that they never went back to dwell with Mouse any more, but remained running up and down over all the earth.

2. Yuki Creation Myth

Taikó-mol, whose name means "Solitude Walker," is the creator god of the Round Valley Yuki Indians of northern California. A *Deus faber*, he divides the primeval waters like the Old Testament Elohim on the second day of creation (Genesis 1:6–8) or the God who asks Job (38:4) where he was "when I laid the foundation of the earth." Taikó-mol uses a rope and then quadrant *lílkae,* or stone crooks, to lay out the world before bringing the earth into existence with a spoken word. Like many artisan creators, Taikó-mol tests his creation, the earth which he has kept separate from the waters by whale-hide. The craft recalls God's questions to Job: "who shut in the sea with doors, / . . . and prescribed bounds for it, / and set bars and doors" (Job 38:8–11).

A. L. Kroeber (1876–1960) summarizes a Yuki version he collected between 1901 and 1906. He (1906–1907:184) glosses Taikomol [*sic*] as "He who goes alone." In the beginning, "on the water, in a fleck of foam, a down feather was circling. From this issued a voice and singing." Coyote is also present. "The creator after a time gradually assumes human physical shape, all the time singing and watched by

Coyote. He thereupon forms the earth from a piece of coiled basket which he makes of materials and with an awl that he takes from his body. The earth is fastened and strengthened with pitch, and the creator thereupon travels over it four times from north to south with Coyote hanging to his body. He then fastens the earth at the four ends and makes the sky from the skin of four whales."

Collector Edward S. Curtis (1868–1952) calls the following text "The Creation" (1924:169). He notes that it was narrated by a Round Valley Yuki and "is patently only an outline."

There was only water, and over it a fog. On the water was foam. The foam moved round and round continually, and from it came a voice. After a time there issued from the foam a person in human form. He had wing-feathers of the eagle on his head. This was Taikó-mol. He floated on the water and sang. He stood on the foam, which still revolved. There was no light. He walked on the water as if it were land. He made a rope and laid it from north to south, and he walked along it, revolving his hands one about the other, and behind him the earth was heaped up along the rope. But the water overwhelmed it. Again he did this, and again the water prevailed. Four times this was done.

Taikó-mol was constantly talking to himself. "I think we had better do it this way. I think we had better try it that way." So now he talked to himself, and he made a new plan. He made four *lílkae,* and planted one in the north and others in the south, west, and east. Then he stretched them out until they were continuous lines crossing the world in the centre. He spoke a word, and the earth appeared. Then he went along the edge and lined it with whale-hide, so that the ocean could not wash away the earth. He shook the earth to see if it was solid, and he still makes this test, causing earthquakes.

3. Uitoto Cosmogony

Paul Radin (1883–1959) calls the following myth a "poetic account" by a monotheist from the Uitoto of Colombia, "an attempt to solve the riddle of creation by postulating something that existed before the beginning, and our primitive philosopher and theologian has quite logically assumed that the appearance of things preceded their actual existence . . . an admirable solution of the much vexed question of how a creator can create something out of nothing" (1954:13–14; also 1957a:355–56). In *Primitive Religion* he terms it "a really complete, in fact an almost redundant, example of . . . a hypothetical history of the earth, the cosmos, consciousness, and even unconsciousness." Radin proclaims, "Assuredly this is a creation *ex nihilo*" (1957b:264–65).

Konrad Theodor Preuss collected the myth and published it in Uitoto with literal and interpretive German translations (1921:166–69). Various translations of the first six (of fifteen) sections, which are those Radin cites, have been anthologized (e.g., Astrov 1962:325–26, Rothenberg 1968:27, Eliade 1974:85, Bierhorst 1976:40–41). The following version is translated literally from the literal German text by Renate Lewis and slightly reworked by David Johnson and Marta Weigle (in Weigle and Johnson 1979:1).

I.

A phantasm. Nothing else was. A phantasm touched the Father. He grasped something mysterious. Nothing existed. Through a dream, the Father Nainuema (He who has or is the vision) held on and explored it.

2.

Not even a tree existed. He held the phantasm with a dream-thread, with breath. He tested for the bottom of the empty phantasm. In testing, there was nothing. "I attached emptiness. I probed it; there was nothing."

3.

Then the Father again sought the bottom of this thing, touched the base of the empty phantasm. The Father tied the dream-thread, pressed it on the emptiness with magic glue. Thus he dreamed, and the magic adhesive held it like tobacco smoke or a fluff of raw cotton.

4.

He seized the bottom of the phantasm and stamped and stamped on it. He seized and held it. Then he sat down on this leveled earth which he had dreamed.

5.

He held the phantasm and thrice spat saliva from his mouth, holding the phantasm. Then he settled on this earth and set the roof of heaven above it. And from this sky he grasped and pulled out blue sky, white sky.

6.

Looking into himself, Rafuema (He who has or is the story) created this story at the foot of heaven, so that we who belong to it may hear it.

4. *The Rape of Philomela, a Greek Myth*

The myth of Philomela's rape by her brother-in-law, Tereus, is one of several in which "the tricky ambivalence ascribed to the speech of women is consonant with the semiotic character of weaving and of graphic art in general, and . . . it finds its intellectual counterpart in the Greek concept of *mētis* or 'transformative intelligence,' itself portrayed as the goddess, Metis" (Bergren 1983:71). Penelope's weaving and unweaving a shroud for Odysseus's father, Laertes, to foil the suitors who think her husband dead (*Odyssey* 19:137–64) is paradigmatic.

More familiar than Philomela's weaving *mētis* is Arachne's hubris in challenging Metis's daughter, Athena, to a weaving contest. Arachne's transformation into what we now know as the spider in the Linnaean classification "arachnid" is only apparently a punishment. In "Dangling Virgins," Eva Cantarella (1986:60, 64) examines the noose as "not only the privileged instrument of female suicide, but also, very often, that with which women were killed," and "the relation between swinging-hanging and the feminine symbolic death of initiation." She suggests that "both in hanging and in rocking on a swing, women are detached from the ground . . . [for] since oldest antiquity, the Western imagination has closely connected women with the earth." Arachne may thus be viewed as a wise initiate, not a pitiful victim.

Philomela's story is found in the same book (VI) of the Roman poet Ovid's *Metamorphoses* (ca. A.D. 8) as Arachne's. According to Michael Simpson (1976:215), "Ovid brings together here two related motifs found throughout the work to make a forceful (perhaps shocking) statement about his vision of art. The first is the motif of the blocked utterance: the inability of a human being to speak to another and its consequences (found, e.g., in the Io, Callisto, and Actaeon episodes). The second is the motif of art *from* pain or *into* pain: art and pain are locked into a cause and effect relationship in which each is now cause, now effect (found, e.g., in the Arachne, Marsyas, and Orpheus episodes . . .). Here blocked utterance (the severing of Philomela's tongue) coincides with and adds to the incredible pain and they together create art (the tapestry). Art does its work well as it sets in motion revenge, more pain, and the horrible death of the innocent Itys."

Ovid ends his tale with Tereus's transformation into a hoopoe, a bird with crested head and a long beak like his drawn sword. According to Morford and Lenardon (1985:412), "In the Greek version of the story it is the nightingale (Procne) that mourns for her dead son, while the tongueless swallow (Philomela) tries to tell her story by her incoherent chatter. The Latin authors, however, changed the names, making Philomela the nightingale and Procne the swallow; it is this version that has survived in later European literature." The nightingale's cry—"Itu! Itu!"—is supposed to mourn the devoured Itys.

The following version of the rape of Philomela (Simpson 1976:205) is from the handbook of Greek mythology known as the *Library* of Apollodorus (3.14.8–14). Although attributed to the Athenian grammarian Apollodorus (180–120 or 110 B.C.), its author (ca. A.D. 120) is unknown.

Pandion married Zeuxippe, the sister of his mother, and by her had two daughters, Procne and Philomela, and twin sons, Erechtheus and Butes. When war broke out with Labdacus over land boundaries, Pandion summoned Tereus, the son of Area, from Thrace as an ally. After winning the war with his help he gave to Tereus his daughter Procne to marry. Tereus had a son, Itys, by her. Tereus fell in love with Philomela and seduced her, saying that Procne, whom he had hidden in the country, was dead. Afterwards he married Philomela and went to bed with her. He also cut out her tongue. But by weaving letters in a robe, Philomela spelled out to Procne the terrible things that had been done to her. After she sought out her sister, Procne killed her son Itys, boiled him, and served him to Tereus without his knowledge. Then she fled at once with Philomela. When Tereus learned what had happened, he seized an axe and pursued them. They were caught at Daulia in Phocis and prayed to the gods to be turned into birds. Procne became a nightingale and Philomela a swallow. Tereus, too, was turned into a bird, becoming a hoopoe.

5. "Novels and Children," a Barthes "Mythology"

Critic Roland Barthes (1915–1980) sees evidence of a mythic pro/creative female in an *Elle* magazine photograph of seventy women novelists who also have borne children.

Jonathan Culler (1983:33) introduces his discussion of Barthes as mythologist thus: "Between 1954 and 1956, Barthes wrote brief monthly feature articles called 'Mythology of the Month' for *Les Lettres nouvelles*. 'I resented seeing Nature and History confused at every turn in accounts of contemporary life,' he reports, and in discussing aspects of mass culture he sought to analyse the social stereotypes passed off as natural, unmasking 'what-goes-without-saying' as an ideological imposition. . . . In many cases, as he reveals the ideological implications of what seems natural, 'myth' means a delusion to be exposed."

In the preface to the 1957 Paris edition of his *Mythologies,* Roland Barthes (1972:11) writes: "The following essays were written . . . on topics suggested by current events. I was at the time trying to reflect regularly on some myths of French daily life. The media which prompted these reflections may well appear heterogeneous (a newspaper article, a photograph in a weekly, a film, a show, an exhibition), and their subject-matter very arbitrary: I was of course guided by my own current interests." He expresses "impatience at the sight of the 'naturalness' with which newspapers, art and common sense constantly dress up a reality which, even though it is the one we live in, is undoubtedly determined by history."

"Novels and Children" is the eleventh essay (Barthes 1972:50–52). It follows a "mythology" of "The Iconography of the Abbe Pierre," whose "fine physiognomy . . . clearly displays all the signs of apostleship," and precedes one of "Toys," as "a microcosm of the adult world" prepared for children viewed as homunculi (Barthes 1972:47, 53).

If we are to believe the weekly *Elle,* which some time ago mustered seventy women novelists on one photograph, the woman of letters is a remarkable zoological species: she brings forth, pell-mell, novels and children. We are introduced, for example, to *Jacqueline Lenoir (two daughters, one novel); Marina Grey (one son, one novel); Nicole Dutreil (two sons, four novels),* etc.

What does it mean? This: to write is a glorious but bold activity; the writer is an "artist", one recognizes that he is entitled to a little bohemianism. As he is in general entrusted—at least in the France of *Elle*—with giving society reasons for its clear conscience, he must, after all, be paid for his services: one tacitly grants him the right to some individuality. But make no mistake: let no women believe that they can take advantage of this pact without having first submitted to the eternal statute of womanhood.

Women are on the earth to give children to men; let them write as much as they like, let them decorate their condition, but above all, let them not depart from it: let their Biblical fate not be disturbed by the promotion which is conceded to them, and let them pay immediately, by the tribute of their motherhood, for this bohemianism which has a natural link with a writer's life.

Women, be therefore courageous, free; play at being men, write like them; but never get far from them; live under their gaze, compensate for your books by your children; enjoy a free rein for a while, but quickly come back to your condition. One novel, one child, a little feminism, a little connubiality. Let us tie the adventure of art to the strong pillars of the home: both will profit a great deal from this combination: where myths are concerned, mutual help is always fruitful.

For instance, the Muse will give its sublimity to the humble tasks of the home; and in exchange, to thank her for this favour, the myth of child-bearing will lend to the Muse, who sometimes has the reputation of being a little wanton, the guarantee of its respectability, the touching decor of the nursery. So that all is well in the best of all worlds—that of *Elle*. Let women acquire self-confidence: they can very well have access, like men, to the superior status of creation. But let men be quickly reassured: women will not be taken from them for all that, they will remain no less available for motherhood by nature. *Elle* nimbly plays a Molieresque scene, says yes on one side and no on the other, and busies herself in displeasing no one; like Don Juan between his two peasant girls, *Elle* says to women: you are worth just as much as men; and to men: your women will never be anything but women.

Man at first seems absent from this double parturition; children and novels alike seem to come by themselves, and to belong to the mother alone. At a pinch, and by dint of seeing seventy times books and kids bracketed together, one would think that they are equally the fruits of imagination and dream, the miraculous products of an ideal parthenogene-sis able to give at once to woman, apparently, the Balzacian joys of creation and the tender joys of motherhood. Where then is man in this family picture? Nowhere and everywhere, like the sky, the horizon, an authority which at once determines and limits a condition. Such is the world of *Elle:* women there are always a homogeneous species, an established body jeal-ous of its privileges, still more enamoured of the burdens that go with them. Man is never inside, femininity is pure, free, powerful; but man is everywhere around, he presses on all sides, he makes everything exist; he is in all eternity the creative absence, that of the Racinian deity: the feminine world of *Elle,* a world without men, but entirely constituted by the gaze of man, is very exactly that of the gynaeceum.

In every feature of *Elle* we find this twofold action: lock the gynaeceum, then and only then release woman inside. Love, work, write, be business-women or women of letters, but always remember that man exists, and that you are not made like him; your order is free on condition that it depends on his; your freedom is a luxury, it is possible only if you first acknowledge the obligations of your nature. Write, if you want to, we women shall all be very proud of it; but don't forget on the other hand to produce children, for that is your destiny. A Jesuitic morality: adapt the moral rule of your condition, but never compromise about the dogma on which it rests.

6. Thompson Indian Creation Myth

The Thompson Indians of British Columbia tell of a male supreme deity who descends to the watery chaos on a cloud. His emanatistic creations of women from five hairs seem both alchemical (Earth Mother, Water, and Fire—with the cloud, or Air, already existent) and allegorical (Good and Bad Mothers).

Collector James A. Teit (1864–1922), first married to a Thompson Indian woman who died in 1899, was active as a political advisor to the British Columbian Indians. He first met Franz Boas (1858–1942) in 1894 and long served as ethnographic fieldworker for the anthropologist. Boas became Teit's mentor and editor, according to Ralph Maud (1982:64), and the former "prepared for publication all of Teit's work printed in his lifetime, so that it is impossible to entirely separate the pupil's contribution from the teacher's. On the other hand, we do have a way of easily distinguishing a Teit story from a Boas story: we are invariably struck, as Dr. Snowden Dunn Scott was, by the simplicity, felicity, and clearness of Teit's language."

The Tcawa'xamux̱ (Nicola Valley) myth below, "The Creation of the Earth by Old-One" (Teit 1912:322–24), was narrated by "a shaman called Nkamtcinê'ɬx, belonging to Sulū's, and probably somewhat over seventy years of age. He stated that he never heard this tale except from his grandfather,—the first time when he was about eight or ten years of age. Other old men who had particular tales were Tcuiê'ska of

Nicola, who had a story of a man who watched the women bathing from the top of a tree; and Ye'luska of Spences Bridge, who had a long tale of women who hung their babies up in trees or bushes. He did not remember the details of these stories, but had heard them narrated only by these men. Tcuiê'ska died a few years ago in Nicola, aged over eighty; and Ye'luska was killed in the Spences Bridge land-slide in August, 1905, when aged about eighty" (Teit 1912:324).

Teit (1912:322, 324) provides two important footnotes (indicated as [fn1] and [fn2] in the following story). Both suggest Christian elements (see the discussion of Teit's work in Ramsey 1977:448–53). The first reads: "The narrator said he was not quite sure whether the hairs were from the head or pubes. He also said he thought they might have been five ribs taken by the chief from his right side." The second is related to the apocalyptic part of the creation myth. On the transformation of the five women to "their original forms": "My informant was vague when questioned as to the nature of this change. He thought people might be conducted to the upper world, or placed on some new earth created for them. He was sure there would be a reunion of the dead and the living, who afterwards would all live together under the same conditions. Both would have human form; and there would be no more sickness, death, misery, and evil. All would be good and happy. Conditions would be an improvement over both the spirit world and this world."

Old-One or Chief came down from the upper world on a cloud, which, when it approached the surface of the great lake, became a bank of fog. He was tired looking at the endless and monotonous expanse of water underneath the sky, and thus had descended to create some kind of a world in the midst of the watery waste which was where the earth is now. The cloud descended until it rested on the surface of the lake. Then Old-One pulled five hairs from his head, [fn1] and, throwing them down on the clouds, they became endowed with life, and sprang up in the form of young women. They were all perfect women endowed with speech, sight, and hearing. He asked the first one to speak and state what she preferred to be. She answered, "I wish to be a woman and to bear children. I shall be bad and foolish, and shall seek after my own pleasure. My descendants will fight, lie, steal, murder, and commit adultery. They will be wicked." The Chief answered her, saying, "I am sorry you have spoken thus, for in this way death and much sorrow will arise."

Now he asked the second woman to state what she wished to be. She answered, "I wish to be a woman and to bear children. I shall be good and virtuous. My descendants will be wise, peaceful, honest, truthful, and chaste." The Chief was glad when he heard her speak thus, and said, "You have spoken well. Wisdom and virtue will eventually triumph over foolishness and evil. The process will be very long, however, and there will be much sorrow and misery meanwhile."

Now the third woman was asked to choose her lot, and she answered, "I wish to be the earth, upon which my sisters will live. They will love me, and draw their life from me. I will make everything fat and happy." The Chief answered, "It is good. From you everything will grow. You will produce, nourish, and give rest. When people die, you will receive them on your breast and will cover them. Trees, plants, grass, flowers, gold, silver, and all that is good and beautiful, will spring from you. You will make your sister's children glad."

Now he asked the choice of the fourth woman, and she answered, "I wish to be fire, and will be in the grass, trees, and in all wood. I shall make people happy by giving them heat and comfort. When they are cold and miserable, they will seek me and obtain warmth and happiness. With my aid they will eat." The Chief answered, "It is good. You will render assistance, and make your sisters' children rejoice."

Then he transformed them. The Earth fell backwards, spread out her legs, and rolled off from the cloud into the lake, where she took the form of the earth we live on. The Chief said, "My daughter, you will be as you have asked. Henceforth you will be the earth in the midst of the great lake, and people will live on you. They will call you their mother." Water he transformed into the present water we see in the shape of lakes, pools, springs, and streams, and it began to run over the top of the earth. Fire he transformed into the present fire, or the heat of fire we see and feel when wood burns. He put the spirit of fire in all woods and plants. The remaining two women he placed on the earth, and, after endowing them with the power to bear offspring, he impregnated them. He told them, "You will be sisters, and from you all people will spring. Your children will be male and female, and your descendants will cover the earth. The offspring of Evil will be most numerous at first, but at last the children of Good will outnumber them. Good will prevail, and Evil finally disappear. Then I will collect all people, both dead and alive. Earth and her sisters will assume their original forms, and all together will become changed and new." [fn2] In this manner will come the end of the world, and this is why both bad and good people are found in the world at the present day. The children of the two women were male and female. They married one another, and from them all people are descended. None of them could live without the earth, fire, and water: therefore these are part of us, and are related to people as if by blood.

7. Iroquoian Creation Myths

A. HURON

An earth-diver myth from the Huron Indians of the Great Lakes woodlands tells how a goddess fell from the sky into a chaos of sea and water animals. She proves to be a *Dea faber* who fashions the earth brought up by the successful toad diver on the tortoise's shell. After her death from an unnatural birth, she becomes an emanatistic culture heroine/vegetation goddess, and the contests of her twin sons (one good and one evil) bring into being the world as it is now.

Collector Horatio Hale (1817–1896) calls this text, only the first part of which is included here, "The Making of the World" (1888:180–81). He writes: "The following is perhaps the most complete account of the Huron cosmogonic myth which has yet been obtained, and may be deemed to represent the primitive belief of the oldest branch of the Huron-Iroquois race. Clarke was about seventy-five years of age in 1874, and as he had heard the myth in his youth from the elders of his people, their joint recollections would carry it back to the middle of the last century, when the customs and traditions of the Wendat were retained in their full vigor." Very likely this is the man described by Hale in a May 14, 1881, letter to Bureau of (American) Ethnology director John Wesley Powell: "The Iroquois myths have been carefully gathered, but less is known of the Hurons. From a very intelligent half breed chief, whose wife is a Frenchwoman, I have obtained a series of their legendary stories, which illustrate both their mythology and their history, and at the same time display a force of imagination and a power of connected narrative, indicative of a high grade of intellectual endowment" (Gruber 1967:36).

In the beginning there was nothing but water, a wide sea, which was peopled by various animals of the kind that live in and upon the water. It happened then that a woman fell down from the upper world. It is supposed that she was, by some mischance, pushed down by her husband through a rift in the sky. Though styled a woman, she was a divine personage. Two loons, which were flying over the water, happened to look up and see her falling. To save her from drowning they hastened to place themselves beneath her, joining their bodies together so as to form a cushion for her to rest on. In this way they held her up, while they cried with a loud voice to summon the other animals to their aid. The cry of the loon can be heard to a great distance, and the other creatures of the sea heard it, and assembled to learn the cause of the summons. Then came the tortoise (or "snapping turtle," as Clarke called it), a mighty animal, which consented to relieve the loons of their burden. They placed the woman on the back of the tortoise, charging him to take care of her. The tortoise then called the other animals to a grand council, to determine what should be done to preserve the life of the woman. They decided that she must have earth to live on. The tortoise directed them all to dive to the bottom of the sea and endeavor to bring up some earth. Many attempted it,—the beaver, the musk-rat, the diver, and others,—but without success. Some remained so long below that when they rose they were dead. The tortoise searched their mouths, but could find no trace of earth. At last the toad went down, and after remaining a long time rose, exhausted and nearly dead. On searching his mouth the tortoise found in it some earth, which he gave to the woman. She took it and placed it carefully around the edge of the tortoise's shell. When thus placed, it became the beginning of dry land. The land grew and extended on every side, forming at last a great country, fit for vegetation. All was sustained by the tortoise, which still supports the earth.

When the woman fell she was pregnant with twins. When these came forth they evinced opposite dispositions, the one good, the other evil. Even before they were born the same characters were manifested. They struggled together, and their mother heard them disputing. The one declared his willingness to be born in the usual manner, while the other malignantly refused, and, breaking through his mother's side, killed her. She was buried, and from her body sprang the various vegetable productions which the new earth required to fit it for the habitation of man. From her head grew the pumpkin-vine; from her breasts the maize; from her limbs the bean and the other useful esculents.

B. Onondaga

Motifs of miraculous conception, parturition, possibly couvade, earth-divers, culture heroines, and dream origins (on the dream ritual see Wallace 1958) are evident in an Onondaga version of the Iroquoian cosmology. Collector J. N. B. Hewitt (1903:136) claims that, "although these legends concerning the beginnings of things are usually called myths, creation stories, or cosmogonies, the terms myth and creation are, in fact, misnomers. In all of these narratives, except such as are of modern date, creation in the modern acceptation of the word is never signified, nor is it even conceived; and when these legends or narratives are called myths, it is because a full comprehension and a correct interpretation of them have to a large extent been lost or because they have been supplanted by more accurate knowledge, and they are related without a clear conception of what they were designed to signify, and rather from custom than as the source of the major portion of the customs and ceremonies and opinions in vogue among the people relating them."

In his history of the Bureau of American Ethnology, Neil M. Judd (1967:50–51) describes J. N. B. Hewitt as "a Tuscarora Indian and a member of the Bear clan (he said it had been founded by a captive white woman), [who] was a conductor on a New Jersey streetcar when hired to assist Mrs. Erminnie A. Smith in her study of the Iroquois language (*1st Ann. Rep.*, 1879–80, *xxii*). Mrs. Smith died June 9, 1886, and thereafter Major Powell engaged Hewitt to complete her manuscript (*7th Ann. Rep.*, 1885–86, *xxxi*)." He did not hurry his work, but produced monographs in *Annual Reports* 21, 32, 43, and 46. "Hewitt was entirely self-educated as an ethnologist, and he was undoubtedly conscious of an inferior education compared with those about him. But he was a stickler for accuracy, and what others have called a procrastinating habit may have been an ancestral [*sic*] unwillingness to be judged careless and inaccurate. His shortcomings sometimes irritated but more frequently amused his colleagues."

The following text (1903:141–86) is entitled "An Onondaga Version: The Manner in Which it Established Itself, in Which it Formed Itself, in Which, in Ancient Time, it Came about that the Earth Became Extant." According to Hewitt (1903:136–37): It was "obtained in 1889 on the Grand River reservation, Canada, from the late chief and fire-keeper, John Buck, of the Onondaga tribe. Afterward, in 1897, it was revised and somewhat enlarged by the aid of Mr. Joshua Buck, a son of the first relator. It is not as long as the Mohawk text printed herewith because the relator seemed averse to telling more than a brief outline of the legend." The text is given in Onondaga with literal and free translations. Portions of the latter are included below, with this editor's summaries in brackets and editorial deletions of the lengthy piece indicated by ellipses.

Hewitt (1903:141) notes of the word *ongwe'*, translated as "Man-being": "The classific conceptual term ongwe' . . . signifies 'mankind, man, human beings; a human being, a person.' But its original meaning was 'man-being' or 'primal being,' which signified collectively those beings who preceded man in existence and exceeded him in wisdom and effective power, the personified bodies and elements of nature, the gods and demigods of later myth and legend, who were endowed by an imputative mode of reasoning with anthropic form and attributes additional to those normally characteristic of the particular bodies or elements that they represented. . . . In this legend, when applied to times previous to the advent of man the word ongwe' usually denotes a man-being that is a personification, one of the gods of the myths, one of that vague class of primal beings of which man was regarded by Iroquoian and other sages as a characteristic type."

In commentary to a Seneca text recorded in 1900, Hewitt (1928: 464–65) says that the first "gigantic anthropic beings" lived in a place "conceived to have been on the upper surface of the visible sky, which was regarded as a solid plane." The first cosmic period ended when "into the sunless and moonless skyland, lighted only by the snowy white flowers of the great tree of light, standing high near the lodge of De'hao^n'hwĕñdjiawă''kho^n' ('He the Earth-holder'), the presiding chief of that realm, jealousy crept. This chief, reputed to be invincible to sorcery, took a young wife by betrothal in fulfillment of a vision of his soul. The name of the young woman was Awĕ^n'hā'i', 'Mature Flowers,' or 'Mature (i.e., fertile) Earth.' Through the crafty machinations of the Fire Dragon of the White Body, the consuming jealousy of the aged presiding chief was kindled against his young spouse. Unfortunately for her welfare, she, by inhaling the breath of her spouse before the completion of their antenuptial ordeals, became parthenogenetically gravid. The betrothed husband, not knowing the cause or source of her condition, questioned her chastity, and with reluctance resolved within himself to expel from his lodge and land his suspected but innocent spouse, and because of inherent inability to aid him, or to change or transform at the same time the nature of all the man-beings who were his neighbors and associates. The disturbed state of his mind caused him to have another vision of his soul. In fulfillment of the requirements of this vision he caused the tree of light, then standing over the supposed aperture through which the sun now shines, to be uprooted, whereby there was formed an abyss into the empyrean of this world. By craft he succeeded in thrusting his unsuspecting young spouse into this abyss."

He who was my grandfather was wont to relate that, verily, he had heard the legend as it was customarily told by five generations of grandsires, and this is what he himself was in the habit of telling. He customarily said: Man-beings dwell in the sky, on the farther side of the visible sky (the ground separating this from the world above it). . . .

Sometime afterward, then, this came to pass. As soon as all the man-beings had severally departed this woman-being came forth and went thither [to the men's house] and, moreover, arrived at the place where the man-being abode, and she carried a comb with her. She said: "Do thou arise; let me disentangle thy hair." Now, verily, he arose, and then, more-over, she disentangled his hair, and straightened it out. It continued in this manner day after day.

Sometime afterward her kindred were surprised. It seems that the life of the maiden was now changed. Day after day it became more and more manifest that now she would give birth to a child. Now, moreover, her mother, the ancient one, became aware of it. Then, verily, she questioned her, saying to the maiden: "Moreover, what manner of person is to be joint parent with thee?" The maiden said nothing in reply. So, now, at that time, the man-being noticed that he began to be ill. For some time it continued thus, when, verily, his mother came to the place where he lay. She said: "Where is the place wherein thou art ill?" Then the man-being said in reply: "Oh, my mother! I will now tell thee that I, alas, am about to die." And his mother replied, saying: "What manner of thing is meant by thy saying, 'I shall die?'"

It is said that they who dwelt there did not know what it is for one to say "I shall die." And the reason of it was that no one living there on the sky had ever theretofore died. [The dying man-being instructs his mother on the proper ritual and place of burial.] . . .

Sometime after they had laid the burial-case in the high place, the maiden, now a woman-being, gave birth to a child, which was a female, a woman-being. Then the ancient one (elder one, the mother of the maiden) said: "Moreover, what manner of person is the father of the child?" The maiden said nothing in reply.

The girl grew rapidly in size. It was not long after this that the girl child was running about. Suddenly, it seems, the girl child began to weep. It was impossible to stop her. Five are the number of days, it is said, that the girl child continued to weep. Then the elder one (her grandmother) said: "Do ye show her the burial-case lying there in the high place." Now, verily, they carried her person, and caused her to stand up high there. Then the girl child looked at it (the corpse), and then she ceased her weeping, and also she was pleased. . . .

[The girl is periodically instructed by the corpse until the time comes for her to marry.]

Now the next day she dressed herself. As soon as she was ready she then again ran, going again to the place where lay the dead man-being. Then she told him, saying: "The time for me to depart has arrived." Now, at that time he told her, saying: "Do thou have courage. Thy pathway throughout its course is terrifying, and the reason that it is so is that many man-beings are traveling to and fro along this pathway. Do not, moreover, speak in reply if some person, whoever he may be, addresses words to thee. And when thou hast gone one half of thy journey, thou wilt come to a river there, and, moreover, the floating log whereon persons cross is maple. When thou dost arrive there, then thou wilt know that thou art halfway on thy journey. Then thou wilt cross the river, and also pass on. Thou must continue to travel without interruption. And thou wilt have traveled some time before thou arrives at the place where thou wilt see a large field. Thou wilt see there, moreover, a lodge standing not far away. And there beside the lodge stands the tree that is called Tooth. [Hewitt's note: "Probably the yellow dog-tooth violet, Erythronium americanum."] Moreover, the blossoms this standing tree bears cause that world to be light, making it light for the man-beings dwelling there.

"Such, in kind, is the tree that stands beside the lodge. Just there is the lodge of the chief whom thou art to marry, and whom his people call He-holds-the-earth. When thou enterest the lodge, thou wilt look and see there in the middle of the lodge a mat spread, and there, on the mat, the chief lying down. Now, at that time, thou shalt lay thy basket [filled with bread made by her mother] down at his feet, and moreover, thou shalt say: 'Thou and I marry.' He will say nothing. When it becomes night, he who is lying down will spread for thee a skin robe at the foot of his mat. There thou wilt stay over night. As soon as it is day again, he will say: 'Do thou arise, do thou work. Customarily one who lives in the lodge of her spouse works.' Then, verily thou must work. He will lay down a string of corn ears and, moreover, he will say: 'Thou must soak the corn and thou must make mush.' At that time there will be a kettle of water set on the fire. As soon as it boils so that it is terrifying, thou must dissolve the meal therein. It must be boiling when thou makest the mush. He himself will speak, saying: 'Do thou undress thyself.' Moreover, thou must there undress thyself. Thou must be in thy bare skin. Nowhere wilt thou have any garment on thy body. Now, the mush will be boiling, and the mush will be hot. Verily, on thy body will fall in places the spattering mush. He will say: 'Thou must not shrink back from it'; moreover, he will have his eyes fixed on thee there. Do not shrink back from it. So soon as it is cooked, thou shalt speak, saying: 'Now, verily, it is cooked; the mush is done.' He will arise, and, moreover, he will remove the kettle, and set it aside. Then, he will say: 'Do thou seat thyself on this side.' Now then, he will say: 'My slaves, ye dogs, do ye two come hither.' They two are very large. As soon as they two arrive he will say: 'Do ye two lick her body where the mush has fallen on it.' And their tongues are like rough bark. They will lick thee, going over thy whole body, all along thy body. Blood will drop from the places where they will lick. Do not allow thy body to flinch therefrom. As soon as they two finish this task he will say: 'Now, do thou again put on thy raiment.' Now, moreover, thou must again dress thyself completely. At that time he will take the basket and set it down, saying, moreover: 'Now, thou and I marry.' So now, so far as they are concerned, the dogs, his slaves, they two will eat." That is what the dead man-being told her. . . .

[The journey and marriage transpire as her father instructed.]

As soon as they two [dogs] completed the task, then he himself took up sunflower oil, and with that, moreover, he annointed her body. As soon as he had finished this task he said: "Now, verily, do thou again dress thyself." Now she redressed herself entirely, and she was again clothed with raiment.

When it became night, he spread a mat for her at the foot of his mat. There they two passed two more nights. And the third day that came to them the chief said to her: "Now thou must again depart. Thou must go again to the place whence thou didst start." Then he took up the basket of the maiden and went then to the place where he kept meat of all kinds hanging in quarters. Now, verily, he took up the dried meat of the spotted fawn and put it into her basket. All the various kinds of meat he placed therein. As soon as the basket was full, he shook the basket to cause its contents to settle down. When he did shake it, there was seemingly just a little room left in it. Seven times, it is said, he shook the basket before he completely filled it. At that time he said: "Now thou must again depart. Do not, moreover, stand anywhere in the course of thy path homeward. And, moreover, when thou dost arrive there, thou must tell the people dwelling there that they, one and all, must remove the roofs from their several lodges. By and by it will become night and I will send that which is called corn. In so far as that thing is concerned, that is what man-beings will next in time live upon. This kind of thing will continue to be in existence for all time." At that time he took up the basket and also said: "Now, verily, thou shouldst bear it on thy back by means of the forehead strap." Now, at that time she departed. . . .

[Events transpire as her husband declares.]

In a short time they were surprised, seemingly, that the maiden was nowhere to be found. She had again departed. They knew that she had again gone to the place where stood the lodge of the chief who was her consort. Now, verily, in reference to him he himself in turn was surprised to see her return home. When it became day again, the chief noticed that seemingly it appeared that the life of the maiden, his spouse, had changed. [Hewitt's note: The expression "life has changed" is employed usually as a euphemism for "is pregnant."] Thus it was that, day after day and night after night, he still considered the matter. The conditions were such that he did not know what thing was the cause that it (his spouse's condition) was thus, so he merely marveled that it had thus come to pass.

It is certain, it is said, that it formed itself there where they two conversed, where they two breathed together; that, verily, his breath is what the maiden caught, and it is that which was the cause of the change in the life of the maiden. And, moreover, that is the child to which she gave birth. And since then, from the time that he (her spouse) let man-beings go here on the earth, the manner in which man-beings are paired has transformed itself. This is the manner in which it will continue to be; this will be its manner of being done, whereby it will be possible for the man-beings dwelling on the earth to produce ohwachiras of posterity. Thus, too, it seems, it came to pass in regard to the beast-world, their bodies all shared in the change of the manner in which they would be able to produce ohwachiras of offspring here on the earth.

Thus it was that, without interruption, it became more and more evident that the maiden would give birth to a child. At that time the chief became convinced of it, and he said: "What is the matter that thy life has changed? Verily, thou art about to have a child. Never, moreover, have thou and I shared the same mat. I believe that it is not I who is the cause that thy life has changed. Dost thou thyself know who it is?" She did not understand the meaning of what he said.

Now, at that time, the chief began to be ill. Suddenly, it seems, she herself now became aware that her life had changed. Then she said, addressing the chief: "I believe that there is, perhaps, something the matter, as my life at the present time is not at all pleasant." He did not make any reply. Not long thereafter she again said: "My thoughts are not at all pleasant." Again he said nothing. So it continued thus that she did nothing but consider the matter, believing that something must be the matter, perhaps, that the condition of her body was such as it was. It became more and more evident that she was pregnant. Now it was evident that she was big with child.

Sometime afterward she again resolved to ask him still once more. She said: "As a matter of fact, there must be something the matter, perhaps, that my body is in this condition. And the thoughts of my mind are not at all pleasant. One would think that there can be no doubt that, seemingly, something is about to happen, because my life is so exceedingly unpleasant." Again he said nothing. When it became night, then, verily, they laid their bodies down and they slept. So now, verily, he there repeatedly considered the matter. Now, in so far as the maiden was concerned, she still did not understand what was about to take place from the changed condition of her body. Sometime afterward the chief spoke to her, saying: "As a matter of fact, a man-being (or rather woman-being) will arrive, and she is a man-being child, and thou must care for her. She will grow in size rapidly, and her name is Zephyrs." [Hewitt's note: This name Zephyrs merely approximates the meaning of the original, which signifies the warm spring-tide zephyrs that sometimes take the form of small whirlwinds or eddies of warm air.] The maiden said nothing, for the reason that she did not understand what her spouse told her. Not long afterward, then, verily, she gave birth to a child. She paid no attention to it. The only thing she did was to lay it on the place where the chief customarily passed the night. After ten days' time she again took it up therefrom.

Sometime afterward the chief became aware that he began to be ill. His suffering became more and more severe. All the persons dwelling in the village came to visit him. There he lay, and sang, saying: "Ye must pull up this standing tree that is called Tooth. The earth will be torn open, and there beside the abyss ye must lay me down. And, moreover, there where my head lies, there must sit my spouse." That is what he, the Ancient One, sang. Then the man-beings dwelling there became aware that their chief was ill.

Now, verily, all came to visit him. They questioned him repeatedly, seeking to divine his Word, what thing, seemingly, was needful for him, what kind of thing, seemingly, he expected through a dream. Thus, day after day, it continued that they sought to find his Word. After a time the female man-being child was of fair size. She was then able to run about from place to place. But it thus continued that they kept on seeking to divine his Word. After a while, seemingly, one of the persons succeeded in finding his Word, and he said: "Now, perhaps, I myself have divined the Word of him, the ordure, our chief." He who is called Aurora Borealis said this. And when he told the chief what manner of thing his soul craved, the chief was very pleased. And when he divined his Word, he said: "Is it not this that thy dream is saying, namely, that it is direful, if it so be that no person should divine thy Word, and that it will become still more direful? And yet, moreover, it is not certain that this is what thy soul craves; that its eyes may have seen thy standing tree, Tooth as to kind, pulled up, in order that the earth be torn open, and that there be an abyss that pierces the earth, and, moreover, that there beside the abyss one shall lay thee, and at thy head thy spouse shall be seated with her legs hanging down into the abyss." At that time the chief said: "Ku'". [Hewitt's note: This is an exclamation expressing gratification at having one's dream or vision divined and satisfied.] I am thankful! Now, verily, the whole matter has been fulfilled by thy divining my Word."

During this time (the duration of the dream feast), a large body of man-beings [Hewitt's note: The relator of this version stated that there was a reputed connection between the visits of these different personages and the presence of their kinds in the new world beneath the sky land, but he had forgotten it.] paid a visit there. . . .

Verily, it did thus come to pass that they did uproot the standing tree, Tooth, that grew beside the lodge of the chief. And all the inhabitants of that place came thither with the intention of looking into the abyss. It did thus come to pass that everyone that dwelt there did look therein. At that time the chief then said, addressing his spouse: "Now, too, let us two look into the abyss. Thou must bear her, Zephyrs, on thy back. Thou must wrap thyself with care." Now, moreover, he gave to her three ears of corn, and, next in order, the dried meat of the spotted fawn, and now, moreover, he said: "This ye two will have for provision." Now he also broke off three fagots of wood, which, moreover, he gave to her. She put them into her bosom, under her garments. Then, verily, they went thither to the place. They arrived at the spot where the earth was torn up, and then he said: "Do thou sit here." There, verily, she sat where the earth was broken off. There she hung both legs severally into the abyss. Now, in so far as he was concerned, he, the chief, was looking into the abyss, and there his spouse sat. Now, at that time he unpraised himself, and said: "Do thou look hence into the abyss." Then she did in this manner, holding with her teeth her robe with its burden. Moreover, there along the edge of the abyss she seized with her hands, and, now, moreover, she bent over to look. He said: "Do thou bend much and plainly over." So she did do thus. As soon as she bent forward very much he seized the nape of her neck and pushed her into the abyss. Verily, now at that time she fell down thence. Now, verily, the man-being child and the man-being mother of it become one again. When she arrived on earth, the child was again born. At that time the chief himself arose and said, moreover: "Now, verily, I have become myself again; I am well again. Now, moreover, do ye again set up the tree."

And the chief was jealous, and that was the cause that he became ill. He was jealous of Aurora Borealis, and, in the next place, of the Fire Dragon with the pure white body. This latter gave him much mental trouble during the time that he, the chief, whom some call He-holds-the-earth, was married.

So now, verily, her body continued to fall. Her body was falling some time before it emerged. Now, she was surprised, seemingly, that there was light below, of a blue color. She looked, and there seemed to be a lake at the spot toward which she was falling. There was nowhere any earth. There she saw many ducks on the lake (sea), whereon they, being waterfowl of all their kinds, floated severally about. Without interruption the body of the woman-being continued to fall.

Now, at that time the waterfowl, called the Loon shouted, saying: "Do ye look, a woman-being is coming in the depths of the water, her body is floating up hither." They said: "Verily, it is even so." Now, verily, in a short time the waterfowl (duck) called Bittern (Whose eyes-are-ever-gazing-upward), said: "It is true that ye believe that her body is floating up from the depths of the water. Do ye, however, look upward." All looked upward, and all, moreover, said: "Verily, it is true." They next said: "What manner of thing shall we do?" One of the persons said: "It seems, then, that there must be land in the depths of the water." At that time the Loon said: "Moreover, let us first seek to find someone who will be able to bear the earth on his back by means of the forehead pack strap." All said, seemingly: "I shall be able to bear the earth by means of the forehead pack strap." He replied: "Let us just try; it seems best." Otter, it seems, was the first to make the attempt.

As soon, then, as a large bulk of them mounted on his back, verily, he sank. In so far as he was concerned, he was not able to do anything. And they said: "Thou canst do nothing." Now many of them made the attempt. All failed to do it. Then he, the Carapace, the Great Turtle, said: "Next in turn, let me make the attempt." Then, verily, a large bulk of them mounted on his back. He was able to bear them all on his back. Then they said: "He it is who will be able to bear the earth on his back." Now, at that time, they said: "Do ye go to seek earth in the depths of the water." There were many of them who were not able to obtain earth. After a while it seems that he, the Muskrat, also made the attempt. He was able to get the ground thence. Muskrat is he who found earth. When he came up again, he rose dead, holding earth in his paws, and earth was also in his mouth. They placed all of it upon the carapace of the Turtle. Now their chief said: "Do ye hurry, and hasten yourselves in your work." Now a large number of muskrats continued to dive into the depths of the water. As fast as they floated to the surface they placed the earth on the back of the Turtle. Sometime thereafter then, verily, they finished covering the carapace with earth. Now, at that time, the carapace began to grow, and the earth with which they had covered it became the Earth.

Now, also, they said: "Now, moreover, do ye go to see and to meet this woman-being whose body is falling hither." At once a great number of the large waterfowl flew hence, joining their bodies together, and there on their joined bodies her person impinged. Then slowly the large waterfowl descended, and also they placed the woman-being there on the carapace. Moreover, the carapace had now grown much in size. Now, moreover, they said: "Now, verily, we are pleased that we have attended to the female man-being who has appeared in the same place with us."

The next day came, and she looked and saw lying there a deer, also fire and firebrands, and also a heap of wood, all of which had been brought thither. At that time she kindled a fire, using for this purpose the three fagots which she had slipt into the bosom of her garment, and of which he (the chief) had said: "Ye two will have this for a provision." At that time she laid hands on the body of the deer. She broke up its body, some of which she roasted for food. She passed three nights there, when she again gave birth, again becoming possessed of a child. The child was a female. That, verily, was the rebirth of Zephyrs. Now the elder woman-being erected a booth, thatching it with grasses. There the mother and daughter remained, one being the parent of the other.

Now the earth was large and was continually increasing in size. It was now plain where the river courses would be. There they two remained, the mother attending to the child, who increased in size very rapidly. Some time afterward she then became a maiden. And they two continued to remain there.

After a while, seemingly, the elder woman-being heard her offspring talking with someone. Now, verily, the elder woman-being was thinking about this matter, wondering: "Whence may it be that a man-being could come to talk with her." She addressed her, saying: "Who is it, moreover, who visits thee?" The maiden said nothing in reply. As soon as it became night and the darkness was complete, he, the man-being, again arrived. And just as the day dawned the elder woman-being heard him say: "I will not come again." Verily he then departed.

Not long after this the life of the maiden was changed. Moreover, it became evident that she was about to give birth to a child. After a time, when, seemingly, the maiden had only a few more days to go, she was surprised, seemingly, to hear two male man-beings talking in her body. One of the persons said: "There is no doubt that the time when man-beings will emerge to be born has now arrived." The other person replied: "Where, moreover, does it seem that thou and I should emerge?" He replied, saying: "This way, moreover, thou and I will go." Now, again, one of them spoke, saying: "It is too far. This way, right here, is near, and, seemingly, quite transparent." At that time he added, saying: "Do thou go then; so be it." Now, he started and was born. The child was a male. Then, so far as the other was concerned, he came out here through her armpit. And now, verily, he killed his mother. The grandmother saw that the child that was born first was unsurpassedly fine-looking. At that time she asked, saying: "Who, moreover, killed your mother, now dead?" Now, he who did it replied, saying: "This one here." Verily, he told a falsehood. Now, the elder woman-being seized the other one by the arm and cast his body far beyond, where he fell among grasses. Now, she there attended to the other one. It is said that they grew rapidly in size. After a while, seemingly, he was in the habit of going out, and there running about from place to place. In like manner they two grew very rapidly.

8. Luiseño Cosmogony

The Luiseños, Shoshonean Indians who lived inland in a territory south of Los Angeles, were named after the mission San Luis Rey de Francia. Their creation myth shows some similarities to Hesiod's

Theogony: chaos as abyss; cosmic hierogamy, here of siblings; Earth Mother hiding the Sun and monstrous Chun-itch'-nish like Gaia hiding the Titans from Ouranus.

More important are the definite similarities between the Luiseño stages of coming-into-being and those in various Oceanic cosmogonies like the Hawaiian Kumulipo (Beckwith 1972). Constance Goddard DuBois (1906:52) notes of these stages: "[Father Geronimo] Boscana alludes to the periods of time in the Creation Myth which he records, the story to-day being analogous to that which he obtained from the Indians eighty years ago. He says: 'We have the six productions of the mother of Ouiot, corresponding to the six days of the creation of the world.' I did not obtain this series thus distinctly stated, but on the other hand the introductory periods of creation were clearly named and defined. Whether these eight periods show any trace of Christian influence I am not as yet prepared to say. The myth in its entirety is strictly primitive. Only the slightest traces of any external influence could be suspected." Boscana's, DuBois's, and others' versions of Luiseño creation myths are analyzed by Sam D. Gill (1987:88–106) in his study of Mother Earth in Native American beliefs.

According to Gill (1987:90–91), Constance Goddard DuBois published four versions of the Luiseño creation between 1904 and 1908. She "was a philanthropist and novelist with strong ethnographic interests. She surveyed and served the needs of the native peoples of southern California as she understood them. She was a highly sympathetic observer of Luiseño culture, and apparently had extensive experience with southern California cultures. She did not know Luiseño language, and there is no way to evaluate the competence of her interpreters or the reliability of her sources, except for the few general comments she made about them. Were it not for the fact that she collected a number of accounts of the original story from different people, her contribution would be of doubtful value." Goddard does not identify her informant, noting only that "this paper has been communicated as part of the Proceedings of the California branch of the American Folk-Lore Society." Her other notes have been incorporated into the text, "San Luiseño Creation Myth" (DuBois 1906:52–54), in brackets.

In the beginning all was empty space. Ké-vish-a-ták-vish was the only being. This period was called Óm-ai-yá-mai signifying emptiness, nobody there. Then came the time called Há-ruh-rúy, upheaval, things coming into shape. Then a time called Chu-tu-taí, the falling of things downward; and after this, Yu-vaí-to-vaí, things working in darkness without the light of sun or moon. Then came the period Tul-múl Pu-shún, signifying that deep down in the heart or core of earth things were working together.

Then came Why-yaí Pee-vaí, a gray glimmering like the whiteness of hoar frost; and then, Mit-aí Kwai-raí, the dimness of twilight. Then came a period of cessation, Na-kaí Ho-wai-yaí, meaning things at a standstill.

Then Ké-vish-a-ták-vish made a man, Túk-mit, the Sky; and a woman, To-maí-yo-vit, the Earth. There was no light, but in the darkness these two became conscious of each other.

"Who are you?" asked the man.

"I am To-maí-yo-vit. And you?"

"I am Túk-mit."

"Then you are my brother."

"You are my sister."

. . . [*sic*]

By her brother the Sky the Earth conceived and became the Mother of all things. Her first-born children were, in the order of their birth, See-vat and Pá-ve-ut [Note 3: Pá-ve-ut is the name given to the sacred pointed stones of chipped flint, etc., used, not for arrow points, but for insertion in the end of the sword-shaped stand carried by the chief in the religious ceremonials. Boscana gives as the second production of Mother Earth "rocks and stones of all kinds, particularly flints for their arrows."], Ush-la and Pik-la, Ná-na-chel and Patch'-ha-yel, Tópal and Tam'·yush. [Note 4: Tam'·yush, or Tam-ish (obscure sound) is the name for the sacred stone bowls, incorrectly called mortars, hollowed out of solid rounded stones, large and small, used in the toloache fiesta for mixing and distributing the drink, and placed upon the ground in the sacred house (called temple by Boscana) during the religious ceremonies. They were painted with bright colors within and without; and when not in use were carefully buried from sight in places known only to the religious leaders.]

Then came forth all other things, people, animals, trees, rocks, and rivers, but not as we see them now. All things then were people.

But at first they were heavy and helpless and could not move about, and they were in darkness, for there was no light. But when the Sun was born he gave a tremendous light which struck the people into unconsciousness, or caused them to roll upon the ground in agony; so that the Earth-Mother, seeing this, caught him up and hid him away for a season; so then there was darkness again.

After the Sun was born there came forth another being called Chun-itch'-nish (spelled Chin-ig-chin-ich by Boscana), a being of power, whose voice sounded as soon as he was born, while all the others rolled helplessly upon the ground, unable to utter a word. The others were so terrified by his appearance that the Earth-Mother hid him away, and ever since he has remained invisible.

The rattlesnake was born at this time, a monster without arms or legs.

When all her children were born, the Earth-Mother left the place and went to Ech'-a-mo Nóy-a-mo. The people rolled, for like newborn babies they could not walk. They began then to crawl on hands and knees, and they talked this way: Chák-o-lá-le, Wá-wa, Tá-ta. This was all that they could say. For food they ate clay. From there they moved to Kak-wé-mai Po-lá-la, then to Po-és-kak Po-lá-lak.

They were growing large now and began to recognize each other. Then the Earth-Mother made the sea so that her children could bathe in it, and so that the breeze from the sea might fill their lungs, for until this time they had not breathed.

Then they moved farther to a place called Na-ché-vo Po-mé-sa-vo, a sort of a cañon which was too small for their abiding-place; so they returned to a place called Tem-ech'-va Tem-eck'-o, and this place people now call Temecula, for the Mexicans changed the Indian name to that.

Here they settled while everything was still in darkness. All this time they had been travelling about without any light.

The Earth-Mother had kept the sun hidden away, but now that the people were grown large enough and could know each other she took the Sun out of his hiding-place, and immediately there was light. They could all see each other; and while the Sun was standing there among them they discussed the matter and decided that he must go east and west and give light all over the world; so all of them raised their arms to the sky three times, and three times cried out Cha-cha-cha (unspellable guttural), and he rose from among them and went up to his place in the sky.

After this they remained at Temecula, but the world was not big enough for them, and they talked about it and concluded that it must be made larger. So this was done, and they lived there as before.

9. Zuni Pueblo Emergence Myth

Frank Hamilton Cushing's 1896 "Outlines of Zuñi Creation Myths" is both typical of nineteenth-century ethnological/folklore texts and exemplary of creation myths for being a much anthologized, analyzed, and anathematized text. Because they contain virtually all the creation and procreation motifs considered in this book, the first eight "outlines" (Cushing 1896:379–84) are reprinted here. They have been numbered for ease of reference, but Cushing's titles are retained.

Cushing (1857–1900) arrived at Zuni Pueblo in New Mexico in 1879 as an ethnologist with the fledgling Bureau of Ethnology's collecting expedition led by James Stevenson. He dropped out of the group and "remained for four and a half years, became proficient in the language, and—partly winning his way through a combination of charm, luck, and stubbornness and partly being pulled along by the Indians' own determination to convert and absorb him—entered so far into the life of the pueblo that he not only was formally initiated into the tribe but became a member of the tribal council and of the Bow Priesthood" (Green 1979:5). As Curtis Hinsley (1983:56) notes: "The stories of Cushing's physical sufferings and gradual acceptance among some groups in the pueblo, his initiation into the Priesthood of the Bow, and the bestowing of his name, Medicine Flower, have become part of the folklore of American anthropology, and have justified the claim that he pioneered the method of participant-observation in North America."

In his introduction, Cushing (1896:374) claims: "Frequently I have occasion to reproduce portions of songs or rituals, or, again, words of the Uanami or 'Beloved Gods.' In the originals these are almost always in faultless blank verse meter, and are often even grandly poetic. I do not hesitate either to reproduce as nearly as possible their form, or to tax to the uttermost my power of expression in rendering the meanings of them where I quote, clear and effective and in intelligible English. Yet in doing this I do not have to depart very far from 'scientific' accuracy, even in the linguistic sense." Jesse Green (1979: 333–34) quotes from Cushing's unpublished "Notes on Myth and Folklore": "It has seemed good to me to tell these tales as I do—not always withholding little touches which do not belong strictly in the places where they occur, yet which are, in the way of understandings, always implied as understood. . . . [The "outlines"] are not to be considered as literally translated, yet nevertheless they are true in word as well as in idea to the originals. As I have presented them, each is a composite of the various accounts I have heard of it and of the large amount of information of one kind and another always vouchsafed me with each repetition or separate telling of it and related myths."

Cushing (1896:375) claims his outlines are "a preliminary rendering . . . , properly speaking, . . . a series of explanation-myths. Now, while such myths are generally disconnected, often, indeed, somewhat contradictory episode-legends with primitive peoples, they are, with the Zunis, already become serial, and it is in their serial or epic form (but merely in outline) that I here give them. . . . These various myths are held in brief and repeated in set form and one sequence as are placed the beads of a rosary or on a string, each entire, yet all making a connected strand." In the introduction to her "Zuñi Origin Myths," Ruth L. Bunzel (1932:547–48) commends him for this insight: "Cushing, however, hints at the true character of Zuñi mythology. There is no single origin myth but a long series of separate myths. Each ceremonial group has a myth which contains, in addition to a general synopsis of early history, the mythological sanction for its own organization and rituals. . . . These separate myths are preserved in fixed ritualistic form and are sometimes recited during ceremonies, and are transferred like any other esoteric knowledge."

Nevertheless, Bunzel, like many other anthropologists and folklorists (notably Dennis Tedlock in, e.g., 1983:31–61, 233–46), is appropriately critical of Cushing. Commenting on Cushing (1896), Stevenson (1904), and Parsons (1923), Bunzel (1932:547) observes: "The three versions placed side by side give one of the most striking examples of the great handicap under which the science of ethnology labors. All ethnological information comes to us through the medium of another mind, and, with data so complex and subtle as those of human civilization, no matter how clear and honest that mind is, it can absorb only what is congenial to it, and must give it out again through such means of expression as it may command. The Zuñis are as much preoccupied with the origins and early history of their people as were, for instance, the ancient Hebrews, and the three accounts are what might be gathered from any people by individuals of varying interests." Bunzel's incisive observations, like Tedlock's, apply as well to all the creation texts and interpretations herein.

Sam D. Gill (1987:79) notes that Cushing intended to follow the preliminary "Outlines of Zuñi Creation Myths" with a second study, which "would present detailed explanations of the Zuni stories, including his authority for framing and translating the stories." He (1987:81) concludes that the outlines are "an interpretive English rendering" and that: "Cushing, in effect, wrote a story incorporating Zuni story elements. He created a myth upon Zuni mythology. He presented a metamyth. His stories are an interpretation of Zuni mythology in literary form. There is not necessarily fault in this approach, nor did Cushing intend to deceive. He stated his intention to explain his interpretive presentation. Still, his approach, while decades ahead of its time, has invited the wide misconception that what he is presenting is an exact record of Zuni creation stories."

I. THE GENESIS OF THE WORLDS, OR THE BEGINNING OF NEWNESS

Before the beginning of the new-making, Áwonawílona (the Maker and Container of All, the All-father Father), solely had being. There was nothing else whatsoever throughout the great space of the ages save everywhere black darkness in it, and everywhere void desolation.

In the beginning of the new-made, Áwonawílona conceived within himself and thought outward in space, whereby mists of increase, steams potent of growth, were evolved and uplifted. Thus, by means of his innate knowledge, the All-container made himself in person and form of the Sun whom we hold to be our father and who thus came to exist and appear. With his appearance came the brightening of the spaces with light, and with the brightening of the spaces the great mist-clouds were thickened together and fell, whereby was evolved water in water; yea, and the world-holding sea.

With his substance of flesh (*yépnane*) outdrawn from the surface of his person, the Sun-father formed the seed-stuff of twain worlds, impregnating therewith the great waters, and lo! in the heat of his light these waters of the sea grew green and scums (*k'yanashótsiyallawe*) rose upon them, waxing wide and weighty until, behold! they became Áwitelin Tsíta, the "Four-fold Containing Mother-earth," and Apoyan Tä'chu, the "All-covering Father-sky."

II. THE GENESIS OF MEN AND THE CREATURES

From the lying together of these twain upon the great world waters, so vitalizing, terrestrial life was conceived; whence began all beings of earth, men and the creatures, in the Four-fold womb of the World (Áwiten Tehu'hlnakwi).

Thereupon the Earth-mother repulsed the Sky-father, growing big and sinking deep into the embrace of the waters below, thus separating from the Sky-father in the embrace of the waters above. As a woman forebodes evil for her first-born ere born, even so did the Earth-mother forebode, long withholding from birth her myriad progeny and meantime seeking counsel with the Sky-father. "How," said they to one another, "shall our children, when brought forth, know one place from another, even by the white light of the Sun-father?"

Now like all the surpassing beings (*píkwaiyin áhâi*) the Earth-mother and the Sky-father were *ʼhlímna* (changeable), even as smoke in the wind; transmutable at thought, manifesting themselves in any form at will, like as dancers may be mask-making.

Thus, as a man and woman, spake they, one to the other. "Behold!" said the Earth-mother as a great terraced bowl appeared at hand and within it water, "this is as upon me the homes of my tiny children shall be. On the rim of each world-country they wander in, terraced mountains shall stand, making in one region many, whereby country shall be known from country, and within each, place from place. Behold, again!" said she as she spat on the water and rapidly smote and stirred it with her fingers. Foam formed, gathering about the terraced rim, mounting higher and higher. "Yea," said she, "and from my bosom they shall draw nourishment, for in such as this shall they find the substance of life whence we were ourselves sustained, for see!" Then with her warm breath she blew across the terraces; white flecks of the foam broke away, and, floating over above the water, were shattered by the cold breath of the Sky-father attending, and forthwith shed downward abundantly fine mist and spray! "Even so, shall white clouds float up from the great waters at the borders of the world, and clustering about the mountain terraces of the horizons be borne aloft and abroad by the breaths of the surpassing of soul-beings, and of the children, and shall hardened and broken be by thy cold, shedding downward, in rain-spray, the water of life, even into the hollow places of my lap! For therein chiefly shall nestle our children mankind and creature kind, for warmth in thy coldness."

Lo! even the trees on high mountains near the clouds and the Sky-father crouch low toward the Earth-mother for warmth and protection! Warm is the Earth-mother, cold the Sky-father, even as woman is the warm, man the cold being!

"Even so!" said the Sky-father; "Yet not alone shalt *thou* helpful be unto our children, for behold!" and he spread his hand abroad with the palm downward and into all the wrinkles and crevices thereof he set the semblance of shining yellow corn-grains; in the dark of the early world-dawn they gleamed like sparks of fire, and moved as his hand was moved over the bowl, shining up from and also moving in the depths of the water therein. "See!" said he, pointing to the seven grains clasped by his thumb and four fingers, "by such shall our children be guided; for behold, when the Sun-father is not nigh, and thy terraces are as the dark itself (being all hidden therein), then shall our children be guided by lights—like to these lights of all the six regions turning round the midmost one—as in and around the midmost place, where these our children shall abide, lie all the other regions of space! Yea! and even as these grains gleam up from the water, so shall seed-grains like to them, yet numberless, spring up from thy bosom when touched by my waters, to nourish our children." Thus and in other ways many devised they for their offspring.

III. THE GESTATION OF MEN AND THE CREATURES

Anon in the nethermost of the four cave-wombs of the world, the seed of men and the creatures took form and increased; even as within eggs in warm places worms speedily appear, which growing, presently burst their shells and become as may happen, birds, tadpoles or serpents, so did men and all creatures grow manifoldly and multiply in many kinds. Thus the lowermost womb or cave-world, which was Ánosin téhuli (the womb of sooty depth or of growth-generation, because it was the place of first formation and black as a chimney at night time, foul too, as the internals of the belly), thus did it become overfilled with being. Everywhere were unfinished creatures, crawling like reptiles one over another in filth and black darkness, crowding thickly together and treading each other, one spitting on another or doing other indecency, insomuch that loud became their murmurings and lamentations, until many among them sought to escape, growing wiser and more manlike.

IV. THE FORTHCOMING FROM EARTH OF THE FOREMOST OF MEN

Then came among men and the beings, it is said, the wisest of wise men and the foremost, the all-sacred master, Póshaiyaŋk'ya, he who appeared in the waters below, even as did the Sun-father in the wastes above, and who arose from the nethermost sea, and pitying men still, won upward, gaining by virtue of his (innate) wisdom-knowledge issuance from that first world-womb through ways so dark and narrow that those who, seeing somewhat, crowded after, could not follow, so eager were they and so mightily did they strive with one another! Alone, then, he fared upward from one womb (cave) to another out into the great breath of daylight. There, the earth lay, like a vast island in the midst of the great waters, wet and unstable. And alone fared he forth dayward, seeking the Sun-father and supplicating him to deliver mankind and the creatures there below.

V. THE BIRTH FROM THE SEA OF THE TWAIN DELIVERERS OF MEN

Then did the Sun-father take counsel within himself, and casting his glance downward espied, on the great waters, a Foam-cap near to the Earth-mother. With his beam he impregnated and with his heat incubated the Foam-cap, whereupon she gave birth to Úanam Achi Píahkoa, the Beloved Twain who descended; first, Úanam Éhkona, the Beloved Preceder, then Úanam Yáluna, the Beloved Follower, Twin brothers of Light, yet Elder and Younger, the Right and the Left, like to question and answer in deciding and doing. To them the Sun-father imparted, still retaining, control-thought and his own knowledge-wisdom, even as to the offspring of wise parents their knowingness is imparted and as to his right hand and his left hand a skillful man gives craft freely surrendering not his knowledge. He gave them, of himself and their mother the Foam-cap, the great cloud-bow, and for arrows the thunderbolts of the four quarters (twain to either), and for buckler the fog-making shield, which (spun of the floating clouds and spray and woven, as of cotton we spin and weave) supports as on wind, yet hides (as a shadow hides) its bearer, defending also. And of men and all creatures he gave them the fathership and dominion, also as a man gives over the control of his work to the management of his hands. Well instructed of the Sun-father, they lifted the Sky-father with their great cloud-bow into the vault of the high zenith, that the earth might become warm and thus fitter for their children, men and the creatures. Then along the trail of the sun-seeking Póshaiyank'ya, they sped backward swiftly on their floating fog-shield, westward to the Mountain of Generation. With their magic knives of the thunderbolt they spread open the uncleft depths of the mountain, and still on their cloud-shield—even as a spider in her web descendeth—so descended they unerringly, into the dark of the underworld. There they abode with men and the creatures, attending them, coming to know them, and becoming known of them as masters and fathers, thus seeking the ways for leading them forth.

VI. The Birth and Delivery of Men and the Creatures

Now there were growing things in the depths, like grasses and crawling vines. So now the Beloved Twain breathed on the stems of these grasses (growing tall, as grass is wont to do toward the light, under the opening they had cleft and whereby they had descended), causing them to increase vastly and rapidly by grasping and walking round and round them, twisting them upward until lo! they reach forth even into the light. And where successively they grasped the stems ridges were formed and thumb-marks whence sprang branching leaf-stems. Therewith the two formed a great ladder whereon men and the creatures might ascend to the second cave-floor, and thus not be violently ejected in after-time by the throes of the Earth-mother, and thereby be made demoniac and deformed.

Up this ladder, into the second cave-world, men and the beings crowded, following closely the Two Little but Mighty Ones. Yet many fell back and, lost in the darkness, peopled the under-world, whence they were delivered in after-time amid terrible earth shakings, becoming the monsters and fearfully strange beings of olden time. Lo! in this second womb it was dark as is the night of a stormy season, but larger of space and higher than had been the first, because it was nearer the navel of the Earth-mother, hence named K'ólin tehuli (the Umbilical-womb, or the Place of Gestation). Here again men and the beings increased and the clamor of their complainings grew loud and beseeching. Again the Two, augmenting the growth of the great ladder, guided them upward, this time not all at once, but in successive bands to become in time the fathers of the six kinds of men (the yellow, the tawny gray, the red, the white, the mingled, and the black races), and with them the gods and creatures of them all. Yet this time also as before, multitudes were lost or left behind. The third great cave-world, whereunto men and the creatures had now ascended, being larger than the second and higher, was lighter, like a valley in starlight, and named Áwisho tehuli—the Vaginal-womb, or the Place of Sex-generation or Gestation. For here the various peoples and beings began to multiply apart in kind one from another; and as the nations and tribes of men and the creatures thus waxed numerous as before, here, too, it became overfilled. As before, generations of nations now were led out successively (yet many lost, also as hitherto) into the next and last world-cave, Tépahaian tehuli, the Ultimate-uncoverable, or the Womb of Parturition.

Here it was light like the dawning, and men began to perceive and to learn variously according to their natures, wherefore the Twain taught them to seek first of all our Sun-father, who would, they said, reveal to them wisdom and knowledge of the ways of life—wherein also they were instructing them as we do little children. Yet like the other cave-worlds, this too became, after long time, filled with progeny; and finally, at periods, the Two led forth the nations of men and the kinds of being, into this great upper world, which is called Ték'ohaian úlahnane, or the World of Disseminated Light and Knowledge or Seeing.

VII. THE CONDITION OF MEN WHEN FIRST INTO THE WORLD OF DAYLIGHT BORN

Eight years made the span of four days and four nights when the world was new. It was while yet such days and nights continued that men were led forth, first in the night, that it might be well. For even when they saw the great star (*móyächun 'hlána*), which since then is spoken of as the lying star (*mókwanosona*), they thought it the Sun himself, so burned it their eyeballs! Men and the creatures were nearer alike then than now: black were our fathers the late born of creation, like the caves from which they came forth; cold and scaly their skins like those of mud-creatures; goggled their eyes like those of an owl; membranous their ears like those of cave-bats; webbed their feet like those of walkers in wet and soft places; and according as they were elder or younger, they had tails, longer or shorter. They crouched when they walked, often indeed, crawling along the ground like toads, lizards and newts; like infants who still fear to walk straight, they crouched, as before-time they had in their cave-worlds, that they might not stumble or fall, or come to hurt in the uncertain light thereof. And when the morning star rose they blinked excessively as they beheld its brightness and cried out with many mouth-motionings that surely now the Father was coming; but it was only the elder of the Bright Ones, gone before with elder nations and with his shield of flame, heralding from afar (as we herald with wet shell scales or crystals) the approach of the Sun-father! And when, low down in the east the Sun-father himself appeared, what though shrouded in the midst of the great world waters, they were so blinded and heated by his light and glory that they cried out to one another in anguish and fell down wallowing and covering their eyes with their bare hands and arms. Yet ever anew they looked afresh to the light and anew struggled toward the sun as moths and other night creatures seek the light of a camp fire; yea, and what though burned, seek ever anew that light!

Thus ere long they became used to the light, and to this high world they had entered. Wherefore, when they arose and no longer walked bended, lo! it was then that they first looked full upon one another and in horror of their filthier parts, strove to hide these, even from one another, with girdles of bark and rushes; and when by thus walking only upon their hinder feet the same became bruised and sore, they sought to protect them with plaited soles (sandals) of yucca fiber.

VIII. THE ORIGIN OF PRIESTS AND OF KNOWLEDGE

It was thus, by much devising of ways, that men began to grow knowing in many things, and were instructed by what they saw, and so became wiser and better able to receive the words and gifts of their fathers and elder brothers, the gods, Twain and others, and priests. For already masters-to-be were amongst them. Even in the dark of the under-worlds such had come to be; as had, indeed, the various kinds of creatures-to-be, so these. And according to their natures they had found and cherished things, and had been granted gifts by the gods; but as yet they knew not the meaning of their own powers and possessions, even as children know not the meanings and right uses of the precious or needful things given them; nay nor yet the functions of their very parts! Now in the light of the Sun-father, persons became known from persons, and these things from other things; and thus the people came to know their many fathers among men, to know them by themselves or by the possessions they had.

Now the first and most perfect of all these fathers among men after Póshaiyaŋk'ya was Yanáuluha, who brought up from the under-world water of the inner ocean, and seeds of life-production and growing things; in gourds he brought these up, and also things containing the "of-doing-powers."

10. Acoma Pueblo Emergence Myth

The Acoma Pueblo "origin myth" below recounts the birth and maturation of culture heroine twin daughters of the sun. Their creative knowledge and eventual emergence from the underworld Shipapu comes from the tutelary spirit Tsichtinako, or Thought Woman (Spider Woman).

Matthew W. Stirling (1942:vii), then director of the Bureau of American Ethnology, reports: "The following information was obtained in September and October 1928 from a group of Pueblo Indians from Acoma and Santa Ana visiting Washington. . . . Dr. C. Daryll Forde, who was in Washington at the time, worked with the writer during the recording of the early part of the myth, a section of which was published by him in Folk-Lore, with my permission." Forde's version is somewhat different. He (1930:370) prefaces it with an account slightly at variance with Stirling's: "The following creation story was obtained from a party of Indians from the Pueblo of Acoma visiting the Bureau of American Ethnology, Washington, D.C., in August 1928. The myth was told in Keresan by the old man of the party and translated by one of his sons."

In his preface Stirling (1942:vii) states: "The Acoma origin and migration myth is presented as it was learned by the chief informant during his initiation in youth into the Koshari, the group of sacred clowns to whom theoretically all religious secrets are divulged. With this myth, according to Acoma ideology, everything in the culture must harmonize. When new practices are adopted, there is an attempt to fit them into the general scheme, although in recounting the tradition, the informant was careful to differentiate between contemporary practice and what was given in the tradition. Frequently after his dictation, when I would question him to bring out more concrete instances, he would say, 'It is not done so any more.' The tradition is couched in archaic language so that in many places the younger interpreters were unable to translate and the elderly informant would have to explain in modern Acoma phraseology. This may account in part for certain obvious paraphrases of Pueblo or even of merely Indian ways of speaking. Other paraphrases may have been made for the benefit of the White man or as interpretation of Acoma religion by one who is an exceptionally good Catholic and no longer a participant in the ceremonial life of Acoma." The text (1942:1–4) is followed by Stirling's notes and his bibliography of sources cited in those notes.

In the beginning[1] two female human beings were born. These two children were born underground at a place called Shipapu. As they grew up, they began to be aware of each other. There was no light and they could only feel each other. Being in the dark they grew slowly.

After they had grown considerably, a Spirit whom they afterward called Tsichtinako[2] spoke to them, and they found that it would give them nourishment. After they had grown large enough to think for themselves, they spoke to the Spirit when it had come to them one day and asked it to make itself known to them and to say whether it was male or female, but it replied only that it was not allowed to meet with them. They then asked why they were living in the dark without knowing each other by name, but the Spirit answered that they were nuk'timi[3] (under the earth); but they were to be patient in waiting until everything was ready for them to go up into the light. So they waited a long time, and as they grew they learned their language from Tsichtinako.

When all was ready, they found a present from Tsichtinako, two baskets of seeds and little images of all the different animals (there were to be) in the world. The Spirit said they were sent by their father. They asked who was meant by their father, and Tsichtinako replied that his name was Ūch'tsiti[4] and that he wished them to take their baskets out into the light, when the time came. Tsichtinako instructed them, "You will find the seeds of four kinds of pine trees, lā'khok, gēi'etsu (dyai'its), wanūka, and lā'nye, in your baskets. You are to plant these seeds and will use the trees to get up into the light." They could not see the things in their baskets but feeling each object in turn they asked, "Is this it?" until the seeds were found. They then planted the seeds as Tsichtinako instructed. All of the four seeds sprouted, but in the darkness the trees grew very slowly and the two sisters became very anxious to reach the light as they waited this long time. They slept for many years as they had no use for eyes. Each time they awoke they would feel the trees to see how they were growing. The tree lanye grew faster than the others and after a very long time pushed a hole through the earth for them and let in a very little light. The others stopped growing, at various heights, when this happened.

The hole that the tree lanye made was not large enough for them to pass through, so Tsichtinako advised them to look again in their baskets where they would find the image of an animal called dyu·p' (badger) and tell it to become alive. They told it to live, and it did so as they spoke, exclaiming, "A'uha! Why have you given me life?" They told it not to be afraid nor to worry about coming to life. "We have brought you to life because you are to be useful." Tsichtinako spoke to them again, instructing them to tell Badger to climb the pine tree, to bore a hole large enough for them to crawl up, cautioning him not to go out into the light, but to return, when the hole was finished. Badger climbed the tree and after he had dug a hole large enough, returned saying that he had done his work. They thanked him and said, "As a reward you will come up with us to the light and thereafter you will live happily. You will always know how to dig and your home will be in the ground where you will be neither too hot nor too cold."

Tsichtinako now spoke again, telling them to look in the basket for Tāwāi'nū (locust), giving it life and asking it to smooth the hole by plastering. It, too was to be cautioned to return. This they did and Locust smoothed the hole but, having finished, went out into the light. When it returned reporting that it had done its work, they asked it if it had gone out. Locust said no, and every time he was asked he replied no, until the fourth time when he admitted that he had gone out. They asked Locust what it was like outside. Locust replied that it was just tsī'ītī (laid out flat). They said, "From now on you will be known as Tsi·k'ă.[5] You will also come up with us, but you will be punished for disobedience by being allowed out only a short time. Your home will be in the ground and you will have to return when the weather is bad. You will soon die but you will be reborn each season."

The hole now let light into the place where the two sisters were, and Tsichtinako spoke to them, "Now is the time you are to go out. You are able to take your baskets with you. In them you will find pollen and sacred corn meal. When you reach the top, you will wait for the sun to come up and that direction will be called ha'nami (east). With the pollen and the sacred corn meal you will pray to the Sun. You will thank the Sun for bringing you to light, ask for a long life and happiness, and for success in the purpose for which you were created." Tsichtinako then taught them the prayers and the creation song, which they were to sing. This took a long while, but finally the sisters followed by Badger and Locust, went out into the light, climbing the pine tree. Badger was very strong and skillful and helped them. On reaching the earth, they set down their baskets and saw for the first time what they had. The earth was soft and spongy under their feet as they walked, and they said, "This is not ripe." They stood waiting for the sun, not knowing where it would appear. Gradually it grew lighter and finally the sun came up. Before they began to pray, Tsichtinako told them they were facing east and that their right side, the side their best aim was on, would be known as kū'ā'mē (south) and the left ti dyami (north) while behind at their backs was the direction pūna'me (west) where the sun would go down. They had already learned while underground the direction nŭk'ŭm (down) and later, when they asked where their father was, they were told tyunami (four skies above).

And as they waited to pray to the Sun, the girl on the right moved her best hand and was named Iatiku which meant "bringing to life." Tsichtinako then told her to name her sister, but it took a long time. Finally Tsichtinako noticed that the other had more in her basket, so Tsichtinako told Iatiku to name her thus, and Iatiku called her Nautsiti which meant "more of everything in the basket."[6]

They now prayed to the Sun as they had been taught by Tsichtinako, and sang the creation song. Their eyes hurt for they were not accustomed to the strong light. For the first time they asked Tsichtinako why they were on earth and why they were created. Tsichtinako replied, "I did not make you. Your father, Uchtsiti made you, and it is he who has made the world, the sun which you have seen, the sky, and many other things which you will see. But Uchtsiti says the world is not yet completed, not yet satisfactory, as he wants it. This is the reason he has made you. You will rule and bring to life the rest of the things he has given you in the baskets." The sisters then asked how they themselves had come into being. Tsichtinako answered saying, "Uchtsiti first made the world. He threw a clot of his own blood into space and by his power it grew and grew until it became the earth. Then Uchtsiti planted you in this and by it you were nourished as you developed. Now that you have emerged from within the earth, you will have to provide nourishment for yourselves. I will instruct you in this." They then asked where their father lived and Tsichtinako replied, "You will never see your father, he lives four skies above,[7] and has made you to live in this world. He has made you in the image of himself." So they asked why Tsichtinako did not become visible to them, but Tsichtinako replied, "I don't know how to live like a human being. I have been asked by Uchtsiti to look after you and to teach you. I will always guide you." And they asked again how they were to live, whether they could go down once more under the ground, for they were afraid of the winds and rains and their eyes were hurt by the light. Tsichtinako replied that Uchtsiti would take care of that and would furnish them means to keep warm and change the atmosphere so that they would get used to it.

At the end of the first day, when it became dark they were much frightened, for they had not understood that the sun would set and thought that Tsichtinako had betrayed them. "Tsichtinako! Tsichtinako! You told us we were to come into the light," they cried, "why, then, is it dark?" So Tsichtinako explained, "This is the way it will always be. The sun will go down and the next day come up anew in the east. When it is dark you are to rest and sleep as you slept when all was dark." So they were satisfied and slept. They rose to meet the sun, praying to it as they had been told, and were happy when it came up again, for they were warm and their faith in Tsichtinako was restored.

NOTES

1. All Keresan pueblo origin myths that have been collected so far begin in the same general way and follow essentially the same pattern: In the beginning the people were in the interior of the earth; there were two women, sisters; the people emerge from an opening in the north, migrate southward, etc.

2. Boas (1928, pt. 1, pp. 221, 222, 228; pt. 2, pp. 10, 11) reports a spirit at Laguna known as Ts'ɩts'te'i·'na·'k'o, "Thought-Woman." Gunn (1917, p. 89) speaks of Sitchtchenako, who is "creator of all." At Sia we find Sûs'sɨstinnako, who is also a creator, and is said to be a spider (Stevenson, 1894, pp. 26–27). A spirit name Tsi'tyostin:nako is reported from Santa Ana (White, ms.).

3. Diacritical marks will be noted only in the first use of a term or in terms quoted from published sources.

4. From kut'tsiti, crammed full (in the basket); the implication being "nothing lacking."

5. At Santa Ana the cicada is called tsi:k'ă. In the Santa Ana origin myth the badger and the cicada assist in preparing for the emergence as they do here (White, ms.).

6. This is the only instance of translations of these names thus far reported. In many

Keresan origin myths Ï'ts'tsʸ'it'i and Nau'ts'itʸ'i are sisters. At Laguna, according to Boas (1928, pt. 1, p. 221), I'ts'ts'itʸ'i has been transformed into a man, "the father of the Whites." He attributes this change to Catholic influence.

7. This may be another instance of adaptation of a Catholic idea to Indian form. Iatik, the great mother-deity of the Keres, lives in the interior of the earth, "four worlds down."

BIBLIOGRAPHY
Boas, Franz
1928.   Keresan texts. Publ. Amer. Ethnol. Soc., vol. 8, pts. 1 and 2.
Gunn, John M.
1917.   Schat-Chen; history, traditions and narratives of the Queres Indians of Laguna and Acoma. Albuquerque.
Stevenson, Matilda Coxe
1894.   The Sia. 11th Ann. Rep. Bur. Ethnol., 1889–1890, pp. 3–157.
White, Leslie A.
MS. The Pueblo of Santa Ana.

11. Navajo Emergence Myth

In characterizing some thirty or more versions of "Navajo Views of Their Origin," Sam D. Gill (1983:502) starts his account: "The origin story begins with a description of a journey of emergence upward through a subterranean domain of unaccounted origin. This domain amounts to worlds described as either platters or hemispheres, numbering variously from 2 to 14, stacked one on top of another. These worlds are identified by number and distinguishing color as well as by the events that transpire on them." In the Hastin Tlo'tsi hee version below, the deepest or first world is black, the second blue, the third yellow, the fourth white, and the fifth, the present world, "changeable." The narrator also refers to the underworlds as "the Four Dark Worlds" and adds that "some medicine men tell us that there are two worlds above us, the first is the World of the Spirits of Living Things, the second is the Place of Melting into One."

Gill (1983:502) notes: "In the beginning, the underworlds are inhabited by insect (usually ant) or animal peoples. There may also be a number of special figures like First Man, First Woman, and Coyote." All these are in the version below.

In his valuable commentary on this text, Gary Witherspoon (1977: 57–58) points out "several significant points," including: "The essential elements from which life forms evolved were four kinds of clouds or gases, differentiated by their color. In the Navajo version the verb stem does not specify that these four elements were clouds but only indicates that they were in a gaseous state. Where the white gas and the black gas conjoined, the first form of life appeared and contained within itself the male principle and was called First Man. Likewise, the yellow and blue gases conjoined, and another form of life came into being, containing within itself the female principle, and was called First Woman. It was from these primordial unions that the earth surface people and other creatures of the fifth world eventually evolved. Although the text refers to the original beings of the first world as mist people, my intellectual friends have always maintained that they were *nilch'i dine'é* 'air people', who evolved in the air where water was undergoing vaporization and were transparent except for their color." This first world is called "first language," and "illustrates how significant the Navajos feel that language was in both the biological and cultural evolution of man; and language, it should be remembered, is made possible by the projection of symbols into the air, both in its crude form found in the first world and in its very sophisticated form found in the present fifth world."

In her preface, written in Santa Fe, New Mexico, in December 1953, Aileen O'Bryan (1956:vii) tells how the following version was performed.

Sandoval, Hastin Tlo'tsi hee (Old Man Buffalo Grass), was the first of the four chiefs of the Navaho People. I had known him for years. In late November 1928, he came to the Mesa Verde National Park, where I was then living, for the purpose of having me record all that he knew about his people.

"You look at me," he said, "and you see only an ugly old man, but within I am filled with great beauty. I sit as on a mountaintop and I look into the future. I see my people and your people living together. In time to come my people will have forgotten their early way of life unless they learn it from white men's books. So you must write down all that I will tell you; and you must have it made into a book that coming generations may know this truth."

This I promised to do. I have recorded it without interpolation, and presented it, in so far as is possible, in the old man's words.

Sam Ahkeah, Sandoval's nephew, now head of the Navaho

Council at Window Rock, as well as First Chief of his people, was the interpreter, as Sandoval spoke only the Athapascan tongue.

Sandoval told us that medicine men know the chants and the ceremonies in detail, but these stories are the origins from which the ceremonies were developed; also, that some medicine men divide the different periods into 12 worlds, whereas the older version holds to 4 darks worlds and the present or changeable world.

During the 17 days of his stay with us on this occasion, he spent the greater part of each day narrating the legends and checking them for correction. He would often stop and chant a short prayer, and sprinkle the manuscript, Sam, and myself with corn pollen.

He believed the Mesa Verde to be the center of the old cultures, and he said that it was fitting that the stories should be reborn, written down, in "the Place of the Ancients."

Sandoval died the following January.

In 1928 Aileen O'Bryan was married to then Mesa Verde National Park director, anthropologist Jesse L. Nusbaum. A native of Las Vegas, New Mexico, O'Bryan (1889–?) had been educated at the Sorbonne, where she first married a musician, Alfred Baehrens. She had published a book, *Zuni Indian Tales* (G. P. Putnam's Sons) in 1926. Presumably, O'Bryan's later experience working to prepare the state guidebook for the New Mexico Federal Writers' Project in the late 1930s also influenced her editing and transcription of the myth.

The texts below (O'Bryan 1956:1–4, 11–12) are part of a section entitled "The Creation or Age of Beginning." O'Bryan's footnotes have been transcribed as endnotes and are followed by appropriate references from her bibliography.

THE FIRST WORLD

These stories were told to Sandoval, Hastin Tlo'tsi hee, by his grand-mother, Esdzan Hosh kige. Her ancestor was Esdzan at a', the medicine woman who had the Calendar Stone in her keeping. Here are the stories of the Four Worlds that· had no sun, and of the Fifth, the world we live in, which some call the Changeable World.

The First World, Ni'hodilqil,[1] was black as wool. It had four corners, and over these appeared four clouds. These four clouds contained within themselves the elements of the First World. They were in color, black, white, blue, and yellow.

The Black Cloud represented the Female Being or Substance. For as a child sleeps when being nursed, so life slept in the darkness of the Female Being. The White Cloud represented the Male Being or Substance. He was the Dawn, the Light-Which-Awakens, of the First World.

In the East, at the place where the Black Cloud and the White Cloud met, First Man, Atse'hastqin,[2] was formed; and with him was formed the white corn, perfect in shape, with kernels covering the whole ear. Dohonot i'ni is the name of this first seed corn,[3] and it is also the name of the place where the Black Cloud and the White Cloud met.

The First World was small in size, a floating island in mist or water. On it there grew one tree, a pine tree, which was later brought to the present world for firewood.

Man was not, however, in his present form. The conception was of a male and a female being who were to become man and woman. The creatures of the First World are thought of as the Mist People; they had no definite form, but were to change to men, beasts, birds, and reptiles of this world.[4]

Now on the western side of the First World, in a place that later was to become the Land of Sunset, there appeared the Blue Cloud, and opposite it there appeared the Yellow Cloud. Where they came together First Woman was formed, and with her the yellow corn. This ear of corn was also perfect. With First Woman there came the white shell and the turquoise and the yucca.[5]

First Man stood on the eastern side of the First World. He represented the Dawn and was the Life Giver. First Woman stood opposite in the West. She represented Darkness and Death.

First Man burned a crystal for a fire. The crystal belonged to the male and was the symbol of the mind and of clear seeing. When First Man burned it, it was the mind's awakening. First Woman burned her turquoise for a fire. They saw each other's lights in the distance. When the Black Cloud and the White Cloud rose higher in the sky First Man set out to find the turquoise light. He went twice without success, and again a third time; then he broke a forked branch from his tree, and, looking through the fork, he marked the place where the light burned. And the fourth time he walked to it and found smoke coming from a home.

"Here is the home I could not find," First Man said.

First Woman answered: "Oh, it is you. I saw you walking around and I wondered why you did not come."

Again the same thing happened when the Blue Cloud and the Yellow Cloud rose higher in the sky. First Woman saw a light and she went out to find it. Three times she was unsuccessful, but the fourth time she saw the smoke and she found the home of First Man.

"I wondered what this thing could be," she said.

"I saw you walking and I wondered why you did not come to me," First Man answered.

First Woman saw that First Man had a crystal for fire, and she saw that it was stronger than her turquoise fire. And as she was thinking, First Man spoke to her. "Why do you not come with your fire and we will live together." The woman agreed to this. So instead of the man going to the woman, as is the custom now, the woman went to the man.

About this time there came another person, the Great-Coyote-Who-Was-Formed-in-the-Water,[6] and he was in the form of a male being. He told the two that he had been hatched from an egg. He knew all that was under the water and all that was in the skies. First Man placed this person ahead of himself in all things. The three began to plan what was to come to pass; and while they were thus occupied another being came to them. He also had the form of a man, but he wore a hairy coat, lined with white fur, that fell to his knees and was belted in at the waist. His name was Atse'hashke', First Angry or Coyote.[7] He said to the three: "You believe that you were the first persons. You are mistaken. I was living when you were formed."

Then four beings came together. They were yellow in color and were called the tsts'na or wasp people. They knew the secret of shooting evil and could harm others. They were very powerful.

This made eight people.

Four more beings came. They were small in size and wore red shirts and had little black eyes. They were the naazo'zi or spider ants. They knew how to sting, and were a great people.

After these came a whole crowd of beings. Dark colored they were, with thick lips and dark, protruding eyes. They were the wolazhi'ni nlchu nigi, meaning that which emits an odor.[8]

And after the wasps and the different ant people there came the beetles, dragonflies, bat people, the Spider Man and Woman, and the Salt Man and Woman,[9] and others that rightfully had no definite form but were among those people who peopled the First World.[10] And this world, being small in

size, became crowded, and the people quarreled and fought among themselves, and in all ways made living very unhappy. . . .

THE FIFTH WORLD

First Man was not satisfied with the Fourth World. It was a small, barren
land; and the great water had soaked the earth and made the sowing of
seeds impossible. He planted the big Female Reed and it grew up to the
vaulted roof of this Fourth World. First Man sent the newcomer, the
badger, up inside the reed, but before he reached the upper world water
began to drip, so he returned and said that he was frightened.

At this time there came another strange being. First Man asked him
where he had been formed, and he told him that he had come from the
Earth itself. This was the locust.[40] He said that it was now his turn to do
something, and he offered to climb up the reed.

The locust made a headband of a little reed, and on his forehead he
crossed two arrows. These arrows were dressed with yellow tail feathers.
With this sacred headdress and the help of all the Holy Beings the locust
climbed up to the Fifth World. He dug his way through the reed as he digs
in the earth now. He then pushed through mud until he came to water.
When he emerged he saw a black water bird[41] swimming toward him. He
had arrows[42] crossed on the back of his head and big eyes.

The bird said: "What are you doing here? This is not your country."
And continuing, he told the locust that unless he could make magic he
would not allow him to remain.

The black water bird drew an arrow from back of his head, and
shoving it into his mouth drew it out his nether extremity. He inserted it
underneath his body and drew it out of his mouth.

"That is nothing," said the locust. He took the arrows from his
headband and pulled them both ways through his body, between his shell
and his heart. The bird believed that the locust possessed great medicine,
and he swam away to the East, taking the water with him.

Then came the blue water bird from the South, and the yellow water
bird from the West, and the white water bird from the North, and everything happened as before. The locust performed the magic with his arrows;
and when the last water bird had gone he found himself sitting on land.

The locust returned to the lower world and told the people that the
beings above had strong medicine, and that he had had great difficulty
getting the best of them.

Now two dark clouds and two white clouds rose, and this meant that two nights and two days had passed, for there was still no sun. First Man again sent the badger to the upper world, and he returned covered with mud, terrible mud. First Man gathered chips of turquoise which he offered to the five Chiefs of the Winds who[43] lived in the uppermost world of all. They were pleased with the gift, and they sent down the winds and dried the Fifth World.

First Man and his people saw four dark clouds and four white clouds pass, and then they sent the badger up the reed. This time when the badger returned he said that he had come out on solid earth. So First Man and First Woman led the people to the Fifth World, which some call the Many Colored Earth and some the Changeable earth. They emerged through a lake surrounded by four mountains. The water bubbles in this lake when anyone goes near.[44]

NOTES

1. Informant's note: Five names were given to this First World in its relation to First Man. It was called Dark Earth, Ni'hodliqil; Red Earth, Ni'haichi; One Speech, Sada hat lui; Floating Land, Ni'ta na elth; and One Tree, De east'da eith.

   Matthews (1897, p. 65): The First World was red. Franciscan Fathers (1912, p. 140): ni, the world or earth; ni' hodiqil, the dark or lowest of the underworlds; (p. 111) lai, one, or first. Franciscan Fathers (1910, p. 81): sad, a word, a language; Sad lai, First Speech.

2. Franciscan Fathers (1912, p. 93): Aste'hastqin, First Man.

3. Informant's note: Where much corn is raised one or two ears are found perfect. These are always kept for seed corn.

   Franciscan Fathers (1912, p. 85): do honot'i ni, the name of a full ear, or seed corn.

4. Informant's note: The Navaho people have always believed in evolution.

5. Informant's note: Five names were given also to the First World in its relation to First Woman: White Bead Standing, Yoigal'na ziha; Turquoise Standing, Doit l'zhi na ziha; White Bead Floating Place, Yolgai'dana eith gai; Turquoise Floating Place, Dolt l'zhi na eith gai; and Yucca Standing, Tasas y ah gai. Yucca represents cleanliness and things ceremonial.

   Franciscan Fathers (1912, p. 181): Tsa'zi ntqe'li, *Yucca baccata*, wide leaf yucca or Spanish bayonet. The roots of this species furnish a rich lather; the plant is frequently referred to as tqalawhush, soap.

6. Informant's note: The Great Coyote who was formed in the water, Mai tqo y eith chili. Franciscan Fathers (1912, p. 117): ma'itso, wolf (big roamer); and ma'ists o'si, coyote (slender roamer).

7. Informant's note: Some medicine men claim that witchcraft came with First Man and First Woman, others insist that devil conception or witchcraft originated with the Coyote called First Angry.

Franciscan Fathers (1912, pp. 140, 175, 351).

8. Informant's note: No English name given this insect. Ants cause trouble, as also do wasps and other insects, if their homes are harmed.

Franciscan Fathers (1910, p. 346): Much evil, disease and bodily injury is due also to secret agents of evil, in consequence of which the belief . . . shooting of evil (sting) is widely spread.

9. Informant's note: Beetle, ntlsa'go; Dragonfly, tqanil ai'; Bat people, ja aba'ni; Spider Man, nashjei hastqin; Spider Woman, nashjei esdza; Salt Man, ashi hastqin; Salt Woman, ashi esdza.

10. Matthews (1897, p. 65); Stevenson (1891, pp. 275–285); Alexander (1916, vol. 10, ch. 8, p. 159); Franciscan Fathers (1910, pp. 346–349); Klah-Wheelwright (1942, pp. 30–41); Haile and Wheelwright (1949, pp. 3–5).

. . .

40. Informant's note: The name of the locust was not given.

Franciscan Fathers (1912, p. 123): locust, nahacha'gi. This also means grasshopper, cicada.

41. Informant's note: The water birds were grebes.

42. Recorder's note: The arrows crossed on the back of the bird's head. See both Navaho and Zuni Arrow Ceremony.

43. The First Chief, Nichi ntla'le, the Left Course Wind: the Second Chief, Nichi lichi, the Red Wind; the Third Chief, Nichi shada ji na'laghail, the Wind Turning from the Sun; the Fourth Chief, Nichi qa'hashchi, the Wind with Many Points; the Fifth Chief, Nichi che do et siedee, the Wind with the Fiery Temper.

44. Informant's note: The place of emergence is said to be near Pagosa Springs, Colo. The white people have put a wire fence around our Sacred Lake.

Matthews (1897, p. 135): place of emergence. Franciscan Fathers (1910, pp. 347–354): The First or Dark World: ants, beetles, dragonflies, locusts, bats, frogs. The Second or Blue World: blue heron, swallow people. They lived in rough, lumpy houses with the entrance in a hole in the top of the roof or in caves. The Third or Yellow World: grasshoppers, etc. The Fourth or Larger World was of All Colors: four snow-covered mountains; the Pueblo People; corn, pumpkins.

Parsons (1933, pp. 611–631); Cushing (1923, p. 164).

BIBLIOGRAPHY

Alexander, Hartley Burr.

1916. North American. *In* "The Mythology of All Races," L. H. Gray, editor, vol. 10, 325 pp. Boston.

Cushing, Frank Hamilton.

1923. Origin myth from Oraibi. Journ. Amer. Folk-Lore, vol. 36, pp. 163–170.

Franciscan Fathers.

1910. An ethnologic dictionary of the Navaho language. 536 pp. Saint Michaels, Ariz.

1912. A vocabulary of the Navaho language. . . . 2 vols. Saint Michaels, Ariz.

Haile, Berard, Father, and Wheelwright, Mary Cabot.

1949. Emergence myth, according to the Hanelthnayhe or upward-reaching rite.

Mus. Navajo Ceremonial Art, Navajo Religion Ser., vol. 3. Santa Fe, N. Mex.

Klah, Hasteen, and Wheelwright, Mary Cabot.
1942.   Navajo creation myth, the story of the emergence. Mus. Navajo Ceremonial Art, Navajo Religion Ser., vol. 1. Santa Fe, N. Mex.

Matthews, Washington.
1897.   Navaho legends. Collected and translated . . . Mem. Amer. Folk-Lore Soc., vol. 5. Boston and New York.

Parsons, Elsie Clews.
1933.   Some Aztec and Pueblo parallels. Amer. Anthrop., n.s., vol. 35, pp. 611–631.

Stevenson, James.
1891.   Ceremonial of Jasjelti Dailjis and mythical sand painting of the Navajo Indians. 8th Ann. Rep. Bur. [Amer.] Ethnol., 1886–87, pp. 229–285.

12. Chukchee Procreation and Creation Myth

A myth from the Chukchee of northeastern Siberia leaves, according to Alan Dundes (1962:1040), "no doubt of the connection between pregnancy envy and anal creation." He also uses the text (1986:363) to bolster his contention "that flood myths are an example of males seeking to imitate female creativity." Citing Donald Tuzin's New Guinea study of Arapesh water symbolism (1977:220): "Anyone witnessing a childbirth cannot fail to notice that the event is accompanied by a forcible discharge of an impressive volume of water," Dundes maintains: "But in male-produced myths, the male must use whatever means he has to create a flood. As the female flood seemingly emerges from her genital area, so it makes (psycho)logical sense for the male flood to come from his genital area. So here we have a rationale for a urinal flood."

In the Chukchee myth, Raven, known as Ku'urkɪl, counters his wife's effortless, transformative gestation and parturition of male twins with a strained, nonmetamorphic defecation and urination of the world and its waters. Refused help by benevolent beings, Raven is attended by male midwives who cannot themselves multiply. Later, as *Deus faber* woodworker, he can only craft males; Spider Woman alone can create females within her body. Finally, Raven must teach the friction-generated men and the spider-procreated women how to copulate and multiply properly.

Waldemar Bogoras (Vladimir Germanovich Bogoraz, 1865–1936) collected the narrative from Aᵍ'ttin·qeu, a Maritime Chukchee man, at Mariinsky Post, on the Pacific Coast of the Chukchee Peninsula, in

October 1900. He recorded other versions during fieldwork in 1900 and 1901 and claims (1910:151) that "variations . . . , with several different episodes, are to be met with everywhere among the Chukchee." He suggests that "some notion of the Flood [which] is also present . . . was probably borrowed from the Russian."

Bogoras (1910:3) says: "The attempt has been made to render the texts as accurately as possible, but it has been found necessary to omit in the translations many of the conjunctions and interjections which are quite numerous in Chukchee and which often appear in extended groups." The following narrative appears in a section called "Creation Tales," which in Chukchee are literally translated "new-creation-limits-tidings." The first version of "Raven-Tale" (Bogoras 1910:151–54), it is one of the few entitled by the Chukchee. Bogoras's footnote is in brackets.

Raven and his wife live together, —the first one, not created by any one, Raven, the one self-created. The ground upon which they live is quite small, corresponding to their wants, sufficient for their place of abode. Moreover, there are no people on it, nor is there any other living creature, nothing at all,—no reindeer, no walrus, no whale, no seal, no fish, not a single living being. The woman says, "Ku'urkıl." —"What?" —"But we shall feel dull, being quite alone. This is an unpleasant sort of life. Better go and try to create the earth!" —"I cannot, truly!" —"Indeed, you can!" —"I assure you, I cannot!" —"Oh, well! since you cannot create the earth, then I, at least, shall try to create a 'spleen-companion.'" —"Well, we shall see!" said Raven.

"I will go to sleep," said his wife. "I shall not sleep," said Ku'urkıl. "I shall keep watch over you. I shall look and see how you are going to be." — "All right!" She lay down and was asleep. Ku'urkıl is not asleep. He keeps watch, and looks on. Nothing! she is as before. His wife, of course, had the body of a raven, just like himself. He looked from the other side: the same as before. He looked from the front, and there her feet had ten human fingers, moving slowly. "Oh, my!" He stretches out his own feet, —the same raven's talons. "Oh," says he, "I cannot change my body!" Then he looks on again, and his wife's body is already white and without feathers, like ours. "Oh, my!" He tries to change his own body, but how can he do so? Although he chafes it, and pulls at the feathers, how can he do such a thing? The same raven's body and raven's feathers! Again he looks at his wife. Her abdomen has enlarged. In her sleep she creates without any effort. He is frightened, and turns his face away. He is afraid to look any more. He says, "Let me remain thus, not looking on!" After a little while he wants to look again, and cannot abstain any longer. Then he looked again, and, lo! there are already three of them. His wife was delivered in a moment. She brought forth male twins. Then only did she awake from her sleep. All three have bodies like ours, only Raven has the same raven's body. The children laugh at Raven, and ask the mother, "Mamma, what is that?" —"It is the father." —"Oh, the father! Indeed! Ha, ha, ha!" They come nearer, push him with their feet. He flies off, crying, "Qa, qa!" They laugh again. "What is that?" —"The father." —"Ha, ha, ha! the father!" They laugh all the time. The mother says, "O children! you are still foolish. You must speak only when you are asked to. It is better for us, the full-grown ones, to speak here. You must laugh only when you are permitted to. You have to listen and obey." They obeyed and stopped laughing.

Raven said, "There, you have created men! Now I shall go and try to create the earth. If I do not come back, you may say, 'He has been drowned in the water, let him stay there!' I am going to make an attempt." He flew away. First he visited all the benevolent Beings (va′ɪrgɪt), and asked them for advice, but nobody gave it. He asked the Dawn, —no advice. He asked Sunset, Evening, Mid-day, Zenith, —no answer and no advice. At last he came to the place where sky and ground come together. There, in a hollow, where the sky and the ground join, he saw a tent. It seemed full of men. They were making a great noise. He peeped in though a hole burnt by a spark, and saw a large number of naked backs. He jumped away, frightened, ran aside, and stood there trembling. In his fear he forgot all his pride in his recent intentions.

One naked one goes out. "Oh! it seemed that we heard some one passing by, but where is he!" —"No, it is I," came an answer from one side. "Oh, how wonderful! Who are you?" —"Indeed, I am going to become a creator. I am Ku′urkɪl, the self-created one." —"Oh, is that so?" "And who are you?" —"We have been created from the dust resulting from the friction of the sky meeting the ground. We are going to multiply and to become the first seed of all the peoples upon the earth. But there is no earth. Could not somebody create the earth for us?" —"Oh, I will try!" Raven and the man who spoke flew off together. Raven flies and defecates. Every piece of excrement falls upon water, grows quickly, and becomes land. Every piece of excrement becomes land, —the continent and islands, plenty of land. "Well," says Raven, "Look on, and say, is this not enough?" —"Not yet," answers his companion. "Still not sufficient. Also there is no fresh water; and the land is too even. Mountains there are none." —"Oh," says Raven, "shall I try again?" He began to pass water. Where one drop falls, it becomes a lake; where a jet falls, it becomes a river. After that he began to defecate a very hard substance. Large pieces of that excrement became mountains, smaller pieces became hills. The whole earth became as it is now.

Then he asks, "Well, how is it now?" The other one looked. "It seems still not enough. Perhaps it would have been sufficient if there had not been so much water. Now some day the water shall increase and submerge the whole land, even the mountain-tops will not be visible."

Oh, Raven, the good fellow, flew farther on. He strains himself to the utmost, creates ground, exhausts himself, and creates water for the rivers and lakes. "Well, now, look down! Is this not enough?" —"Perhaps it is enough. If a flood comes, at least the mountain-tops will remain above water. Yes, it is enough! Still, what shall we feed upon?"

Oh, Raven, the good fellow, flew off, found some trees, many of them, of various kinds, —birch, pine, poplar, aspen, willow, stone-pine, oak. He took his hatchet and began to chop. He threw the chips into the water, and they were carried off by the water to the sea. When he hewed pine, and threw the chips into the water, they became mere walrus; when he hewed oak, the chips became seals. From the stone-pine the chips became polar bears; from small creeping black birch, however, the chips became large whales. Then also the chips from all the other trees became fish, crabs, worms, every kind of beings living in the sea; then, moreover, wild reindeer, foxes, bears, and all the game of the land. He created them all, and then he said, "Now you have food! hm!" His children, moreover, became men, and they separated and went in various directions. They made houses, hunted game, procured plenty of food, became people. Nevertheless they were all males only. Women there were none, and the people could not multiply. Raven began to think, "What is to be done?" A small Spider-Woman (Ku'rgu-ñe'ut) is descending from above on a very slender thread. "Who are you?" —"I am a Spider-Woman!" —"Oh, for what are you coming here?" —"Well, I thought, 'How will the people live, being only males, without females?' Therefore I am coming here." —"But you are too small." —"That is nothing. Look here!" Her abdomen enlarged, she became pregnant, and then gave birth to four daughters. They grew fast and became women. "Now, you shall see!"

A man came, —that one who was flying around with Raven. He saw them, and said, "What beings are these, so like myself and at the same time quite different? Oh, I should like to have one of them for a companion! We have separated, and live singly. This is uncomfortable. I am dull, being alone. I want to take one of these for a companion." —"But perhaps it will starve!" —"Why should it starve? I have plenty of food. We are hunters, all of us. No, I will have it fed abundantly. It shall not know hunger at all."

He took away one woman. The next day Raven went to visit them, made a hole in the tent-cover, and peeped through. "Oh," says he, "they are sleeping separately in opposite corners of the sleeping-room! Oh, that is bad! How can they multiply?"

He called softly, "Halloo!" —"Halloo!" The man awoke and answered him. "Come out here! I shall enter." He entered. The woman lay quite naked. He drew nearer. He inhaled the odor [instead of kissing] of her arm. His sharp beak pricked her. "Oh, oh, oh!" —"Be silent! We shall be heard." He pushed her legs apart and copulated with her. Then he repeated it again. The other one was standing outside. He felt cold, and said, "It seems to me that you are mocking me." —"Now, come in! You shall know it too. This is the way for you to multiply." The other one entered. The woman said, "It is a good thing. I should like to repeat it once more." The man answered, "I do not know how." —"Oh, draw nearer!" He says, "Oh, wonderful!" — "Do this way, and thus and thus." They copulated.

Therefore girls understand earlier than boys how to copulate. In this manner human kind multiplied.

13. Midwifery: A Netsilik Eskimo Delivery

The Netsilik Eskimo woman Nâlungiaq was about forty-five years old when Danish anthropologist Knud Rasmussen (1879–1933) lived with her and her husband Inũtuk between April and early November 1923. A native of Greenland, Rasmussen grew up "speaking the Eskimo language as my native tongue," began ethnographic work among the Eskimos in 1902, and in 1910 established "a station for trading and for study in North Greenland, and to it I gave the name of 'Thule,' because it was the most northerly post in the world,—literally, the Ultima Thule." From it he launched various expeditions to study the Eskimo. He stayed with Nâlungiaq and Inũtuk during the fifth expedition, organized "to attack the great primary problem of the origin of the Eskimo race" from Greenland to the Pacific and officially entitled "The Fifth Thule Expedition,—Danish Ethnographical Expedition to Arctic North America, 1921–24" (Rasmussen 1927:vi–viii).

According to a summer 1923 census Rasmussen (1931:84, 86) made of the isolated "little handful of people calling themselves Netsilingmut (the Seal Eskimos)," twenty-two men and fifteen women lived "at

Kuggup pa (i.e. on the ice outside the mouth of Murchison River [between the Gulf of Boothia and McClintock Channel, near King William Island, in the Northwest Territories of Canada])." Among the seven households was one comprising "ino·tuk (the one who is too short), his wife na·luni·aq (the infant) and their sons hatlАre· (?) and norquat (that used for hitting the eye)." Nâlungiaq herself had delivered two stillborn sons and a son and a daughter who were then still living (Rasmussen 1931:141; photos of Nâlungiaq: facing 377, 408; of Inūtuk: facing 377; of daughter: facing 182).

Rasmussen (1931:258–59) describes Netsilik childbirth in the beginning of his seventh chapter, "Precepts and Taboo."

A woman must never be confined in the ordinary dwelling house or tent. As soon as she begins to feel the birth pangs a very small temporary snow hut must be built for her or, in summer, a tiny tent. This is called ЕRnivik. There she must remain four or five days, the period in which she is considered to be unclean in the sight of game and men and therefore must submit to the most strict taboo.

As soon as these first days are over she is removed to an ordinary, better built snow hut or to a spacious tent, where she must likewise remain isolated from her husband and family. This house is called the kinЕrsЕrvik. The meaning of the word is somewhat vague. It may be translated by: the place where one places something unclean and dirty in water to be softened and cleaned. The woman living in it is called kinЕrsЕrtoq.

She brings her child into the world while on her knees and alone, without help. If it is winter, she allows the child to glide down into a small hollow in the snow on the platform itself. No skin lining is placed in the hollow for the child, which falls straight into the snow.

The woman's husband must never stay in the ЕRnivik. Sometimes her mother or some elderly woman may be in the ЕRnivik while the birth is proceeding, but never for the purpose of actually assisting, for no one must touch the woman. Should anyone do so they must submit to the same strict taboo as the mother of the child. For she is a dangerous tЕqinАrtoq, an unclean one. Such great care is taken that her taboo is observed because she not only exposes herself to danger but the whole village too, and especially all men who hunt.

There must be no skin or sleeping rugs in the ЕRnivik while the woman is being confined, as they would all be infected and therefore unusable later, for it is believed that children give off an unclean and dangerous vapour at the moment they are born.

If a woman has difficulty in delivery, a shaman may be summoned; in return for payment in the form of some article of great value—the value being in proportion to the worth of the wife in the eyes of her husband—the shaman must summon his helping spirits to assist the woman; for it is always thought that it is some evil spirit that wants to delay the birth. As a rule the shaman is content to merely qilavɔq. The payment he receives usually consists of a gun, a kayak, an ulo, a dog or some similar precious object.

Naming is also an important ceremony during the birth itself, and in fact it is with this in view that an elderly woman is sometimes allowed to be present: for she names all the dead people she can think of who may want to take up residence in the new person. . . .

Sometimes, when the confinement nevertheless proceeds slowly, a more direct method is resorted to than merely conjuring up spirits; a seal thong is tied round the waist of the woman above the foetus, and they then try to encourage the birth by pulling on it.

Particular attention must be paid to the after-birth. If it will not come normally, one who is especially skilled in magic must say an Erinalio·t. As soon as the after-birth has come it is buried in the snow of the snow platform below where the woman sits, for it must remain in the house as long as the woman herself is isolated. Only when she is allowed to return to her house and husband is it taken out, and then it must be placed somewhere on the ice or on land where there are no footprints.

Nâlungiaq also participated in another "delivery," this one attended by ethnographer/"shaman" Rasmussen, who begins his fourth chapter, "Religion and Views of Life," with the following account (1931: 206–9) of the woman's own mythology, which here includes creation by the word, couvade, and emergence, as well as the performance context for this cross-sexual midwifery of creation myths.

*"We believe that people can live
a life apart from real life."*

Nâlungiaq.

It was a most difficult matter to obtain a coherent account of the beliefs of the Netsilingmiut. They never think of reasoning with themselves about them, but simply react to what some event or other may force upon their notice. And they have traditional rules of life to follow for any unusual situation. As a consequence, our talks on religious subjects were always split up on account of all the questions I had to put in order to learn anything at all. This applies to both men and women.

However, an evening came when Nâlungiaq suddenly, and quite without any solicitation on my part, began to tell me everything about the very things in their lives that she knew I took such a passionate interest in. The whole thing started so casually. A sunset revived memories of her childhood, and, once her recollections began to stream over her, she became chatty and, without fear of interrupting her, I was then able to interject various questions, with the result that all unconsciously she gave me a connected account of the views they hold of life. I admit that this had scarcely been possible if an intimate knowledge of her temperament had not enabled me to put my questions in the right way, psychologically. While she talked I could make no notes, for then she would quickly have discovered my intention and her free, almost pert delivery would have stiffened. Therefore it has been necessary to reconstruct our conversation as well as I could immediately after it took place.

For half a year Nâlungiaq and her husband Inûtuk had been my housemates and all that we had gone through in the time we lived together had made them most trustful towards me. I suppose Nâlungiaq was about forty-five years old. Her life had not been entirely the usual one. In her young days she had been very pretty, and clever into the bargain, and consequently an unusually courted woman. Her present marriage was her third. Her first husband, Pualrina, had been murdered out of jealousy by her second husband Pujatoq, who in his turn had been killed by her present husband Inûtuk with the same motive. For a time Inûtuk had first been husband number two, for then Nâlungiaq had always had two husbands, but he had finally made up his mind to be her one and only. And indeed since then she had been content with only the one.

She turned out to be extremely well versed in all the traditions of her tribe. Yet she was no outstanding teller of folk tales, for as yet she had too lively a mind to occupy herself with spiritual entertainment. But once in the mood, her words came easily and naturally, and all the mystic things that concerned her not one jot in the ordinary run of things would suddenly seize her and make her eloquent. In this respect her narration gives a good idea of what a slender foundation Eskimo belief requires.

It is said that it is so, and therefore it is so.

The same credulity is extended to the folk tales; and Nâlungiaq had an excellent opportunity to show how in many respects their religion is entirely based upon the tales. For all that is described in them did really happen once, when everything in the world was different to what it is now. Thus these tales are both their real history and the source of all their religious ideas.

BELIEFS AND VIEWS OF LIFE.

Nâlungiaq speaks:

"I am just an ordinary woman, knowing nothing from myself. I have never been ill and seldom dream. So I have never seen visions. When I sometimes go up country to gather fuel I am only happy in feeling the heat of the sun, and many are the memories that rush over me from the parts I see again and where I have wandered ever since I was a little girl. I experience nothing but that when I am alone, I have to be content to listen when others tell. So all that I know I have from an old uncle, Unarâluk the shaman. His helping spirits were his dead father and mother, the sun, a dog, and a sea scorpion. These spirits enabled him to know everything about what was on the earth and under the earth, in the sea and in the sky.

"But what you have asked me about, and what I am going to tell you about, is something that is known to every child, every child that has been hushed to sleep with a story by its mother. Children are full of life, they never want to sleep. Only a song or monotonous words can make them quieten down so that at last they fall asleep. That is why mothers and grandmothers always put little children to sleep with tales. It is from them we all have our knowledge, for children never forget. And now my story begins:

The hare makes the earth to be light.

In the very first times there was no light on earth. Everything was in darkness, the lands could not be seen, the animals could not be seen. And still, both people and animals lived on the earth, but there was no difference between them. They lived promiscuously: A person could become an animal, and an animal could become a human being. There were wolves, bears, and foxes but as soon as they turned into humans they were all the same. They may have had different habits, but all spoke the same tongue, lived in the same kind of house, and spoke and hunted in the same way.

That is the way they lived here on earth in the very earliest times, times that no one can understand now. That was the time when magic words were made. A word spoken by chance would suddenly become powerful, and what people wanted to happen could happen, and nobody could explain how it was.

From those times, when everybody lived promiscuously, when some-

times they were people and other times animals, and there was no difference, a talk between a fox and a hare has been remembered:

"tʌ·q-tʌ·q-tʌ·q!: Darkness, darkness, darkness," said the fox; it liked
the dark when it was going out to steal from the caches of the humans.

"uɓlɔq-uɓlɔq-uɓlɔq: Day, day, day," said the hare; it wanted the light
of day so that it could find a place to feed.

And suddenly it became as the hare wished it to be; its words were the
most powerful. Day came and replaced night, and when night had gone day
came again. And light and dark took turns with each other.

The earliest times on earth.

In those times there were no animals in the sea; people knew nothing
of burning blubber in their lamps. At that time newly drifted snow would
burn, the soft, chalky-white heaps of very fine snow that gather in the
shelter of the firm, hard drifts, the kind we call apɛrlɔrqʌ·q. No one needed
blubber then. This story, people say, is a distant memory of the very first
days, the time when the first people lived on earth and had to travel far from
one place to another. For they had to go far to get something to live on. But
at that time they knew magic words that could move houses; they just sat
still in their houses and said magic words, and then they rushed through the
air with house and everything in it, to a new settlement where they started
at once to break up the ground to find food.

That was the time people lived in darkness, in the very first beginning,
when there were only men and no women. Then forests grew on the
bottom of the sea, and it is the remains of those forests that to this day tear
themselves loose when the storms blow, so that we find driftwood on our
shores.

And in the first days there was no ice on the sea. The sea was always
open and never closed by ice. Sea ice came from an angry old witch-woman.
She wanted to kill a man. The man was Kivioq, the one you know from the
story. The witch was angry because she had not got him to eat, and when he
got down into his kayak she threw her ulo at him; it made "ducks and
drakes" over the water and turned to ice. That is where the sea ice came
from, the story says.

Woman was made by man. It is an old, old story, difficult to understand. They say that the world collapsed, the earth was destroyed, that great
showers of rain flooded the land. All the animals died, and there were only
two men left. They lived together. They married, as there was nobody else,
and at last one of them became with child. They were great shamans, and

when the one was going to bear a child they made his penis over again so that he became a woman, and she had a child. They say it is from that shaman that woman came.

That is all I know about people. I have also heard that the earth was here before the people, and that the very first people came out of the ground from tussocks. But these are hard things to understand, difficult things to talk about, all this about where something began, where the first people came from. It is sufficient for us to see that they are here and that we ourselves are here.

And there are those who say that the children of the earth were not the first people, and that they only came to make people many. Women who happened to be out wandering found them sprawling in the tussocks and took them and nursed them; in that way people became numerous.

And the earth. Here we only know our land. It has become habitable because the Tunrit first came here and found out how to hunt the game. But we know that our land is not the whole earth, for the earth has no boundaries, and he who wants to can keep on travelling on and on. The earth was as it is at the time when our people began to remember.

14. Midwifery: A Maya Birth Event

Doña Juana, a Maya Indian widow of about sixty, serves as *partera empirica,* or native lay midwife, in a rural Yucatan, Mexico, community. She provides prenatal and postpartum care, both of which include massage, and supervises the birth event. Her mother was a midwife. According to Brigitte Jordan (1980:13–14), "It is not clear how much of her knowledge was handed down by her mother. Doña Juana says that she learned how to attend women in childbirth from a Doctor Sanchez who gave her a course and provided her with her equipment. Doctor Sanchez is long dead but he functions for her somewhat like a mythical ancestor who can be called upon to legitimize what she does . . . (cf. McClain 1975 for similar claims by indigenous midwives). . . . Doña Juana also attended a course for midwives given by a governmental agency in Mexico City some years ago. She is generally considered the best midwife in town and is on mutually respectful terms with the chief of the town's small hospital."

Medical anthropologist Brigitte Jordan and her collaborator Nancy Fuller met Doña Juana when they first began fieldwork in 1972. During their second stay in 1974, Jordan "became proficient in the formal role of 'helper,' " and thereafter: "During births, Nancy Fuller, seated on a low stool or in an extra hammock to one side of the birth area, would run the tape recorder and take detailed notes regarding the setting, the interaction of people, and the movement of objects. Brigitte Jordan would sit next to the midwife, relieving her from time to time, and taking turns with the other helpers in assisting the woman in labor. Sometimes she would mention details that were not visible to the notetaker in a low and casual voice." They claim that birth participants soon became accustomed to the tape recorder (and after 1976 the videorecording equipment) and that "at births we always did a play-back of the baby's first cry for the family, and that re-experiencing was invariably an occasion for relief, laughter, and satisfied remarks about the successful outcome of the birth" (Jordan 1980:15, 16).

The godsiblingship and gossip of midwifery is evident in the Maya birth event. It takes place in an area set apart from the public space where ordinary family and community life continues as usual. "A blanket may be hung from the rafters, screening the woman's ham-mock from the rest of the room, or the entire house may be held off limits to all but the midwife and the expectant mother's 'helpers' " (Jordan 1980:18). *All* in attendance are participants, "who are engaged in the common task of producing an event and making it visible as the business at hand, as doing a birth. . . . That, in the particular events on which this investigation is based, participants sometimes come from different cultural backgrounds or speak different native languages, that some of them have never been present at a birth before, that others had themselves borne children or witnessed births in various kinds of settings or had managed births as professional specialists, should not provide motivation for questioning a person's full participant status (there are no 'apprentice participants') but should rather be seen as providing the resources for producing the birth as a locally sensible event" (Jordan 1980:9).

The following account of "The Birth Event" was written jointly by Brigitte Jordan and Nancy Fuller, whose notes are numbered as in the original text and reprinted after the selection (Jordan 1980:22–29, 91–93). The larger study was part of Jordan's doctoral research (University of California at Irvine, Ph.D., 1975), which included the crosscultural comparison of birthing systems in Yucatan, Holland, Sweden, and the United States. This part of the work also had an applied dimension, and "the videotapes of traditional births and perinatal practices in

Yucatan proved invaluable for educating physicians and nurses in the local ways of doing birth . . . [and] also served as excellent and culturally appropriate discussion stimulators for the midwives themselves" (Jordan 1980:iii).

When a messenger (most likely the woman's husband) arrives at Doña Juana's compound to tell her that one of her *enfermeras*[8] is in labor, she picks up her case of equipment and walks to the woman's house to assess the situation. In her case she carries a sheet of clear plastic to place under the expectant mother; a heavy clear plastic apron which she will put on during the later stages of the birth event; a gown, cap, and face mask acquired during the Mexico City course; a metal box with a syringe and two needles; and two stainless steel bowls, one for washing her hands and the other for "sterilizing" the scissors used to cut the umbilical cord. Also stored in the case are a rubber squeeze bulb for extracting mucus from the newborn's nose and mouth, eye drops, a glass jar of cotton balls, a metal soap box, a small hand brush, and a closed glass jar in which the waxed thread for tying the umbilical cord is soaking in alcohol.

When she arrives at the woman's house, there is a friendly exchange of greetings with the family. Doña Juana asks about the frequency and strength of contractions and has the mother lie down for a massage, during which she feels for the baby's head to see if it is engaged or still moving freely. If she decides that it isn't time yet, she may return home or go on to visit another *enfermera* in the neighborhood, stopping on the way to make a purchase or to chat with someone she knows. If it appears, on the other hand, that labor has begun in earnest, she arranges her case on a chair, washes her hands, and settles down on a wooden chair in front of the woman's hammock. . . .

If, initially, it appears that progress will be slow, we may have time to go home briefly, or we may have a meal of frijoles and tortillas with the family in their cooking hut, possibly joined by the expectant mother. The woman may get up every once in a while during early labor, not only to eat, but also to urinate, or to feed a child, or to take care of pressing household business. Most of this time, however, she rests in her hammock, chatting with her helpers. While the contractions are weak and far apart, the talk which fills the long hours of waiting has to do with everyday concerns, rambling perhaps from divorce to the high cost of living, or from community affairs (like the upcoming fiesta) to building a new house for the growing family ("There are ten hammocks in here at night, we're packed like sardines").

When contractions become stronger and more frequent, talk begins to focus on the business at hand. Stories are told about such things as miscarriages, abortions, the horrors of hospital deliveries, and, especially, the birth experiences of the women present.[10] Some instruction will take place at this time if this is a first child for the couple. In that case neither husband nor wife will know much about labor and birth since men are allowed only at the birth of their own children and women can attend other women only after they have given birth themselves. Typically, explanations and directions are given *during* labor, in the situation where they are relevant, rather than hypothetically.

Doña Juana, at some time during the early stages, will explain the progress of labor; she will describe how contractions will come closer and closer together, how the woman will finally have to push, and how the baby will be born. Whenever possible, her teaching is demonstrative rather than merely verbal. She will, for example, lay a chair on its side, sit down on its legs and hold on to an imaginary rope, demonstrating birthing position; or she will get into a hammock and show the couple how the woman should throw her arms around her husband's neck for support. She not only *tells* the woman that she will have to push with all her strength but *shows* her, and so realistic is her performance that invariably somebody will make a joke about Doña Juana being the one who is having the baby. Often the woman's attendants join in, too, each one of them demonstrating her own favorite method of giving birth. Doña Juana says that every woman must *buscar la forma* (find her own style). For her, the midwife's function is to assist with whatever method the woman comes to find best.

In Yucatan, the woman's husband is expected to be present during labor and birth. They say he should see "how a woman suffers." This rule is quite strong and explicit and we heard of cases where the husband's absence was blamed for the stillbirth of a child. In addition to the husband, the woman's mother should also be there, and mothers sometimes travel considerable distances for daughters' births. If the labor turns out to be long and difficult, other women will appear: mothers-in-law, godmothers, sisters, sisters-in-law, close friends and neighbors. This group of "helpers" substantially contributes to a successful birth. Jointly and by turns they give the woman the mental and physical support she needs. They encourage her, urge her on, scold her when necessary, always letting her know that she is not alone, that the business of getting this baby born will get done. It will take time and work and pain, to be sure, but "we have all done this before and this baby will arrive, soon now."

During this time, the expectant mother is lying crosswise in her matrimonial hammock, her feet propped in its folds, her legs slightly drawn up and comfortably apart.[11] She is wearing a short, loose *huipil* and is covered from the waist down with a cloth. Doña Juana has arranged the sheet of heavy plastic under her. If the woman complains of backache, a short length of cloth-covered board or a folded blanket or perhaps a rolled up pair of stiff jeans may be tucked under her back.

As the mother begins to feel some discomfort, one helper takes her or his place on a chair behind the hammock, at the woman's head. (In what follows we will use the feminine personal pronoun because, especially during a difficult birth where there is much turn-taking this position is most frequently taken by women. It should be noted, however, that the husband also takes an active part.) With her arms under the woman's shoulders, the "head helper" supports her hammock-encased body on her lap. Its flexible compactness permits her to pull up at the height of a contraction, raising her almost to a sitting position. As the contraction fades away, she gently lets her down again to rest. Meanwhile, the midwife and another helper are occupied with rubbing her abdomen, her back, her legs, and pressing down on the thighs whenever a contraction comes on.

From time to time the midwife feels the vaginal area with a cloth over her hand, checking for indications of progress, such as blood stained mucus, or, especially, the breaking of the water. When the water does break, the fluid collects in the plastic sheet and is sponged up with dry cloths. Doña Juana never ruptures the membranes, and it is frequently the case that before the baby's head is born, the fluid-filled membranes appear externally as a bubble about the size of a tennis ball. This bubble fills up at the height of a contraction and recedes as the contraction subsides, thereby cushioning the baby's head and allowing a gradual stretching of the perineal area. Tearing, in fact, is very rare; none occurred with the women in whose births we participated though several were having their first baby. Doña Juana says she would call a doctor in such a case but she gave none of her usual case histories.

When it looks like the time of birth is approaching, the midwife asks for boiling water which one of the women brings from the cooking hut. Doña Juana then takes out her stainless steel bowls and pours the hot water over the tongs, rubber bulb, and scissors, to "sterilize" them. She also puts on her gown, cap, and mask, as well as the plastic apron which she has swabbed with alcohol.

If the midwife and helpers become concerned about a drawn-out, desultory labor, the question of whether a problem exists and what should be done about it is discussed at length. If it appears after a while that some stimulation is needed, a common remedy is to give the woman a raw egg to swallow. Her mother gets it from the cooking hut, breaks it, and the woman swallows it with a shudder of revulsion. She immediately throws it up again and the retching usually brings on powerful contractions.

If this method fails, injections will be considered in due course. They consist of the same vitamin B complex that the midwife has prescribed prenatally. She says that injections should be unnecessary during labor if the mother had taken her vitamins earlier. In fact, she would rather not use them at all. If, however, the labor continues to be difficult and no progress is apparent, consensus will edge towards administering the injection. We saw her give an injection twice, and in those cases contractions did, in fact increase, and the baby was born a short time later.

When a woman needs encouragement to renew her flagging strength, helpers respond to her with what we came to call "birth talk." At the onset of a contraction, casual conversation stops. A rising chorus of helpers' voices pours out an insistent rhythmic stream of words whose intensity matches the strength and length of the contraction. *"Ence, ence, mama,"* *"jala, jala, jala,"* *"tuuchila,"* *"ko'osh, ko'osh"*[12] come from all sides of the hammock. With the "head helper" behind her, not only holding her but physically matching every contraction, the laboring woman is surrounded by intense urging in the touch, sound and sight of those close to her.

Midwife and helpers watch for signs that the birth is imminent, such as trembling legs, blood-spotting, and increased pain and bulging in the vaginal area. At this time the mother may move from her hammock to sit on the legs of a wooden chair which has been laid on its side. A rag may be used to cushion its hard legs. The woman's feet are planted firmly on the dirt floor and when a contraction comes on, she can pull herself up by holding on to a rope or a *rebozo* (the traditional Maya shawl) slung from a roof beam. As before, she is supported by the arms and body of the "head helper" who sits behind her on another chair. Doña Juana, of course, occupies the low stool in front of her; on each side there is probably a helper keeping up a steady flow of encouraging talk and squatting down with each contraction to steady and brace the mother's feet and knees in order to enable her to push more effectively. The house is filled with sounds of "birth talk," rising and ebbing with the exertions of mother and helpers.

The baby may be born while the woman is on the chair or in the hammock, and we saw one baby born while the mother was sitting on her husband's lap. Although Doña Juana will defer to the woman's wishes in this as well as other respects, she prefers the chair which, she says, makes for an easier delivery. For us, the chair had the added advantage that, squatting on the floor with the midwife, we could see the baby emerge. In a hammock birth, visual access is restricted, and Doña Juana gauges progress by what she feels with her cloth-covered hand ("the baby is at the door") rather than by what she sees.

While the mother is on the chair, the physical involvement of the "head helper" is at its most intense. Most of the weight of the woman giving birth rests on her. When a contraction comes on and the woman begins to push, there is a matching exertion visible in the helper's body. She covers the laboring woman's nose and mouth with her hand, holds her own breath, and pushes herself until they both run out of air. She may also, for the length of a contraction, press her mouth on top of the woman's head and blow into her hair to give her strength and endurance, or stuff a cloth (or the woman's own hair) into her mouth to force her to push.

The intense physical and emotional involvement of the helpers in a long and demanding birth is mirrored in the strain on their faces and in the signs of fatigue that become evident in them as well as the mother. It is our impression that compared to western practices where the pushing is delayed until the cervix is completely dilated, Maya women are encouraged to push too early. Consequently, in a long labor a woman may endure more pain and exhaustion than necessary.[13]

As everybody becomes weary, the helpers' involvement may take the form of scolding in response to the expectant mother's crying or lack of strength. At one of the births we attended, the woman in labor irritably pushed her mother's hand from her nose and mouth, wailing and twisting her head. For an instant, her mother's hand lifted as though she were about to swat an exasperating child. Immediately, the other helpers moved in. One came up on one side and firmly clamped down on the woman's nose and mouth; another approached on the other side so that she found herself completely surrounded by helpers, urging, encouraging, scolding—demanding that she get back to work.

Having a baby is clearly regarded as work. The mother is always expected to do her part, though she may become discouraged, even somewhat panicked. Although the expectation is of a quick, fairly easy birth, at least some pain is recognized as a normal part of bearing a child. It figures in the birth stories which have been told all along, preparing the mother for what is to come. Consequently, she receives little sympathy if she complains. In a typical instance, late in one of the births we attended, the mother cried wearily that she just couldn't push any more; surely she was going to die. Her mother and the midwife laughed, "Listen, if you're not lazy, how could you possibly die? You push hard enough and the baby will come out all right." A woman's pain and weariness are more likely to be seen as indications of progress, since the baby, it is said, is born "in the very center of the pain."[14]

As the baby's head begins to show (sometimes still covered by the unbroken membranes), the excitement in the little house reaches a new pitch. Birth talk is continuous, punctuated only by the midwife's progress reports. She will tell the mother that the baby is "at the door" and ready to be born, she might make an estimate of how many more pushes will be required, and she might report that she can see the baby's beautiful hair. Finally, the head crowns, and with the next contraction or two the product of all this effort emerges in a splash of blood-tinged fluid. Sometimes the baby begins to cry as soon as the head is born, but in any case Doña Juana is quick to suction the mucus from its nose and mouth to facilitate breathing.

If the mother is on the chair, Doña Juana slides the baby into her plastic-aproned lap. If she is in the hammock, she lays the newborn on its mother's abdomen. The mother, smiling and weary, looks down at her baby. Doña Juana announces whether it is a boy or a girl. After a few minutes when the cord has stopped pulsating, the midwife ties and cuts it, though usually she waits for the afterbirth to pass first. When it comes, she shows it to the mother and to anybody else who is interested. She examines it to make sure it is complete before letting it slide into a bowl in which most of the blood and waste has been caught. If the placenta is not expelled in about half an hour, or is expelled incomplete, she says she would send for a doctor to remove it manually.[15]

When the afterbirth has passed, the midwife sponges the mother off with hot water and packs cotton between her legs. The women help her into a fresh *huipil,* she settles back in her hammock in a lengthwise position, and is covered with a blanket.

Then Doña Juana turns her attention back to the newborn, who has probably been lying in her lap or in the arms of its grandmother. . . .

Neither the midwife nor the family treat this newborn as particularly delicate. It is handled matter-of-factly and familiarly as Doña Juana gives it the routine bath. When holding it, neither she nor the helpers make any special attempt to support its head. After swaddling it, someone may give it a little water to drink from a gourd dipper before handing it to its mother. . . .

The mood now in the small house is light with talk and laughter. The baby having been pronounced normal, dressed, and laid in its mother's arms, attention returns once again to more ordinary concerns. . . . A meal appears for the midwife and helpers if the time of day is appropriate; during its course, Doña Juana and the women may discuss the mother's first meal. . . . As we prepare to leave, the mother thanks us for assisting (*"muchas gracias para ayudarme"*) and after a last satisfied look at the baby, we say our good-byes. The payment of Doña Juana's fee (usually 100 to 120 pesos) will be negotiated with the family, depending on their circumstances.

NOTES

8. We want to caution here against interpreting the use of the term *enferma* (which comes from *enfermedad,* illness) as indicative of an illness view of pregnancy among Maya Indian women. Experientially this is simply not the case. The parallel with illness may lie, rather, in the fact that both illness and birth are stressful times associated with ritual and physical danger. A detailed investigation of local notions of the relationship between pregnancy and illness remains for further research.

. . .

10. The question of the nature of the topics which are admissible during the birth process deserves detailed investigation since such talk can be expected to convey not only pragmatic and instructional information but is also likely to contain symbolic messages regarding the meaning of the event. It seems to be the case that one topic that needs to be dealt with in such situations is the topic of death. In our own culture, it is hardly ever permitted to be addressed directly. It nevertheless crops up regularly, in more or less disguised form. For example, in one homebirth recently videotaped by Brigitte Jordan in Michigan, the topic shifts from encyclopedia salesmen to a funny rendering of a promotional scheme for cemetery plots. The story ends with the intended buyer replying to the salesman's pitch: "Oh, that's just great. You'll never believe this, but my uncle just died today." This introduced (and dismissed in the participants' joint laughter) the question of "dying today" which is a pervasive unspoken issue in every birth.

11. Yucatecan matrimonial hammocks stretch out to a width of eight feet and are designed to sleep several people. The term "matrimonial" is, actually, a misnomer. Husband and wife do not normally sleep together at night, rather, each has one or more small children in the hammock with her or him.

12. Ence (Maya): make it go down.
    Jala (Spanish): haul, like a laboring woman pulling down on a rope or someone hauling on the rope to draw water from the well.
    Tuuchila (Maya): meaning unclear, possibly derived from Maya tuch, navel.
    Ko'osh (Maya): come on, let's go.

13. Doña Juana had some notion of this. Though she would sometimes ask directly what we thought of this or that practice when we were sitting around talking at

her compound, she never asked for our opinion during a birth. We had, however, worked out an ingenious way of communicating about such things. At crucial times, for example when the question of pushing was about to come up, Doña Juana would nod off. Sitting next to her in front of the woman, Brigitte Jordan would take that not only as a signal to take over with the usual pressing down on the woman's thighs with each contraction, but also as an occasion to explain to the woman that she should not push until she absolutely had to, etc. After a while Doña Juana would wake up refreshed and take over again. That her sleep was not deep enough to prevent her from hearing was evident at the next birth where she used almost the exact same words to explain to the woman that she should not push until she felt she absolutely had to, etc. We used the same device to communicate about relaxing, breathing techniques, and massage. Clearly, this method had the advantage that, as her assistant, Brigitte Jordan could be seen as speaking *for* her if she chose to validate what she said. At the same time, the midwife retained the option to simply ignore her opinion without the necessity to argue the merits of the case. This way of communicating allowed us to offer what we knew and thought might be beneficial for alleviating some of the suffering while leaving to her the decision of what to do with the information conveyed.

14. *En el centro del dolor.* The Spanish word *dolor* means both "pain" and "contraction" (cf. German *Webe*).

15. This "half hour" is not to be taken literally. Until a couple of years ago, Doña Juana did not even have a watch. It is rather more likely that the need for a doctor would become clear after "too much time" had passed. In the case of serious postpartum hemorrhage the doctor would probably be too late anyway.

Notes

Chapter One

1. According to Emile Grillot de Givry (1973:211–12, fig. 177), "From these two substances of the Godhead [cloud, Word] proceeds the third—the Dove of the Holy Ghost, which flies like a breath of Ruach Elohim, the Spirit of God, and circles the Cosmos. . . . The famous Oxford doctor [Fludd] considers God as the principle of Light beyond which there is only nothingness—that is to say, non-existence—represented by Darkness. The Breath of God draws a luminous circular furrow in the Darkness, agreeably to the theory accepted by Plato, Cicero, and the Alexandrians, who pronounced that spirits must move in circles. Thus the universe contains an evil part, of which God is not the author, bathed in the Divine light with which it is in constant antagonism. The theory propounded thus accords with the fact of the presence of evil in the world and with the incorruptible purity of God, which the theologians by no means wished to see disputed."
2. All subsequent references to the Bible are to the Revised Standard Version unless otherwise indicated.
3. For the full text of Cushing's first eight outlines, see Appendix 9.
4. Freund (1975), Maclagen (1977), Farmer (1979), Weigle and Johnson (1980), and Sanday (1981:239–44) suggest categories similar to those in studies and collections mentioned in this section. Other collections, for example, Sproul (1979) and Van Over (1980), are simply organized geographically. Texts in O'Brien and Major (1982) are presented chronologically, as are those in Brandon (1963), whose subtitles are nontheless suggestive: "Egypt: Cosmogonies of Rival Sanctuaries," "Mesopotamia: Creation by Divine Intention or by Conquest of Primordial Chaos," "Israel: Cosmogony as a Factor in an Ethnic Religion," "Greece: The Intuitions of Mythology and of a Dawning Rationalism," and "Iran: Dualism in Creation."
5. See Appendix 1 for an Ekoi metanarrative folktale about "How All Stories and All History Came Among Men"—as the multi-colored, woven "story-children" of Mouse, who "had no children of her own."
6. On the place of this article and others in "Karen Horney's Critique of Freud," see Westkott (1986:53–65).
7. "God as Architect of the Universe" is reproduced in Watts (1968:39), who notes it shows God in the form of Christ or Logos; in Maclagen (1977:38); and in color in Leeming (1976:152), where it precedes an anthology of texts entitled "In the Beginning: Creation Myths Around the World" (153–84). See Appendix 2 for a Yuki creation myth with a *Deus faber* who measures the deep with a rope.

Chapter Two

1. On his translation from the Keres language of his native Laguna Pueblo, Anthony F. Purley (1974:31) notes: "Some confusion is sometimes created concern-

ing Tse che nako and Old Spider Woman, especially in secular discussions. Keres holy men hesitate to mention Tse che nako's name, especially for purely secular discussions; Thought Woman's name is reserved for use only in sacred ceremonies. In secular discussions and teachings, Tse che nako is often symbolically referred to as Old Spider Woman or Spider Woman. As to the reason for the change, it is believed that only the holy men have the answer." See also Appendix 10.

2. Von Franz here refers to the *Rig-Veda*. For a pertinent discussion of East Indian speculations about the Cosmic Spider and Primordial Weaver, see Eliade (1979: 170–77). It is part of a chapter entitled "Ropes and Puppets," in which Eliade explores various (primarily Eastern and Old World) cosmological and shamanic images and beliefs to illuminate the "rope-trick" of Indian fakirs.

   On mythographer and theogonist Pherecydes of Syros, who lived in the sixth century B.C., and his prose book about the gods, see Kirk and Raven (1964:48–72), West (1971:28–75), Doria and Lenowitz (1976:95–98). Three deities always exist: Chronos (Time), who produces fire, wind, and water by his own seed; Zas (Zeus); and Chthonie, who subsequently receives the name Ge (Earth) during her wedding to Zas, who presents her with a cloth he has woven with designs of Ge and Ogenos (apparently Oceanos). According to West (1971:11), Chthonie "was established by his time as an epithet of gods who are in the earth. 'Earth,' then, for Pherecydes, is 'Goddess-inside-the-earth' plus a robe, and the robe . . . has the visible outer surface of the earth depicted on it." In discussing Zas's weaving, West (1971:54) notes: "In sixth-century Greece weaving probably was an 'unmasculine task'; but what is more important here is the idea of the world as a work of art done by a god. In Greek, Chronos sometimes appears as a craftsman. . . . Empedocles (31 B 23) likens the formation of things from elements under the influence of Love and Strife to the mixing of colours by painters, and elsewhere he represents Aphrodite as a moulder of animal forms. Outside Greece we meet the idea of cosmic *weaving*, in particular by the sun, who is given the name 'Weaver' in the Talmud. An Estonian ballad represents the sky with its bright hues of sunrise and sunset as a mantle woven by Tara, the Old Father, the Old and Wise."

3. The Pima Indians tell a similar creation myth about Earth Doctor, who at first "made a gray spider, which he commanded to spin a web around the unconnected edges of earth and sky" (Russell 1975:207).

4. See Appendix 3 for the full text of the Uitoto cosmogony.

5. John M. Gunn is a mother's uncle of Paula Gunn Allen (1986:282–83).

6. Susan J. Scarberry (1983:100) emphasizes this harmonious relationship in "Grandmother Spider's Lifeline": "Grandmother Spider's web is an expression of her love for the people, binding various life forms together. . . . Whereas most non-Indian cultures have stressed the negative power of Spider Woman, seeing the web as a net or weapon that she uses to entrap unwary men and her loom as a symbol of fate and death, many Indian cultures have stressed her positive life-creating power, recognizing that she uses her power to protect her people." The range of spider imagery is sampled in "Spiders & Spinsters: Myth and Symbol" (Weigle 1982:1–44).

7. See Appendix 4 for Apollodorus's version of Philomela's rape.

Chapter Three

1. See Appendix 5 for the full text of Roland Barthes, "Novels and Children."
2. Carolyn Merchant (1980:11) includes this de Bry engraving, which she entitles "The Female Soul of the World," as an example of how "Renaissance Neoplatonism illustrates the image of the macrocosm enlivened by the female soul. The Neoplatonic alchemist Robert Fludd (1574–1637) pictured the world soul as a woman connected by her right hand to God, represented by the Hebrew tetragrammaton—the four consonants JHVH—transmitted by a golden chain to the terrestrial world below." She notes that the engraving "shows the Western identification of the right hand with masculinity, God the Father, the sun and dominance; the left hand is traditionally associated with the feminine and subordinate moon, earth, and water" (1980:12). See also Economou (1972), Griffin (1978).
3. In Åke Hultkrantz's overview of American Indian tribal religions (1979), for example, only two women are mentioned in passing in the chapter "The Concept of the High God," and no women creators are included in the next chapter, "The World Picture and the Deities of Cosmogonic Myths." Female deities do not figure until the second half of the next chapter, "Gods and Spirits of Nature." Only the Kagaba goddess appears in the fifteen selections anthologized as "Divinities of Primitives (Pre-Literate Societies)" in Mircea Eliade's *From Primitives to Zen* (1974:3–20).
4. According to Richard M. Dorson in "The Eclipse of Solar Mythology" (1965:31), Max Müller advocated finding the "true nature" of the gods by tracing the deities' names back to Sanskrit equivalents: "All the Indo-European peoples belonged to a common Aryan stock; after the migration of the European groups from their Indic homeland, the parent language, and the mythology it related, splintered into various offshoots. A time came when the original meanings of the names of the Vedic gods were forgotten, and survived only in mythical phrases and proverbs of uncertain sense. Stories then developed to explain these phrases. From this 'disease of language' myths were born." Quoting Müller's 1883 *India: What Can It Tell Us? A Course of Lectures Delivered before the University of Cambridge,* Dorson (1965:32) illustrates the result of the former's clearly identifying "similar gods and heroes with etymological proof": "Clearly, mythopoeic man constructed his pantheon around the sun, the dawn, and the sky. How could it be otherwise?, Müller asked, 'What we call the Morning, the ancient Aryans called the Sun or the Dawn. . . . What we call Noon, and Evening, and Night, what we call Spring and Winter, what we call Year, and Time, and Life, and Eternity—all this the ancient Aryans called *Sun*. And yet wise people wonder and say, How curious that the ancient Aryans should have had so many solar myths. Why, every time we say "Good morning," we commit a solar myth. Every poet who sings about "the May driving the Winter from the field again" commits a solar myth. . . . Be not afraid of solar myths.' "
5. Paul Radin's 1924 lecture, "Monotheism among Primitive Peoples," was published in London that year, and parts were incorporated into the eighteenth chapter, "Monotheistic Tendencies," in Part II, "The Higher Aspects of Primitive Thought," of his *Primitive Man as Philosopher* (1927). His somewhat modi-

fied views on the subject were published later as the twelfth chapter, "Monolatry and Monotheism," of his *Primitive Religion* (1937). "On the insistence of friends and colleagues," the 1924 lecture was reprinted in Switzerland in 1954, with a preface summarizing the by then "enormous literature" since his earlier discussion.

6. A major contributor to the discussion of monotheism is the Austrian Jesuit anthropologist, Father Wilhelm P. Schmidt, whose twelve-volume *Der Ursprung der Gottesidee* was published in Münster, 1926–55. Schmidt's, Radin's, and archeologist James Breasted's theories of the origin of high gods are discussed by sociologist Guy E. Swanson in his comparative study of monotheism in thirty-nine societies (1960:55–81). Also see the overview of such theorists as they treat Native American studies in Hultkrantz (1983:39–46).

7. Of the nineteen societies Swanson identifies as displaying "clear evidence" of a high god, only the Iroquois have a female figure, identified as the grandmother of the major creator gods. Among the "11 ambiguous cases" is a clearly female high god: "4. Lepcha—The accounts describe a Creative Mother who, together with her husband, lives under the world. Her children are representatives of the various aspects of reality. Since, among the Lepcha the father is never important in mythology, it is possible that this Creative Mother may be considered the source of reality. The accounts are not clear on this point" (Swanson 1960:69). In her comparative study of thirty-nine creation stories, Peggy Reeves Sanday (1981:241) finds only six with a female creator or ancestress (rather than a sexless creator, couple creators or ancestors, male culture-hero or ancestor, animal creator or ancestor, or supreme being or force) as creative agent: the Shilluk and Tuareg in Africa, the Semang and Lepcha in South Asia, the Copper Eskimo in North America, and the Nambicuara in South America.

8. Hultkrantz (1979:53) does not treat the All-Mother in his chapters on high gods or cosmogonies, but considers the Kagaba deity as an earth goddess or mother goddess who is sometimes in agricultural communities "the all-powerful divinity." He cities a 1951 ethnography by Gerardo Reichel-Dolmatoff on the Kagaba: "Woman is the most elementary expression of fertility and the most exalted deity of culture; she is the Mother, the creator. From her are born mankind, the good black earth, the edible plants, the animals, and all of nature. All these elements are 'Children of the Mother' and are subject to her 'law.' "

9. For the complete historic context of this famous assertion, "among the most quoted of all Native American statements," see Gill (1987:40–68).

10. James A. Teit conducted fieldwork among the Okanagan of British Columbia between 1907 and 1917. According to Ralph Maud (1982:75–76), "Kwelweltaxen (Red-Arm), who told practically all these stories, was a real find. His repertoire is not extensive, but everything he tells has a twinkle to it. For instance, his Origin Myth includes the Garden of Eden and Jesus Christ, but Jesus is something of a failure: 'He taught them no arts, nor wisdom about how to do things, nor did he help to make life easier for them. Neither did he transform or destroy the evil monsters which killed them, nor did he change or arrange the features of the earth in any way.' Coyote was sent down by the Chief to rectify these deficiencies (pp. 81–82)." Gill (1987:57–61) compares the Okanagan and

a Nespelim version as contributing to "the Earth-Woman doctrine" in the Prophet Dance "among tribes throughout the interior plateau area."

    For a similar account of Old-Man's emanatistic creation of the Earth Mother from a woman called Earth, who was in the beginning wife of the Sun, see the Thompson Indian myth also collected by Teit, "The Old-One and the Earth, Sun, and People" (1912:321–22; partially in Long 1963:36; paraphrased and condensed in Eliade 1974:136). See Appendix 6 for another similar Thompson Indian, emanatistic, Earth Mother creation myth.

11. Gill (1987:115–18) discusses Eliade's concept of Mother Earth in the latter's "major works on religion."

12. The Aztec goddess of earth, Coatlicue's origin is recounted in a myth compiled by Spanish missionaries in 1543 but since lost and now available only in a sixteenth-century French translation by André Thévet. John Bierhorst (1976:50) notes of his own English translation of Thévet's version: "Quetzalcoatl and Tezcatlipoca represent the bright and dark aspects of the Creator. The earth herself is the nourisher of life; but she also the burial ground of the dead. One purpose of this myth is to validate the Aztec custom of sacrificing live human hearts."

13. Anthropologist Sherry B. Ortner cities this de Beauvoir quote in her classic article, "Is Female to Male as Nature Is to Culture?" (1974:75). In "Nature, Culture and Gender: A Critique," anthropologist Carol P. MacCormack (1980:17) notes that in formulations such as de Beauvoir's, Ortner's, and Claude Lévi-Strauss's: "The statement that women are doomed by their biology to be natural, not cultural, is of course a mythic statement, and both Ortner and Lévi-Strauss retreat from it. Of course woman cannot be consigned fully to the category of nature, 'for it is perfectly obvious that she is a full-fledged human being endowed with human consciousness just as man is; she is half the human race, without whose cooperation the whole enterprise would collapse' (Ortner 1974:75–6). Or, as expressed by Lévi-Strauss, 'women could never become just a sign and nothing more, since even in a man's world she is still a person, and since insofar as she is defined as a sign she must be recognized as a generator of signs' (1969:496)." See also Rosemary Radford Ruether's discussion of Ortner's article in her "Woman, Body, and Nature: Sexism and the Theology" (1983:72–92).

14. In *A Feminist Dictionary* (1985), Cheris Kramarae and Paula Treichler give no definition for procreate/ion, five for birth, seven for birthing, and one for creation: "Creation of the universe was envisioned by polytheistic religions 'as a process and product of sexual unions between goddesses and gods. . . . The primary divine source of life was presented as a female' (Judith Ochshorn 1981, 1939)" (Kramarae and Treichler 1985:110). They cite one definition for "creative," from Dale Spender, *Women of Ideas and What Men Have Done to Them* (1982). In her introduction Spender (1983:24) maintains: "That women have not been treated as serious intellectual beings is an understanding that is central to my explanation for women's disappearance. . . . Almost all the women in this book . . . have argued that men have taken away women's creativity and intelligence, that they have denied our ability to reason and think, and that they have

supported a division of labour in which mental work is seen as the province of men, and service as the province of women." Spender (1983:28) claims: "We must begin to accept what Berenice Carroll [1981] points out, that the terms *original, innovative, creative, first rank, excellent,* are *political* terms, in that they are terms used by the gatekeepers to exclude women from entry in the 'worthwhile' records of our society. They are unsubstantiated terms used to maintain and justify a male monopoly on intelligence. They are based not on the contribution itself, but on the *sex* of the contributor, and they permit the 'superior' sex to be the producers of 'superior' work."

15. For the development of Christian attitudes toward Genesis 1–3 in the first four centuries, see Pagels (1988). She (1988:xx–xxi) notes: "I have not, by any means, written a history of early Christianity; instead, I am interested in a process of intellectual history—how these ideas of sexuality and moral equality, among others, came about; and I am interested in the hermeneutical process—how Christians read the story of Adam and Eve, and often projected themselves into it, as a way of reflecting upon such matters as sexuality, human freedom, and human nature." For a classic, feminist, hermeneutical perspective on Genesis, see Trible (1976).

Chapter Four

1. On the wind's fertilization, Robert Graves notes Pliny's *Natural History,* iv, 35, and viii, 67, and Homer's *Iliad,* xx, 223. He explains: "In this archaic religious system there were . . . only a universal goddess and her priestesses. . . . Fatherhood was not honoured, conception being attributed to the wind, the eating of beans, or the accidental swallowing of an insect; inheritance was matrilineal and snakes were regarded as incarnations of the dead. Eurynome ('wide wandering') was the goddess's title as the visible moon; her Sumerian name was Iahu ('exalted dove'), a title which later passed to Jehovah as the Creator. It was as a dove that Marduk symbolically sliced her in two at the Babylonian Spring Festival, when he inaugurated the new world order" (1975:28).

2. See the deBry/Fludd engraving in Chapter 1 above for a representation of "Fiat" as a bird enlightening chaos in Genesis 1.

3. Róheim (1954:67–68) has also analyzed the inverse of the bird-soul earth-diver—the shaman's soaring ascent to the heavens. Summing up "the unconscious meaning" of the "whole" of Hungarian-Vogul mythology, he claims, "Manifestly it centers around origin myths of a totemic type, around the shaman's flight to heaven in bird form, around supernatural beings, who represent migrating birds and are projections of the flying shaman. The waterfowl fly south, and return. The path is the quiet Milky Way (the path of birds, of souls, etc.). But something is happening up in the sky that is far from quiet. There is the chase of the pregnant elk (Ostyak), or a doe (Hungarian . . .). There is elopement (Hungarian, Yenisei-Ostyak), battles (Hungarian, Yenisei-Ostyak), and permanent warring of male against female (Yenisei-Ostyak)." Latently, however, "*It is obvious that the nucleus of all these beliefs and myths is the primal scene, or rather a dream of the primal scene.* The quiet path over the sky at

night is violent movement, hunting, fighting, etc. In this dream, the shaman overcomes his anxiety and reacts libidinally to the primal scene—by flying, by an erection. Then by a characteristic mechanism of dreams, a fission takes place—the shaman is there with his guardian spirit, a bird, a god." The shaman thus becomes like the Vogul's triumphant, all-powerful God, World-Surveyor-Man, of whom it is said: "*Up to the present day it is owing to his power that the world continues to exist. . . . When he moves the whole earth moves, that is why we have myths and songs about him.*" Róheim notes "that the primal scene takes place at night. To survey is to see, and to see is projected from the child to the father in the super-ego situation."

4. See Appendix 7 for the Iroquois (Onondaga) text as well as a related Huron one.

5. For a World-Parent creation myth with some similarities to Hesiod, see the Luiseño text in Appendix 8. For a Jungian interpretation of such myths, which concentrates on the Babylonian, see Harding (1965).

6. For a discussion of Hultkrantz's notions of Mother Earth, see Gill (1987:118–28).

7. For an analysis of male parthenogenesis among the Sambia of the New Guinea Highlands, see Herdt (1987:255–94). In the foreword Robert A. LeVine writes: "Dr. Herdt shows us a people who believe that the oral insemination of boys is necessary for them to grow into men, and he describes the cultural beliefs and rituals that encourage homosexual practices for all men before marriage" (p. ix).

8. In Phibionite belief and practice menstrual blood is the women's ritual equivalent of male sperm, according to Epiphanius: "Similarly also with the woman: when she happens to be in the flowing of the blood they gather the blood of menstruation of her uncleanness and eat it together and say: 'This is the blood of Christ'" (trans. Benko 1967, as in Eliade 1976:110). This pro/creative power for menstruating women is also suggested in a Southeast Yuchi Indian creation myth collected by W. O. Tuggle in the late nineteenth century. Various animals have dived for and arranged the land, and both the stars and moon have contributed some light, "but it was still dark" when "T-cho, the Sun, said: 'You are my children, I am your mother, I will make the light. I will shine for you.'

"She went to the east. Suddenly the light spread over all the earth. As she passed over the earth a drop of blood fell from her to the ground, and from this blood and earth sprang the first people, the children of the Sun, the Uchees" (Swanton 1929:84; variants in Speck 1909:105–7).

9. Here Eliade (1976:140) notes: "One must also keep in mind that in the Greek translation of the Old Testament God's *pneuma* hovered over the waters; thus, the *pneuma hagion* was the divine sperm, generator of life; cf. [H.] Leisegang, *La Gnose* [trans. Jean Gouillard, Paris, 1951], p. 134, and esp. his *Pneuma Hagion* (Leipzig, 1922), pp. 71–72, where the Greek medical and philosophical conceptions are also discussed."

10. Erich Neumann (1963:329) sees two "Archetypal Feminine" symbols—"the form of the virgin goddess (lily) with the character of engendering transformation and cure (the caduceus)"—in the Bruyn painting, which he includes as plate 172: "Both symbols recur in a late painting of the Annuciation. Here the angel bears the staff of saving fecundation, which is at the same time a staff of

transformation and healing. But beside Mary stands the vessel that is herself. The body of this vessel bears the host with the name of the divine son, and above it towers the lily of the Cretan virgin goddess. This means that this vessel is the goddess herself bearing the divine sun-child, and Mary—without any conscious intention on the part of the artist—becomes once more the goddess of the beginning. The feminine vessel as vessel of rebirth and higher transformation becomes Sophia and the Holy Ghost."

11. Alan Dundes (1980:184–85, 191–92) cites psychoanalyst Ernest Jones's essay, "A Psycho-analytic Study of the Holy Ghost Concept," in which the latter "argues that the Holy Ghost is a male substitute for the mother figure (1951:360)" and "abundantly illustrates the phallic symbolism of birds with special reference to the dove (1951:322–41). He concludes that it is a phallic organ which expels the fertilizing gas, asserting that he has come across the fantasy in individual psychoanalyses in which a person in childhood 'considered the male organ to be a continuation of the rectum or its contents' (1951:329)."

12. The editor notes: "The following interesting document was given to Col. Gudgeon some years ago, by Tiwai Paraone, of the Maru-tuahu tribes of Hauraki." Translator Hare Hongi says of Io: "This term is here used in a sacred sense. Ordinarily, *io* speaks of a circular hollow centre or tube, from which the solid contents, core or pitch (*ngana*) have been withdrawn. Of this personification *speaking,* it may be urged that it is reminiscent of the biblical creation-myth. That, however, does not necessarily follow. The story of the separation of Rangi ['Space' or 'Sky-father'] and Papa ['Matter' or 'Earth-mother'] is undoubtedly original, and by many versions, Rangi is made therein to *speak* to his children, notably to Tane ['the Sun']. So that this fact of *Io* being made to speak is not singular, or necessarily an imitation" (Hongi 1907:109, 118).

13. See Appendix 9.i for the full text of Cushing's outline.

14. Dennis Tedlock (1979:499) notes, ʔa·wona·wilʔona, 'The One Who Holds the Roads,' can be used as an epithet for either *yatokka tačču,* 'Sun Father,' or *yaʔonakka citta,* 'Moonlight-Giving Mother,' who at Zuni are both considered "the ultimate givers of light and life." He cites Ruth L. Bunzel (1932:486): "This term [a·wona·wi'lona 'the ones who hold our roads'] Mrs. Stevenson erroneously interprets as referring to a bisexual deity; creator and ruler of the universe. The term is never used in this sense, nor was I able to find any trace of such a concept among them. The confusion seems to be due to the fact that the missionaries have hit upon their term as the nearest equivalent to 'God.' The Zunis, accordingly, always translate the term 'God.' When asked if a·wona·wi'lona is man or woman they say, 'Both, of course,' since it refers to a great class of supernaturals."

15. Paul Friedrich (1978:72–103) examines eighteen dimensions of the complex of myth, ritual, and belief about the four Greek queens—Hera, Athena, Artemis, and Aphrodite. He (1978:76) asserts: "Most people have assumed that the term mediating between Athena and the owl is wisdom, but the more likely connection is simply one of locale; as [Martin P.] Nilsson has pointed out, the little owls in question nest in the Acropolis of Athens and the rocky slopes nearby." See also Weigle (1982:77–79). On the dimensions of intelligence and nature

versus culture, Friedrich (1978:90–91) says: "Athena, with her 'masculine' intellect is also the least marked for feminine sexuality; many people—Walter Otti, for example—feel that she basically *is* male, and her physical stance and inevitable helmet do indeed suggest this." Her "*mētis* is mainly . . . a combination of rationality with astuteness, political sagacity, and practical skills. . . . Later her key term becomes *sophia,* in the sense of 'wisdom,' including the philosopher's." Athena is related to culture (versus Artemis, who is related to nature), and her "*mētis* implies arts and crafts (including women's domestic ones), masculine skills, such as shipbuilding and carpentry, and, more generally, all manner of skill, persuasiveness, and courteous or appropriate deceit in conversation or public debate or other types of verbal exchange. This idea of skill in word and deed was one of the most integral values in the civilization of the ancient Greeks, who contrasted themselves with both barbarian people and wild nature by virtue of possessing it."

16. Edmund Leach (1969) stimulated this controversy in "Virgin Birth," the 1966 Henry Myers Lecture at the annual meeting of the Royal Anthropological Institute of Great Britain and Ireland. John A. Saliba, S.J. (1975), presents a useful overview from the theological perspective, a good complement to Delaney's anthropological critique (1986).

Chapter Five

1. Ruth L. Bunzel conducted fieldwork in New Mexico and Arizona Pueblos during the summers of 1924 and 1925. The comment, "Anyone can make a good shape, but you have to use your head in putting on the design" (1972:49), was heard from a number of potters. Bunzel (1972:51) claims: "They all speak of sleepness nights spent in thinking of designs for the pot to be decorated in the morning, of dreams of new patterns which on waking they try and often fail to recapture, and above all, the constant preoccupation with decorative problems even while they are engaged in other kinds of work." She (1972:52) emphasizes: "To say, 'We paint our thoughts,' is common in the villages where designs are clothed with symbolic meaning. But even where symbolism plays no role in decoration, as for instance, among the Acoma and the Hopi, there is nevertheless a strong feeling that each pot is an individual and a significant creation. The condemnation of copying the designs of other women is unanimous."

2. Peter J. Bowler (1971:222) defines various terms connected with seventeenth- and eighteenth-century embryology: "All theories based upon the belief that organisms have been in existence in the form of miniatures since the creation of the world will be called pre-existence theories. . . . The term 'preformation' will be retained only for the belief that the miniature which grows into the full organism is actually formed within the body of the parent."

3. Handy quotes from Tewira Henry, "History and traditions of Tahiti, compiled with notes of J. M. Orsmond, manuscript in preparation for publication by Bernice P. Bishop Museum" (1927:334). He (1927:9) claims the Society Island accounts, like the New Zealand Maori ones, are "a legacy of teachings direct from the mouths of initiated priests"—an example of "the ancient esoteric

teaching in cosmology [which] postulated the pre-existence of a self-created World Soul which evolved the world and the universe out of itself, and called manifest existence out of nothingness by the power of the Word."

4. Carolyn Merchant illustrates and explores many of these themes in a chapter on "Nature as Female" in sixteenth-century Europe, especially sections entitled "The Geocosm: The Earth as a Nurturing Mother" and "Normative Constraints against the Mining of Mother Earth" (1980:20–41).

5. Russell A. Lockhart (1978:4) begins his "Words as Eggs" with an exhortation to re-examine "therapy in words" and not to dismiss it as "just a head trip." He (1978:31) notes that "a fundamental discussion of this image" of the psyche/head is in Onians (1951:93–122). Lockhart's investigations were prompted by a dream and by passages from Gaston Bachelard, *The Poetics of Reverie,* including: "When I was fortunate enough to have a dictionary, I would let myself be enchanted for hours on end by the feminine of words"; and "Words, in our scholarly cultures, have so often been defined, redefined and pigeonholed with so much precision in our dictionaries that they have become instruments for thought. They have lost their power for internal oneirism" (1971:30–31, 35). Lockhart (1978:8–9) discusses Humpty Dumpty as "master of the word," and explores various dictionary definitions, including the egg as female. Wondering "why throwing eggs at someone was such a sign of disdain," he also "realized that the same thing was true of masculine seed, that semen is called 'scum.' . . . And I realized then, too, how much of our language of sexuality, in which the eggs and seeds of life come together, is used for denigration, cursing, and belittling" (Lockhart 1978:28).

6. According to Kurt Seligmann (1971:85), a "colossal amount of writing [was] ascribed to Hermes Trismegistus," little of which is extant. "The Hermetic books were considered by the alchemists as Hermes's bequest to them of the secrets which were veiled in allegories to prevent the precious wisdom from falling into the hands of the profane. Only the wise were able to find their way in this mystical labyrinth. The passage of Hermes most frequently cited, the credo of the adepts, was the inscription found on an emerald tablet 'in the hands of Hermes's mummy, in an obscure pit, where his interred body lay,' situated, according to tradition, in the great pyramid of Gizeh." The so-called *Emerald Tablet* relates to the Maier picture reproduced here: "'Tis true, without falsehood, and most real: that which is above is like that which is below, to perpetrate the miracles of one thing. And as all things have been derived from one, by the thought of one, so all things are born from this thing, by adoption. The sun is its father, the moon is its mother. Wind has carried it in its belly, the earth is its nurse. Here is the father of every perfection in the world. His strength and power are absolute when changed into earth; thou wilt separate the earth from fire, the subtle from the gross, gently and with care. It ascends from earth to heaven, and descends again to earth to receive the power of the superior and the inferior things. By this means, thou wilt have the glory of the world. And because of this, all obscurity will flee from thee. Within this is the power, most powerful of all powers. For it will overcome all subtle things, and penetrate every solid thing. Thus the world was created. From this will be, and

will emerge, admirable adaptations of which the means are here. And for this reason, I am called Hermes Trismegistus, having the three parts of the philosophy of the world. What I have said of the sun's operation is accomplished."

7. The image suggests Caroline Walker Bynum's study of *Jesus as Mother*. She discusses Cistercian authors of the High Middle Ages in whose works "breasts and nurturing are more frequent images than conceiving or giving birth. And where birth and the womb are dominant metaphors, the mother is described as one who conceives and carries the child in her womb, not as one who ejects the child in order to give life. Conceiving and giving birth, like suckling, are thus images primarily of return to, union with, or dependence upon God, not images of Christ's sacrifice or of human alienation. . . . Moreover, other physiological images, such as Guerric's references to the bowels of God or Aelred's to hiding inside Christ, express not merely the compassion or love that God offers man but also the closest possible binding of self to God. As an extreme case of this stress on union, Isaac of Stella goes beyond images of souls drawn into the womb or bowels or side of Christ to develop a theory of the mystical body that claims that Christ himself is not complete until we are all incorporated into him" (Bynum 1982:150).

   A similar, contemporary painting by Ellen Going Jacobs is in the December 1985 issue of *Omni*, accompanying Dick Teresi and Kathleen McAuliffe's article, "Male Pregnancy" (1985), which is heralded: "Can men have babies? Research indicates they can, and volunteers are already lining up." This issue contains a special section entitled "New Birth Technologies" and uses as its cover image a cosmogonic egg painting by New Age artist Ingo Swann. I am grateful to University of New Mexico American Studies graduate student Daniel Moore for calling my attention to this publication.

8. Alice C. Fletcher and Francis La Flesche, a member of the Omaha tribe, call this an "explanation of the teachings of the Pebble society, which may be a paraphrase of a ritual" (1911:570). They include a photograph (567, fig. 125) of the narrator, a "former leader, Waki'dezhi^{n}ga . . . , who is now dead." The literal translation of the I^n'kugthi Athi^n, or Pebble Society, is "They who have the translucent pebble." "Membership was gained by virtue of a dream, or vision, of water or its representative, the pebble, or the water monster, received when fasting. The water monster was said to be a huge creature in animal form that lashed the water with its mighty tail. It was generally spoke of as living in a lake" (1911:565). Fletcher and La Flesche (1911:571) note: "Among the Osage there is a similar myth, on which the elk figures as a helper of mankind to find a place to dwell." They also give the Osage text (p. 63).

9. In *Hamlet's Mill: An Essay on Myth and the Frame of Time,* Giorgio de Santillana and Hertha von Dechend cite the eighteenth-century Charles Dupuis' *L'Origine de tous les cultes,* in which Dupuis claims that myth is the work of science, which science alone will explain. They (1969:2) begin their scientific explication with Amlodhi of Icelandic legend: "Amlodhi was identified, in the crude and vivid imagery of the Norse, by the ownership of a fabled mill which, in his own time, ground out peace and plenty. Later, in decaying times, it ground out salt; and finally, having landed at the bottom of the sea, it is grinding rock and sand,

creating a vast whirlpool, the Maelstrom (i.e., the grinding stream, from the verb *mala*, 'to grind'), which is supposed to be a way to the land of the dead. This imagery stands, as the evidence develops, for an astronomical process, the secular shifting of the sun through the signs of the zodiac which determines world-ages, each numbering thousands of years. Each age brings a World Era, a Twilight of the Gods. Great structures collapse; pillars topple which supported the great fabric; floods and cataclysms herald the shaping of a new world."

10. For the complete text, see Appendix 9.iii.

11. Pregnancy taboos (e.g., in Kitzinger 1980:78–81; Meltzer 1981:73–80, 96–99) express anxieties and active plans about the expected child, the expectant mother, and society at large, and these should be examined in this context.

Chapter Six

1. Artist Judy Chicago (1985:34) calls this statue "an exquisite example" of "the crowning"—along with "creation of the world" and "birth" the three basic images in her needlework and textile arts exhibition. The Birth Project (1980–1985). See also the Aztec "poem to ease birth" addressed to the goddess May-ahuel, a pulque deity with four hundred sons (Vaillant 1966:184, 188). The translation by Anselm Hollo (Rothenberg 1972:50) includes the lines: "on your way on your way / child be on your way to me here / you whom I made new."

2. See Appendix 13 for the full text and Rasmussen's ethnographic account of Netsilik Eskimo childbirth practices.

3. See Appendix 12 for the full text of the Chukchee myth.

4. See Appendix 13 for the full account.

5. In the order of appearance in Martin's text the quotes are from: Jack A. Pritchard, Paul C. MacDonald, and Norman F. Gant, *Williams Obstetrics,* 17th ed. (Norwalk, Connecticut: Appleton-Century-Crofts, 1985), 311; Kieran O'Driscoll and Michael Foley, "Correlation of Decrease in Perinatal Mortality and Increase in Cesarean Section Rates," *Journal of the American College of Obstetricians and Gynecologists* 61, 1 (1983):5; Kenneth R. Niswander, *Obstetrics: Essentials of Clinical Practice,* 2d ed. (Boston: Little, Brown, 1981), 207. Friedman is quoted in Pritchard et al. (1985:314).

6. As part of her chapter entitled "The Creation of New Birth Imagery," Martin quotes from (in order): Nancy Wainer Cohen and Lois J. Estner, *Silent Knife: Cesarean Prevention and Vaginal Birth After Cesarean (VBAC)* (South Hadley, Massachusetts: Bergin and Garvey, 1983), 120–21; and Rahima Baldwin, *Special Delivery: The Complete Guide to Informed Birth* (Millbrae, California: Les Femmes, 1979), 81, 135.

7. Dellenbaugh (1982:46–47) does assert the "biological fact of parthenogenesis" from a reproductive standpoint. The ovum does not need the sperm to reach the full "complement" of forty-six chromosomes, and "all parthenogenetic off-spring should be daughters." She cites Dr. Helen Spurway, a lecturer in the Department of Biometry at London University, who is quoted in *New Statesman and Nation,* November 19, 1955: "Males could only be produced [par-thenogenetically] by a . . . disturbance, by an incomplete restitution of maternal

chromosomes which approximated to the male-producing balance, and they could not have obtained any organizers peculiar to normal males. Therefore males could be expected to be rare and defective [i.e., sterile]. In one at least of the Buddhist theologies the last incarnation before enlightenment is a virgin birth. Therefore it is surprising that Guatama, the Buddha, was a man; it is more surprising that his wife bore him a son. . . . [I] find it difficult to accept that the physiological processes that permitted Guatama to be fertile, would have altered the organizers, or perpetuated the defect, that caused him to develop male."

8. Sumerologist Samuel Noah Kramer maintains that many of the problematic aspects of the Garden of Eden can be illuminated by historical study of its antecedents. Dilmun is the Sumerian paradise, a garden sacred to the goddess Ninhursag, who curses the water-god Enki for eating her eight precious plants. Enki languishes until the fox persuades the goddess to return and heal him. She asks which organ hurts him and then brings to life a healing deity from each afflicted part. Enki's rib is among them, and Nin-ti, "the lady of the rib," was thus created to heal it. In Sumerian, *ti,* or "rib," also means "to make live," and so Nin-ti, "the lady of the rib," by word play also signifies "the lady who makes live." Kramer claims that "it was this, one of the most ancient literary puns, which was carried over and perpetuated in the Biblical paradise story, although here, of course, it loses its validity, since the Hebrew word for 'rib' and that for 'who makes live' have nothing in common." Also associated with the Sumerian myth is "the painless and effortless birth of the goddess after only nine days, instead of nine months of bearing." In one of the extant fragments, the goddess Ninmu takes Enki's seed into her womb for nine days and then gives birth to the goddess Ninkurra "like good, princely cream" (Kramer 1959:145–48).

9. In her analysis of Tiamat, Dellenbaugh (1982:55) draws on Jane Caputi's interpretation of the movie *Jaws*: "Caputi [1978a:78–79; also 1978b] . . . builds on the connections between the sea, the unconscious, and the female. She quotes Jung: 'The sea is the favorite symbol for the unconscious, the mother of all that lives,' and Erich Neumann: 'The Terrible Female is a symbol for the unconscious. And the dark side of the Terrible Mother takes the form of monster.' The message of 'Jaws' is that the 'unconscious,' which is, as Caputi says, 'in essence mysterious, primitive, even wild,' is deadly. ' "Jaws" . . . implants the suggestion that these depths of the mind and of the self are, in fact, deadly. It floods us with the image of a zone inhabited by terrifying creatures where we are out of our element, completely vulnerable, and ultimately subject to destruction. . . . The purpose of fish stories such as "Jaws" is to instill relentless terror, embedding a paralyzing image of an inevitably vanquished female.' 'Jaws' would teach women to be terrified of the depths of our own minds, fearing that if we venture into the oceanic deep we, too, will become vanquished females." Clearly, this contrasts with the earth-diver (Chapter 4).

10. White gives no source for this text, entitled "Emergence and Migration"—the first in the "Myths and Tales" section. See also Appendix 10.

11. See Appendix 9.vi for the full text.

12. On the Red Antway ceremony, which is associated with powerful beings in the undermost world, see Wyman (1973). Also see Appendix 11.

Chapter Seven

1. The Greek relief is the tenth figure in the fourth chapter, "Birth Scenes," of Harold Speert's excellent pictorial resource, *Iconographia Gyniatrica*, "the first attempt to record the history of obstetrics and gynecology primarily through pictures, . . . in broad perspective, extending back to prehistory, topics relating to woman and her role in reproduction, including female anatomy, early midwifery, embryology, scenes of pregnancy and birth, labor and its complications, obstetric instruments, cesarean section, the newborn infant, monsters, nursing, control of contraception, and gynecologic surgery" (1973:vii). Of particular interest to folklorists are the chapters entitled "Monsters and Myths" (14) and "Multiple Pregnancy and Birth" (15).

   The birth scenes in Speert's chapter 4 are "grouped to show (1) births in various ages and cultures, (2) births of Biblical and religious characters, (3) royal births, (4) births in legend, (5) birth as a source of joy and grief, and (6) the puerperium." Speert (1973:79–80) asserts: "In almost all early birth scenes the attendants are depicted as women. Males were usually barred from the birth chamber. Not until the eighteenth century did men begin to achieve recognition as accoucheurs. In most birth scenes the midwife stands, sits, or kneels before the parturient, while one or more additional attendants lend support from behind. In primitive societies the parturient usually assumed one of several positions to enhance her expulsive efforts, which were often augmented by abdominal pressure applied manually by the attendants. After delivery, while the newborn was being bathed and swaddled, food and drink were brought to the mother; but flowers never were to be seen in the parturient's room."

   This picture and reference were found in Chicago (1985:116). In the pictorial credits and sources to Speert (1973:525), the figure (4–10) is identified as by Guido Calzo. Correspondence with Dr. Speert yielded a reference—Docteur Laignel-Lavastine, *Histoire générale de la médecine, de la pharmacie, de l'art dentaire et de l'art vétérinaire* (Paris, 1936), vol. I, p. 374—which was, however, that for figure 4–11 (Speert 1973:84). Other attempts to identify this image, which contrasts so nicely with that of the solitary parturient Tlazolteotl (Chapter 6), have proved fruitless.

2. See Appendix 14 for the full account of this Maya birth event.

3. Francis Huxley presents a good account of "The Sacred" in the first chapter of his *The Way of the Sacred*. In discussing Otto, he (1974:16) notes: "The sacred is by no means single or simple emotion. It is better understood as what grammarians call an oxymoron—a figure of speech that combines contradictory terms, such as *cruel kindness,* or *falsely true.* Oxymorons are useful to straddle the effects caused by the sacred in the mind, to describe which we can use such paradoxical phrases as 'joyful fear,' or 'fascinating terror.' "

4. Meltzer cites Leo Frobenius, *Der Kopf als Schicksal* (Munich: K. Wolff, 1924).

5. A similar distinction between shaman's dreams and women's stories is made by Nâlungiaq (and Knud Rasmussen). See Appendix 13.

6. See Appendix 9.vi for the full text.

7. Ehrenreich and English's 1973 pamphlet is quoted here because its succinct,

vivid narrative is appropriately "myth-like." The two have elaborated their earlier insights in Ehrenreich and English (1979), notably in this context in the second section, "The Rise of the Experts," in which they call "the story of the rise of the psychomedical experts . . . an allegory of science versus superstition: on the one side, the clear-headed, masculine spirit of science; on the other side, a dark morass of female superstition, old wives' tales, rumors preserved as fact . . . [in which] the triumph of science was as inevitable as human progress or natural evolution: the experts triumphed because they were *right*." They claim the conflict "centered on the right to heal," since, "for all but the very rich, healing had traditionally been the prerogative of women," and note that "the women who distinguished themselves as healers were not only midwives caring for other women, but 'general practitioners,' herbalists, and counselors serving men and women alike" (Ehrenreich and English 1979:33–34).

8. On the wisdom of the crone, see, e.g., Walker (1985:41–68).

9. Martin cites (in order): Helen I. Marieskind, "Cesarean Section," *Women and Health* 7, 3–4 (1983):189; Leroy R. Weekes, "Cesarean Section: A Seven-Year Study," *Journal of the American Medical Association* 75, 5 (1983):476; O. Hunter Jones, "Cesarean Section in Present-day Obstetrics," *American Journal of Obstetrics and Gynecology* 126, 5 (1976):521–30; Sandra Blakeslee, "Doctors Debate Surgery's Place in the Maternity Ward," *New York Times,* March 24, 1985; Lester T. Hibbard, quoting Kroener, "Changing Trends in Cesarean Section," *American Journal of Obstetrics and Gynecology* 125, 6 (1976):804.

10. H. R. Ellis Davidson (1964:191, 192, 193) calls "the World Tree, the symbol of universality." It "was renewed continually: thus it became a symbol of the constant regeneration of the universe, and offered to men the means of attaining immortality." It is also associated with "a great gate, called by various names . . . , which cut off the realm of the living from that of the dead. . . . When the dead return to visit the earth, this gate is said to stand open for their passage." Also see Cook (1974).

11. This definition and the one beginning the section "Mouths—Birthing Speech," below, is from Word-Web Two of the *Wickedary*: "In this Word-Web, Journeyers Dis-cover the inhabitants of the Background, observing and participating in their activities and characteristics. The words and phrases of this Web Name the Wild Reality of Hags and Nags, Gorgons and Grimalkins, together with Other Friends and Familiars. This Web can be read as a Guidebook for travelers into the Background. It introduces the reader to the Natives, their world view and customs, describes places of interest, and provides words and phrases necessary for communication in the Country of the Strange" (Daly and Caputi 1987:102).

12. See Appendix II for the emergence part of this Navajo origin myth.

13. Hesiod recounts two versions of the origin of women. The more familiar tale of Pandora and her jar is part of *Works and Days* (lines 54–105); the other appears in *Theogony* (lines 565–612). On the evolution of Pandora imagery, see Panofsky and Panofsky (1962); on Pandora and Eve, see Phillips (1984).

14. The quotation is used out of context, as it might (and probably does) appear in collections of sayings, maxims, and proverbs. It comes from Emerson's first

lecture, "Uses of Great Men," of a series delivered in 1845 and published in 1850 as *Representative Men*. Great *men* are clearly the subject of this and the other lectures (on Plato, Swedenborg, Montaigne, Shakespeare, Napoleon, and Goethe), but in this paragraph women are at least backhandedly included in the discourse. Emerson continues: "Is it not a rare contrivance that lodged the due inertia in every creature, the conserving, resisting energy, the anger at being waked or changed? Altogether independent of the intellectual force in each, is the pride of opinion, the security that we are right. Not the feeblest grandame, not a mowing idiot, but uses what spark of perception and faculty is left, to chuckle and triumph in his or her opinion over the absurdities of all the rest. Difference from me is the measure of absurdity. Not one has a misgiving of being wrong. . . . But, in the midst of this chuckle of self-gratulation, some figure goes by, which Thersites too can love and admire. This is he that should marshal us the way we were going. There is no end to his aid. Without Plato, we should almost lose our faith in the possibility of a reasonable book. . . . We are all wise in capacity, though so few in energy. There needs but one wise man in a company, and all are wise, so rapid is the contagion."

15. Miller quotes (in order): William Buchan, *Advice to Mothers* (Philadelphia 1804), 70; Pye H. Chavasse, *Advice to a Wife* (London 1866).

16. *Papago Woman,* first published in 1936, is narrated by Maria Chona, who was ninety years old in the summer of 1930, when anthropologist Ruth M. Underhill recorded and edited her autobiography with help from fourteen-year-old translator-interpreter Ella Lopez Antone. For a good discussion of the book, Chona, Antone, and Underhill, see the chapter, "Maria Chona: An Independent Woman in Traditional Culture" (Bataille and Sands 1987:47–68).

17. Tedlock refers to Boas's 1914 "Folk-Tales of the North American Indians" (Boas 1940:468–69): "Many California tribes possess origin tales which are expressions of the will of a powerful being who by his thoughts established the present order. When this type of tale became first known to us through the collections of Jeremiah Curtin, it appeared so strange, that the thought suggested itself that we might have here the expression of an individual mind rather than of tribal concepts, resulting either from the recorder's attitude or from that of an informant affected by foreign thought. Further collections, however, have corroborated the impression; and it now seems certain that in northern California there exists a group of true creation tales." Boas gives no sources for the tales, which Tedlock identifies as Maidu and Kato.

18. Wenda R. Trevathan (1987:37), who quotes this from Mead, calls the latter's 1956 discussion "one of the richest, most complete accounts of childbirth in the anthropological literature, not otherwise devoted entirely to birth." In it, Mead "not only notes the activities of the mother, the midwives, and the other attendants but describes in detail the rhythmic sounds of the first few minutes of the infant's life, a rhythm that she then follows and develops for the individual's entire life."

Bibliography

Alderink, Larry J. 1981. *Creation and Salvation in Ancient Orphism*. American Philosophical Association, American Classical Studies, no. 8. Chico, California: Scholars Press.

Alexander, Hartley Burr. 1953. *The World's Rim: Great Mysteries of the North American Indians*, with a foreword by Clyde Kluckhohn. Lincoln: University of Nebraska Press.

Allen, Paula Gunn. 1978. *Coyote's Daylight Trip*. Albuquerque, New Mexico: La Confluencia.

———. 1986. *The Sacred Hoop: Recovering the Feminine in American Indian Traditions*. Boston: Beacon Press.

Allen, Sally G., and Joanna Hubbs. 1980. Outrunning Atalanta: Feminine Destiny in Alchemical Transmutation. *Signs* 6:210–29.

Aston, W. G. 1956 [1924]. *Nihongi; Chronicles of Japan from the Earliest Times to* A.D. *697*. London: Allen and Unwin.

Astrov, Margot, ed. 1962 [1946]. *American Indian Prose and Poetry: An Anthology*. New York: Capricorn Books.

Bachelard, Gaston. 1971 [1969, 1960]. *The Poetics of Reverie: Childhood, Language, and the Cosmos*, trans. Daniel Russell. Boston: Beacon Press.

Bachofen, Johann Jakob. 1967 [1954]. *Myth, Religion, and Mother Right: Selected Writings of J. J. Bachofen*, trans. Ralph Manheim. Bollingen Series 84. Princeton: Princeton University Press.

Bahr, Donald M. 1977. On The Complexity of Southwest Indian Emergence Myths. *Journal of Anthropological Research* 33:317–49.

Barnes, J. A. 1973. Genetrix : Genitor : : Nature : Culture. In *The Character of Kinship*, ed. Jack Goody, pp. 61–73. Cambridge: Cambridge University Press.

Barthes, Roland. 1972 [1957]. *Mythologies*, trans. Annette Lavers. New York: Hill and Wang.

Bataille, Gretchen M., and Kathleen Mullen Sands. 1987 [1984]. *American Indian Women: Telling Their Lives*. Lincoln: University of Nebraska Press.

Beckwith, Martha Warren, ed. and trans. 1972 [1951]. *The Kumulipo: A Hawaiian Creation Chant*, with a new foreword by Katharine Luomala. Honolulu: University Press of Hawaii.

Begg, Ean. 1985. *The Cult of the Black Virgin*. London: Arkana.

Benko, Stephen. 1967. The Libertine Gnostic Sect of the Phibionites According to Epiphanius. *Vigilae Christianae* 2:103–19.

Bergren, Ann L. T. 1983. Language and the Female in Early Greek Thought. *Arethusa* 16:69–95.

Best, Elsdon. 1922. *Some Aspects of Maori Myth and Religion*. Museum Monograph no. 1. Wellington, New Zealand: Dominion Museum.

Bettelheim, Bruno. 1962 [1954]. *Symbolic Wounds: Puberty Rites and the Envious Male*. New York: Macmillan, Collier Books.

Bierhorst, John, ed. 1976. *The Red Swan: Myths and Tales of the American Indians.* New York: Farrar, Straus and Giroux.

Boas, Franz. 1940. *Race, Language and Culture.* New York: The Free Press.

———, ed. 1917. *Folk-Tales of Salishan and Sahaptin Tribes.* Memoirs of the American Folk-Lore Society, vol. 11. Lancaster, Pennsylvania: American Folk-Lore Society.

Bogoras, Waldemar. 1910. *I. Chukchee Mythology.* Memoir of the American Museum of Natural History, New York, The Jesup North Pacific Expedition, ed. Franz Boas, vol. 8, pt. 1. Leiden: E. J. Brill, and New York: G. E. Stechert.

Bowler, Peter J. 1971. Preformation and Pre-existence in the Seventeeth Century: A Brief Analysis. *Journal of the History of Biology* 4:221–44.

Brandon, S. G. F. 1963. *Creation Legends of the Ancient Near East.* London: Hodder and Stoughton.

Brinton, Daniel G. 1976 [1896, 1868]. *Myths of the New World: The Symbolism and Mythology of the Indians of the Americas,* intro. Paul M. Allen. Blauvelt, New York: Multimedia Publishing.

Bruns, J. Edgar. 1973. *God as Woman, Woman as God.* New York: Paulist Press.

Bunzel, Ruth L. 1932. Zuñi Origin Myths. In *47th Annual Report of the Bureau of American Ethnology for the Years 1929–1930,* pp. 545–609. Washington: Government Printing Office.

———. 1972 [1929]. *The Pueblo Potter: A Study of Creative Imagination in Primitive Art.* New York: Dover Publications.

Burland, Cottie. 1980 [1975]. *The Aztecs: Gods and Fate in Ancient Mexico,* with photographs by Werner Forman. Clifton, New Jersey: Golden Press.

Burn, A. R., ed. 1972 [1954]. Herodotus, *The Histories,* trans. Aubrey de Selincourt, rev. ed. New York: Penguin Books.

Bynum, Caroline Walker. 1982. *Jesus as Mother: Studies in the Spirituality of the High Middle Ages.* Berkeley: University of California Press.

Cady, Susan, Marian Ronan, and Hal Taussig. 1986. *Sophia: The Future of Feminist Spirituality.* San Francisco: Harper & Row.

Calisher, Hortense. 1971 [1970]. No Important Woman Writer. In *Women's Liberation and Literature,* ed. Elaine Showalter, pp. 223–30. New York: Harcourt Brace Jovanovich.

Callaway, Helen. 1978. "The Most Essentially Female Function of All": Giving Birth. In *Defining Females: The Nature of Women in Society,* ed. Shirley Ardener, pp. 163–85. New York: John Wiley & Sons.

Campbell, Joseph. 1972 [1968, 1949]. *The Hero with a Thousand Faces.* Bollingen Series 17. Princeton: Princeton University Press.

Cantarella, Eva. 1986. Dangling Virgins: Myth, Ritual, and the Place of Women in Ancient Greece. In *The Female Body in Western Culture: Contemporary Perspectives,* ed. Susan Rubin Suleiman, pp. 57–67. Cambridge: Harvard University Press.

Canto, Monique. 1986. The Politics of Women's Bodies: Reflections on Plato, trans. Arthur Goldhammer. In *The Female Body in Western Culture: Contemporary Perspectives,* ed. Susan Rubin Suleiman, pp. 339–53. Cambridge: Harvard University Press.

Caputi, Jane. 1978a. "Jaws": Fish Stories and Partiarchal Myth. *Sinister Wisdom* 7:66–79.

———. 1978b. *Jaws* As Partiarchal Myth. *Journal of Popular Film* 6 (1978):305–25.

Carroll, Berenice A. 1981. The Politics of "Originality": Women Scholars and Intellectuals. Paper presented at session on "Women Scholars and Intellectuals," Berkshire Conference on Women's History, Vassar College, 17 June.

Carson, Rachel. 1961. *The Sea Around Us.* New York: Mentor.

Chamberlain, Mary. 1981. *Old Wives' Tales: Their History, Remedies and Spells.* London: Virago Press.

Chicago, Judy. 1985. *The Birth Project.* Garden City, New York: Doubleday & Company.

Clark, Alice. 1968 [1919]. *Working Life of Women in the Seventeenth Century.* New York: Augustus M. Kelley.

Clifton, Lucille. 1974. *An Ordinary Woman.* New York: Random House.

Cohen, Percy S. 1969. Theories of Myth. *Man* 4:337–53.

Colum, Padraic. 1930. *Orpheus.* New York: Macmillan. (Ed. used here is reprinted as *Myths of the World,* New York: Universal Library, Grosset & Dunlap, n.d.)

Cook, Roger. 1974. *The Tree of Life: Image for the Cosmos.* Art and Cosmos Series. London: Thames and Hudson.

Corea, Gena. 1985. *The Mother Machine: Reproductive Technologies from Artificial Insemination to Artificial Wombs.* New York: Harper & Row.

Count, Earl W. 1952. The Earth-Diver and the Rival Twins: A Clue to Time Correlation in North-Eurasiatic and North American Mythology. In *Indian Tales of Aboriginal America: Selected Papers of the 29th International Congress of Americanists,* ed. Sol Tax, pp. 55–62. Chicago: University of Chicago Press.

Culin, Stewart. 1975 [1907]. *Games of the North American Indians.* New York: Dover Publications.

Culler, Jonathan. 1983. *Roland Barthes.* New York: Oxford University Press.

Curtis, Edward S. 1924. *The North American Indian.* Vol. 14. Norwood, Massachusetts: Plimpton Press.

Cushing, Frank Hamilton. 1896. Outlines of Zuñi Creation Myths. In *13th Annual Report of the Bureau of [American] Ethnology for the Years 1891–1892,* pp. 321–447. Washington: Government Printing Office.

Daly, Mary. 1984. *Pure Lust: Elemental Feminist Philosophy.* Boston: Beacon Press.

———, conjurer, in cahoots with Jane Caputi. 1987. *Websters' First New Intergalactic Wickedary of the English Language.* Boston: Beacon Press.

Davidson, H. R. Ellis. 1964. *Gods and Myths of Northern Europe.* Baltimore, Maryland: Penguin Books.

de Beauvoir, Simone. 1961 [1953, 1949]. *The Second Sex,* trans. H. M. Parshley. New York: Bantam Books.

de Givry, Emile Grillot. 1973 [1931, 1929]. *The Illustrated Anthology of Sorcery, Magic and Alchemy,* trans. J. Courtenay Locke. New York: A & W Visual Library.

Delaney, Carol. 1986. The Meaning of Paternity and the Virgin Birth Debate. *Man,* n.s. 21:494–513.

Dellenbaugh, Anne G. 1982. She Who Is and Is Not Yet: An Essay on Parthenogenesis. *Trivia: A Journal of Ideas* 1:43–63.

Detienne, Marcel, and Jean-Pierre Vernant. 1978. *Cunning Intelligence in Greek Culture and Society,* trans. Janet Lloyd-Hassocks. Atlantic Highlands, New Jersey: Harvester Press. (Trans. of *Les ruses d'intelligence: la Metis des grecs.* Paris: Flammarion, 1974.)

Doria, Charles, and Harris Lenowitz, eds. and trans. 1976. *Origins: Creation Texts from the Ancient Mediterranean, A Chrestomathy.* Garden City, New York: Anchor Press/Doubleday.

Dorsey, J. Owen. 1894. A Study of Siouan Cults. In *llth Annual Report of the Bureau of [American] Ethnology for the Years 1889–1890,* pp. 351–544. Washington: Government Printing Office.

Dorson, Richard M. 1965 [1955]. The Eclipse of Solar Mythology. In *Myth: A Symposium,* ed. Thomas A. Sebeok, pp. 25–63. Bloomington: Indiana University Press.

DuBois, Constance Goddard. 1906. Mythology of the Mission Indians. *Journal of American Folklore* 19:52–60.

Dundes, Alan. 1962. Earth-Diver: Creation of the Mythopoeic Male. *American Anthropologist* 64:1032–51.

———. 1980 [1976]. A Psychoanalytic Study of the Bullroarer. In Dundes, *Interpreting Folklore,* pp. 176–98. Bloomington: Indiana University Press.

———. 1983. Couvade in Genesis. In *Studies in Aggadah and Jewish Folklore,* ed. Issachar Ben-Ami and Joseph Dan, pp. 35–53. Jerusalem: Magnes Press.

———. 1986. The Flood as Male Myth of Creation. *Journal of Psychoanalytic Anthropology* 9:359–72.

———, ed. 1984. *Sacred Narrative: Readings in the Theory of Myth.* Berkeley: University of California Press.

Economou, George D. 1972. *The Goddess Natura in Medieval Literature.* Cambridge: Harvard University Press.

Ehrenreich, Barbara, and Deirdre English. 1973. *Witches, Midwives, and Nurses: A History of Women Healers.* Glass Mountain Pamphlet no. 1. Old Westbury, New York: The Feminist Press.

———. 1979 [1978]. *For Her Own Good: 150 Years of the Experts' Advice to Women.* Garden City, New York: Anchor Press/Doubleday.

Eliade, Mircea. 1958 [1949]. *Patterns in Comparative Religion,* trans. Rosemary Sheed. New York: World Publishing, Meridian Books.

———. 1960 [1957]. *Myths, Dreams and Mysteries: The Encounter between Contemporary Faiths and Archaic Realities,* trans. Philip Mairet. New York: Harper & Row.

———. 1961 [1959, 1957]. *The Sacred and the Profane: The Nature of Religion,* trans. Willard R. Trask. New York: Harper & Row.

———. 1962 [1956]. *The Forge and the Crucible,* trans. Stephen Corrin. New York: Harper & Row.

———. 1963. *Myth and Reality,* trans. Willard R. Trask. New York: Harper & Row.

———. 1969. *The Quest: History and Meaning in Religion.* Chicago: University of Chicago Press.

———. 1971 [1949]. *The Myth of the Eternal Return or, Cosmos and History,* trans. Willard R. Trask. Bollingen Series 46. Princeton: Princeton University Press.

————. 1972 [1970]. *Zalmoxis The Vanishing God: Comparative Studies in the Religions and Folklore of Dacia and Eastern Europe*, trans. Willard R. Trask. Chicago: University of Chicago Press.

————. 1974 [1967]. *Gods, Goddesses, and Myths of Creation: A Thematic Source Book of the History of Religions, Part 1 of "From Primitives to Zen."* New York: Harper & Row.

————. 1976. *Occultism, Witchcraft, and Cultural Fashions: Essays in Comparative Religions*. Chicago: University of Chicago Press.

————. 1978a. *A History of Religious Ideas, Vol. 1: From the Stone Age to the Eleusinian Mysteries*, trans. Willard R. Trask. Chicago: University of Chicago Press.

————. 1978b. The Myth of Alchemy. *Parabola* 3, 3:6–23.

————. 1979 [1965, 1962]. *The Two and the One*, trans. J. M. Cohn. Chicago: University of Chicago Press.

Engelsman, Joan Chamberlain. 1979. *The Feminine Dimension of the Divine*. Philadelphia: Westminster Press.

Evans, Myfanwy. 1937. *The Painter's Object*. New York: G. Howe.

Farmer, Penelope, ed. 1979. *Beginnings: Creation Myths of the World*. New York: Antheneum.

Fewkes, Jesse Walter. 1973 [1919]. *Designs on Prehistoric Hopi Pottery*. New York: Dover Publications.

Firth, Raymond. 1973. Hair as Private Asset and Public Symbol. In Firth, *Symbols: Public and Private*, pp. 262–98. Ithaca, New York: Cornell University Press.

Fletcher, Alice C., and Francis La Flesche. 1911. The Omaha Tribe. In *27th Annual Report of the Bureau of American Ethnology for the Years 1905–1906*, pp. 16–672. Washington: Government Printing Office.

Folkard, Richard, Jr. 1884. *Plant Lore, Legends, and Lyrics: Embracing the Myths, Traditions, Superstitions, and Folk-Lore of the Plant Kingdom*. London: Sampson Law, Marston, Searle, and Rivington.

Forde, C. Daryll. 1930. A Creation Myth from Acoma. *Folk-Lore* 41:370–87.

Frazer, James George. 1909. Some Primitive Theories of the Origin of Man. In *Darwin and Modern Science*, ed. A. C. Seward, pp. 152–70. Cambridge: Cambridge University Press.

Freud, Sigmund. 1952 [1935, 1920]. *A General Introduction to Psychoanalysis*, trans. Joan Riviere. New York: Washington Square Press.

————. 1959 [1924, 1909, 1908]. On the Sexual Theories of Children. In *The Standard Edition of the Complete Psychological Works of Sigmund Freud*, trans. James Strachey, vol. 9 (1906–1908). London: Hogarth Press and Institute of Psycho-Analysis.

————, and D. E. Oppenheim. 1958. *Dreams in Folklore*. New York: International Universities Press.

Freund, Philip. 1975. *Myths of Creation*. Levittown, New York: Transatlantic Arts.

Friedman, Susan Stanford. 1987. Creativity and the Childbirth Metaphor: Gender Difference in Literary Discourse. *Feminist Studies* 13:49–82.

Friedrich, Paul. 1978. *The Meaning of Aphrodite*. Chicago: University of Chicago Press.

Ghiselin, Brewster, ed. 1952. *The Creative Process: A Symposium*. New York: Mentor Books.

Gill, Sam D. 1977. The Trees Stood Deep Rooted. *Parabola* 2, 2:6–12.

———. 1983. Navajo Views of Their Origin. In *Handbook of North American Indians*, vol. 10: Southwest, ed. Alfonso Ortiz, pp. 502–5. Washington: Smithsonian Institution.

———. 1987. *Mother Earth: An American Story*. Chicago: University of Chicago Press.

Gimbutas, Marija. 1982 [1974]. *The Goddesses and Gods of Old Europe, 6500–3500 B.C.: Myths and Cult Images*, rev. ed. Berkeley: University of California Press.

Grahn, Judy. 1978. *The Work of a Common Woman: The Collected Poetry of Judy Grahn, 1964–77*. Trumansburg, New York: Crossing Press.

Graves, Robert. 1966 [1948]. *The White Goddess: A Historical Grammar of Poetic Myth*, amended and enlarged ed. New York: Farrar, Straus and Giroux.

———. 1975 [1960, 1955]. *The Greek Myths*, vol. 1. Baltimore, Maryland: Penguin.

Green, Jesse, ed. 1979. *Zuñi: Selected Writings of Frank Hamilton Cushing*. Lincoln: University of Nebraska Press.

Griffin, Susan. 1978. *Woman and Nature: The Roaring Inside Her*. New York: Harper & Row.

———. 1982. *Made from This Earth: An Anthology of Writings*. New York: Harper & Row.

Grillot de Givry, Emile. 1973 [1929]. *The Illustrated Anthology of Sorcery, Magic and Alchemy*, trans. J. Courtenay Locke. New York: A&W Visual Library, Causeway Books.

Gruber, Jacob W. 1967. Horatio Hale and the Development of American Anthropology. *Proceedings of the American Philosophical Society* 3:5–37.

Gunn, John M. 1917. *Schat Chen: History, Traditions and Narratives of the Queres Indians of Laguna and Acoma*. Albuquerque, New Mexico: Albright and Anderson.

Haile, Father Berard, O.F.M. 1981. *The Upward Moving and Emergence Way: The Gishin Biye' Version*, ed. Karl W. Luckert. American Tribal Religions, vol. 7. Lincoln: University of Nebraska Press.

Hale, Horatio. 1888. Huron Folk-Lore. *Journal of American Folk-Lore* 1:177–83.

Hall, Manly Palmer. 1947 [1932]. *Man: Grand Symbol of the Mysteries*, 5th ed. Los Angeles: The Philosophical Research Society.

Hamilton, Edith, and Hamilton Cairns, eds. 1961. *The Collected Dialogues of Plato, Including the Letters*. Bollingen Series 71. New York: Pantheon Books.

Handy, E. S. Craighill. 1927. *Polynesian Religion*. Bernice P. Bishop Museum Bulletin 34. Honolulu, Hawaii.

Harding, M. Esther. 1965. *The Parental Image: Its Injury and Reconstruction: A Study in Analytical Psychology*. New York: G. P. Putnam's Sons, for the C. G. Jung Foundation for Analytical Psychology.

Harrington, M. R. 1921. *Religion and Ceremonies of the Lenape*. Museum of the American Indian, Heye Foundation, Indian Notes and Monographs, Misc. 19. New York, New York.

Harris, Marvin. 1968. *The Rise of Anthropological Theory: A History of Theories of Culture*. New York: Thomas Y. Crowell.

Harrison, Jane Ellen. 1980 [1908, 1903]. *Prolegomena to the Study of Greek Religion*, 2d ed. London: Merline Press.

Heidel, Alexander. 1951. *The Babylonian Genesis: The Story of Creation*. 2d ed. Chicago: University of Chicago Press.

Hellbom, Anna-Britta. 1963. The Creation Egg. *Ethnos* 28:63–105.

Herdt, Gilbert H. 1987 [1981]. *Guardians of the Flute: Idioms of Masculinity*. New York: Columbia University Press.

Hewitt, J. N. B. 1903. Iroquoian Cosmology, first part. In *21st Annual Report of the Bureau of American Ethnology for the years 1899–1900*, pp. 127–339. Washington: Government Printing Office.

————. 1928. Iroquoian Cosmology, second part. In *43rd Annual Report of the Bureau of American Ethnology for the Years 1925–1926*, pp. 449–819. Washington: Government Printing Office.

Hinsley, Curtis. 1983. Ethnographic Charisma and Scientific Routine: Cushing and Fewkes in the American Southwest, 1879–1893. In *Observers Observed: Essays on Ethnographic Fieldwork*, ed. George W. Stocking, Jr., pp. 53–69. Madison: University of Wisconsin Press.

Hongi, Hare. 1907. A Maori Cosmogony. *Journal of the Polynesian Society* 16:109–19.

Horny, Karen. 1967. *Feminine Psychology*, ed. Harold Kelman. New York: W. W. Norton.

Horowitz, Maryanne Cline. 1976. Aristotle and Woman. *Journal of the History of Biology* 9, 2:183–213.

Hultkrantz, Åke. 1979. *The Religions of the American Indians*, trans. Monica Setterwall. Berkeley: University of California Press.

————. 1983. *The Study of American Indian Religions*, ed. Christopher Vecsey. American Academy of Religion, Studies in Religion 29. New York: Crossroad Publishing, and Chico, California: Scholars Press.

Huxley, Francis. 1974. *The Way of the Sacred*. Garden City, New York: Doubleday and Company.

Johnson, David. 1977. The Wisdom of Festival. *Parabola* 2, 2:20–23.

Jones, Ernest. 1951. *Essays in Applied Psycho-Analysis*. Vol. 2: Essays in Folklore, Anthropology and Religion. London: Hogarth Press.

Jong, Erica. 1979. Creativity vs. Generativity: The Unexplained Lie. *New Republic* 13 January:27–30.

Jordan, Brigitte. 1980. *Birth in Four Cultures: A Crosscultural Investigation of Childbirth in Yucatan, Holland, Sweden and the United States*. Montreal, Canada: Eden Press Women's Publications.

Judd, Neil M. 1967. *The Bureau of American Ethnology: A Partial History*. Norman: University of Oklahoma Press.

Jung, Carl G. 1968 [1953, 1952, 1944]. *Psychology and Alchemy*, rev. ed., trans. R. F. C. Hull. Bollingen Series 20. Princeton: Princeton University Press.

————, and Marie-Louise von Franz, Joseph L. Henderson, Jolande Jacobi, Aniela Jaffé. 1968 [1964]. *Man and His Symbols*. Laurel Edition. New York: Dell Publishing.

Kirk, G. S., and J. E. Raven. 1964 [1957]. *The Presocratic Philosophers: A Critical History with a Selection of Texts*. Cambridge: University Press.

Kittay, Eva Feder. 1983. Womb Envy: An Explanatory Concept. In *Mothering: Essays in Feminist Theory,* ed. Joyce Trebilcot, pp. 94–128. Totowa, New Jersey: Rowman & Allanheld.

————, and Adrienne Lehrer. 1981. Semantic Fields and the Structure of Metaphor. *Studies in Language* 5, 1:31–63.

Kitzinger, Sheila. 1980 [1978]. *Women as Mothers.* New York: Vintage Books.

Köngäs, Elli Kaija. 1960. The Earth-Diver (Th.A 812). *Ethnohistory* 7:151–80.

Kramarae, Cheris, and Paula A. Treichler, with assistance from Ann Russo. 1985. *A Feminist Dictionary.* Boston: Pandora Press.

Kramer, Samuel Noah. 1959 [1956]. *History Begins at Sumer.* Garden City, New York: Doubleday Anchor Books.

Kris, Ernst, and Otto Kurz. 1979 [1934]. *Legend, Myth, and Magic in the Image of the Artist: A Historical Experiment,* trans. Alastair Laing and rev. Lottie M. Newman. New Haven: Yale University Press.

Kroeber, A. L. 1906–1907. Indian Myths in South Central California. In *University of California Publications in American Archaeology and Ethnology,* ed. Frederick Ward Putnam, vol. 4, no. 4, pp. 167–250. Berkeley: The University Press.

Kroeber, Henriette Rothschild. 1912. Traditions of the Papago Indians. *Journal of American Folklore* 25:95–105.

Lakoff, George, and Mark Johnson. 1980. *Metaphors We Live By.* Chicago: University of Chicago Press.

Landes, Ruth. 1971 [1938]. *The Ojibwa Woman.* Columbia University Contributions to Anthropology. New York: W. W. Norton.

Lattimore, Richmond, trans. and ed. 1953. Aeschylus, *Oresteia.* Chicago: University of Chicago Press.

————. 1959. *Hesiod.* Ann Arbor: University of Michigan Press.

Leach, Edmund R. 1958. Magical Hair. *Journal of the Royal Anthropological Institute of Great Britain and Ireland* 88:147–64.

————. 1969 [1966]. Virgin Birth. In E. Leach, *Genesis as Myth and Other Essays,* pp. 85–112. London: Jonathan Cape.

Leach, Maria, ed. 1972 [1950, 1949]. *Funk & Wagnalls Standard Dictionary of Folklore, Mythology, and Legend.* New York: Funk & Wagnalls.

Leavitt, Judith Walzer. 1986. *Brought to Bed: Childbearing in America, 1750 to 1950.* New York: Oxford University Press.

————, ed. 1984. *Women and Health in America: Historical Readings.* Madison: University of Wisconsin Press.

Leeming, David. 1976. *Mythology,* with pictorial narrative by Edwin Bayrd. New York: Newsweek Books.

Lehner, Ernst. 1969 [1950]. *Symbols, Signs & Signets.* New York: Dover Publications.

Lerner, Gerda. 1986. *The Creation of Patriarchy.* New York: Oxford University Press.

Lévi-Strauss, Claude. 1967 [1963, 1958]. *Structural Anthropology,* trans. Claire Jacobson and Brooke Grundfest Schoepf. Garden City, New York: Anchor Books.

————. 1969 [1949]. *The Elementary Structures of Kinship.* Boston: Beacon Press.

Lincoln, Bruce. 1986. *Myth, Cosmos, and Society: Indo-European Themes of Creation and Destruction.* Cambridge: Harvard University Press.

Lockhart, Russell A. 1978. Words as Eggs. *Dragonflies: Studies in Imaginal Psychology* Fall:3–32.

Long, Charles H. 1963. *Alpha: The Myths of Creation*. New York: George Braziller.

Lubbock, John. 1870. *The Origins of Civilization and the Primitive Condition of Man; Mental and Social Condition of Savages*. London: Longmans, Green.

Luckert, Karl W. 1984. Coyote in Navajo and Hopi Tales. In Father Berard Haile, O.F.M., *Navajo Coyote Tales: The Curly Tó Aheedlíinii Version*, pp. 3–19. Lincoln: University of Nebraska Press.

Lungberg, Ferdinand, and Marynia F. Farnham. 1947. *Modern Woman: The Lost Sex*. New York: Grosset & Dunlap.

MacCormack, Carol P. 1980. Nature, Culture and Gender: A Critique. In *Nature, Culture and Gender*, ed. MacCormack and Marilyn Strathorn, pp. 1–24. Cambridge: Cambridge University Press.

Maclagan, David. 1977. *Creation Myths: Man's Introduction to the World*. Art and Imagination Series. London: Thames and Hudson.

Martin, Emily. 1987. *The Woman in the Body: A Cultural Analysis of Reproduction*. Boston: Beacon Press.

Matthews, Washington. 1902. Myths of Gestation and Parturition. *American Anthropologist* 4:737–42.

Maud, Ralph. 1982. *A Guide to B. C. Indian Myth and Legend: A Short History of Myth-Collecting and a Survey of Published Texts*. Vancouver, British Columbia: Talonbooks.

McClain, Carol. 1975. Ethno-Obstetrics in Ajijic. *Anthropological Quarterly* 48:38–56.

McNeley, James Kale. 1981. *Holy Wind in Navajo Philosophy*. Tucson: University of Arizona Press.

Mead, Margaret. 1956. *New Lives for Old*. New York: William Morrow.

Meltzer, David, ed. 1981. *Birth: An Anthology of Ancient Texts, Songs, Prayers, and Stories*. San Francisco: North Point Press.

Merchant, Carolyn. 1980. *The Death of Nature: Woman, Ecology, and the Scientific Revolution*. San Francisco: Harper & Row.

Michell, John. 1975. *The Earth Spirit: Its Ways, Shrines and Mysteries*. Art and Cosmos Series. London: Thames and Hudson.

Miller, Henry. 1941. *The Wisdom of the Heart*. New York: New Directions.

Miller, John Hawkins. 1978. "Temple and Sewer": Childbirth, Prudery and Victoria Regina. In *The Victorian Family: Structure and Stress*, ed. Anthony S. Wohl. London: Croom Helm.

Moon, Sheila. 1970. *A Magic Dwells: A Poetic and Psychological Study of the Navaho Emergence Myth*. Middletown, Connecticut: Wesleyan University Press.

Mooney, James. 1896. The Ghost-dance Religion and the Sioux Outbreaks of 1890. In *14th Annual Report of the Bureau of [American] Ethnology for the Years 1892–1893*, pt. 2, pp. 641–1110. Washington: Government Printing Office.

Morford, Mark P. O., and Robert J. Lenardon. 1985. *Classical Mythology*. 3d ed. New York: Longman.

Moss, Leonard W., and Stephen C. Cappannari. 1982. In Quest of the Black Virgin: She Is Black Because She Is Black. In *Mother Worship: Theme and Variations*, ed. James J. Preston, pp. 53–74. Chapel Hill: University of North Carolina Press.

Murphy, Yolanda, and Robert F. Murphy. 1974. *Women of the Forest.* New York: Columbia University Press.

Naylor, Maria, ed. 1975. *Authentic Indian Designs: 2500 Illustrations from Reports of the Bureau of American Ethnology.* New York: Dover Publications.

Needham, Joseph. 1934. *A History of Embryology.* Cambridge: Cambridge University Press. (Note too the 2d ed., New York: Abelard-Schuman, 1959, not used here.)

Neumann, Erich. 1963 [1955]. *The Great Mother: An Analysis of the Archetype,* trans. Ralph Manheim. 2d ed. Bollingen Series 47. Princeton: Princeton University Press.

Newall, Venetia. 1971. *An Egg at Easter: A Folklore Study.* Bloomington: Indiana University Press.

Nilsson, Martin P. 1961 [1940]. *Greek Folk Religion.* New York: Harper & Row.

Oakley, Ann. 1976. Wisewoman and Medicine Man: Changes in the Management of Childbirth. In *The Rights and Wrongs of Women,* ed. Juliet Mitchell and Ann Oakley, pp. 17–58. New York: Penguin Harmondsworth.

O'Brien, Joan, and Wilfred Major. 1982. *In the Beginning: Creation Myths from Ancient Mesopotamia, Israel and Greece.* American Academy of Religion, Aids for the Study of Religion Series, no. 11. Chico, California: Scholars Press.

O'Bryan, Aileen. 1956. *The Diné: Origin Myths of the Navajo Indians.* Smithsonian Institution, Bureau of American Ethnology Bulletin 163. Washington: Government Printing Office.

Ochshorn, Judith. 1981. *The Female Experience and the Nature of the Divine.* Bloomington: Indiana University Press.

Onians, Richard Broxton. 1951. *The Origins of European Thought About the Body, the Mind, the Soul, the World, Time and Fate.* Cambridge: Cambridge University Press.

Ortner, Sherry B. 1974. Is Female to Male as Nature Is to Culture? In *Woman, Culture, and Society,* ed. Michelle Zimbalist Rosaldo and Louise Lamphere, pp. 67–87. Stanford, California: Stanford University Press.

Pagels, Elaine. 1988. *Adam, Eve, and the Serpent.* New York: Random House.

Panofsky, Dora, and Erwin Panofsky. 1962. *Pandora's Box: The Changing Aspects of a Mythical Symbol.* Bollingen Series 52. Princeton: Princeton University Press.

Parsons, Elsie Clews. 1923. The Origin Myth of Zuñi. *Journal of American Folklore* 36:135–62.

———. 1939. *Pueblo Indian Religion.* Vol. 1. Chicago: University of Chicago Press.

Patai, Raphael. 1978. *The Hebrew Goddess.* New York: KTAV Publishing House.

Pearson, Carol, and Katherine Pope, eds. 1976. *Who Am I This Time?: Female Portraits in British and American Literature.* New York: McGraw-Hill.

Peck, A. L., trans. 1963 [1953, 1942]. Aristotle, *Generation of Animals.* Loeb Classical Library. Cambridge: Harvard University Press.

Petchesky, Rosalind Pollack. 1987. Fetal Images: The Power of Visual Culture in the Politics of Reproduction. *Feminist Studies* 13:263–92.

Peterson, Gayle. 1984. *Birthing Normally: A Personal Growth Approach to Childbirth*. Berkeley, California: Mindbody Press.

Phillips, John A. 1984. *Eve: The History of an Idea*. San Francisco: Harper & Row.

Phipps, William E. 1976–1977. Adam's Rib: Bone of Contention. *Theology Today* 33:263–73.

Pomeroy, Sarah B. 1975. *Goddesses, Whores, Wives, and Slaves: Women in Classical Antiquity*. New York: Schocken Books.

Pope, Barbara Corrado. 1985. Immaculate and Powerful: The Marian Revival in the Nineteenth Century. In *Immaculate & Powerful: The Female in Sacred Image and Social Reality*, ed. Clarissa W. Atkinson, Constance H. Buchanan, and Margaret R. Miles, pp. 173–200. The Harvard Women's Studies in Religion Series. Boston: Beacon Press.

Poston, Carol H. 1978. Childbirth in Literature. *Feminist Studies* 4:18–31.

Powers, Marla N. 1986. *Oglala Women: Myth, Ritual, and Reality*. Chicago: University of Chicago Press.

Powers, William K. 1986. *Sacred Language: The Nature of Supernatural Discourse in Lakota*. Norman: University of Oklahoma Press.

Preuss, Konrad T. 1921. *Religion und Mythologie der Uitoto*. Vol. 1. Göttingen: Vandenhoeck and Ruprecht.

Pritchard, James B., ed. 1969 [1955, 1950]. *Ancient Near Eastern Texts Relating to the Old Testament*. 3d ed. with supplement. Princeton: Princeton University Press.

Purce, Jill. 1980 [1974]. *The Mystic Spiral: Journey of the Soul*. Art and Imagination Series. New York: Thames and Hudson.

Purley, Anthony F. 1974. Keres Pueblo Concepts of Deity. *American Indian Culture and Research Journal* 1, 1:29–32.

Radin, Paul. 1954 [1924]. *Monotheism Among Primitive Peoples*. Basel, Switzerland: Ethnographical Museum.

———. 1957a [1955, 1927]. *Primitive Man as Philosopher*. 2d ed. rev. New York: Dover Publications.

———. 1957b [1937]. *Primitive Religion: Its Nature and Origin*. New York: Dover Publications.

Ramsey, Jarold. 1977. The Bible in Western Indian Mythology. *Journal of American Folklore* 90:442–54.

Rasmussen, Knud. 1927. *Across Arctic America: Narratives of the Fifth Thule Expedition*. New York: G. P. Putnam's Sons.

———. 1931. *The Netsilik Eskimos: Social Life and Spiritual Culture*, trans. W. E. Calvert. Report of the Fifth Thule Expedition 1921–24, vol. 8, no. 1–2. Copenhagen, Denmark: Gyldendalske Boghandel, Nordisk Forlag.

Reichard, Gladys A. 1968 [1936]. *Navajo Shepherd and Weaver*. Glorieta, New Mexico: Rio Grande Press.

———. 1974 [1963, 1950]. *Navaho Religion: A Study of Symbolism*. 2d ed. in 1 vol. Bollingen Series 18. Princeton: Princeton University Press.

Rich, Adrienne. 1978. *The Dream of a Common Language: Poems 1974–1977*. New York: W. W. Norton.

Richardson, Herbert W. 1969. Three Myths of Transcendence. In *Transcendence*, ed. Richardson and Donald R. Colter, pp. 98–113. Boston: Beacon Press.

Rieu, E. V., trans. 1959. Apollonius of Rhodes, *The Voyage of the Argo*. Harmondsworth: Penguin.

Róheim, Géza. 1952. *The Gates of the Dream*. New York: International Universities Press.

———. 1954. *Hungarian and Vogul Mythology*. Monographs of the American Ethnological Society 23. Seattle: University of Washington Press.

Rooth, Anna Birgitta. 1957. The Creation Myths of the North American Indians. *Anthropos* 52:497–508.

Rothenberg, Jerome, ed. 1968. *Technicians of the Sacred: A Range of Poetries from Africa, America, Asia & Oceania*. Garden City, New York: Anchor Books Doubleday.

———. 1972. *Shaking the Pumpkin: Traditional Poetry of the Indian North Americas*. Garden City, New York: Doubleday & Company.

Ruether, Rosemary Radford, 1975. *New Woman New Earth: Sexist Ideologies and Human Liberation*. New York: The Seabury Press.

———. 1983. *Sexism and God-Talk: Toward a Feminist Theology*. Boston: Beacon Press.

———. 1985. *Womanguides: Readings Toward a Feminist Theology*. Boston: Beacon Press.

———, ed. 1974. *Religion and Sexism: Images of Women in the Jewish and Christian Traditions*. New York: Simon and Schuster.

Russell, Frank. 1975 [1908]. *The Pima Indians,* ed. Bernard L. Fontana. Tucson: University of Arizona Press.

Saliba, John A., S.J. 1975. The Virgin-Birth Debate in Anthropological Literature: A Critical Assessment. *Theological Studies* 36:428–54.

Sanday, Peggy Reeves. 1981. *Female Power and Male Dominance: On the Origins of Sexual Inequality*. Cambridge: Cambridge University Press.

Santillana, Giorgio de, and Hertha von Dechend. 1969. *Hamlet's Mill: An Essay on Myth and the Frame of Time*. Boston: Gambit.

Saunders, E. Dale. 1961. Japanese Mythology. In *Mythologies of the Ancient World,* ed. Samuel Noah Kramer, pp. 411–42. Garden City, New York: Anchor Books, Doubleday.

Scarberry, Susan J. 1983. Grandmother Spider's Lifeline. In *Studies in American Indian Literature: Critical Essays and Course Designs,* ed. Paula Gunn Allen, pp. 100–107. New York: Modern Language Association of America.

Schafer, R. Murray. 1980. *The Tuning of the World: Toward a Theory of Soundscape Design*. Philadelphia: University of Pennsylvania Press.

Seligmann, Kurt. 1971 [1948]. *Magic, Supernaturalism and Religion*. New York: Pantheon Books.

Silko, Leslie Marmon. 1977. *Ceremony*. New York: Viking/Penguin.

Simpson, Michael, trans. and ed. 1976. *Gods and Heroes of the Greeks: The "Library" of Apollodorus*. Amherst: University of Massachusetts Press.

Sjöö, Monica, and Barbara Mor. 1987. *The Great Cosmic Mother: Rediscovering the Religion of the Earth*. San Francisco: Harper & Row.

Spacks, Patricia Meyer. 1985. *Gossip*. Chicago: University of Chicago Press.

Speck, Frank G. 1909. *Ethnology of the Yuchi Indians*. University of Pennsylvania, Anthropological Publications of the University Museum 1, 1. Philadelphia.

————. 1931. *A Study of the Delaware Indian Big House Ceremony*. Publications of the Pennsylvania Historical Commission, vol. 11. Harrisburg.

Speert, Harold, M.D. 1973. *Iconographia Gyniatrica: A Pictorial History of Gynecology and Obstetrics*. Philadelphia: F. A. Davis.

Spender, Dale. 1983 [1982]. *Women of Ideas and What Men Have Done to Them: From Aphra Behn to Adrienne Rich*. London: Ark Paperbacks.

Spretnak, Charlene. 1987. Knowing Gaia. *Anima* 14, 1:12–18.

Sproul, Barbara C. 1979. *Primal Myths: Creating the World*. San Francisco: Harper & Row.

Standing Bear, Chief Luther. 1933. *Land of the Spotted Eagle*. New York: Houghton Mifflin.

Stanworth, Michelle, ed. 1987. *Reproductive Technologies: Gender, Motherhood and Medicine*. Minneapolis: University of Minnesota Press.

Stephen, A[lexander] M. 1930. Navajo Origin Legend. *Journal of American Folklore* 43:88–104.

Stevenson, (Margaret) Sinclair, Mrs. 1920. *The Rites of the Twice-Born*. London: Oxford University Press.

Stevenson, Matilda Coxe. 1904. The Zuñi Indians: Their Mythology, Esoteric, Fraternities, and Ceremonies. In *23rd Annual Report of the Bureau of American Ethnology for the Years 1901–1902*, pp. 1–608. Washington: Government Printing Office.

Stirling, Matthew W. 1942. *Origin Myth of Acoma and Other Records*. Bureau of American Ethnology Bulletin 135. Washington: Government Printing Office.

Strouse, Jean, ed. 1974. *Women & Analysis: Dialogues on Psychoanalytic Views of Femininity*. New York: Grossman Publishers.

Swanson, Guy E. 1960. *The Birth of the Gods: The Origin of Primitive Beliefs*. Ann Arbor: University of Michigan Press.

Swanton, John R. 1908. Social Condition, Beliefs, and Linguistic Relationship of the Tlingit Indians. In *26th Annual Report of the Bureau of American Ethnology for the Years 1904–1905*, pp. 391–485. Washington: Government Printing Office.

————. 1929. *Myths and Tales of the Southeastern Indians*. Bureau of American Ethnology Bulletin 88. Washington: Government Printing Office.

Swentzell, Rina, and Tito Naranjo. 1986. Nurturing: The *Gia* at Santa Clara Pueblo. *El Palacio* 92, 1:35–39.

Talbot, Percy Amaury. 1912. *In the Shadow of the Bush*. London: William Heinemann.

Tedlock, Dennis. 1979. Zuni Religion and World View. In *Handbook of North American Indians,* vol. 9: Southwest, ed. Alfonso Ortiz, pp. 499–508. Washington: Smithsonian Institution.

————. 1983. *The Spoken Word and the Work of Interpretation*. Philadelphia: University of Pennsylvania Press.

————, trans. 1985. *Popol Vuh: The Mayan Book of the Dawn of Life*. New York: Simon & Schuster.

Teit, James A. 1912. *Mythology of the Thompson Indians*. Publications of the Jessup

North Pacific Expedition, vol. 8, pt. 2. Leiden and New York: Brill and Stechert.

Teresi, Dick, and Kathleen McAuliffe. 1985. Male Pregnancy. *Omni* 8, 3 (December):50–56, 118.

Thompson, Stith, ed. 1955–1958. *Motif-Index of Folk-Literature: A Classification of Narrative Elements in Folktales, Ballads, Myths, Fables, Mediaeval Romances, Exempla, Fabliaux, Jest-Books, and Local Legends.* 6 vols. Bloomington: Indiana University Press.

———. 1966 [1929]. *Tales of the North American Indians.* Bloomington: Indiana University Press.

Toelken, Barre. 1976a. A Circular World: The Vision of Navajo Crafts. *Parabola* 1, 1:30–37.

———. 1976b. Seeing with a Native Eye: How Many Sheep Will It Hold? In *Seeing with a Native Eye: Essays on Native American Religion,* ed. Walter Holden Capps with Ernst F. Tonsing, pp. 9–24. New York: Harper & Row.

———. 1979. *The Dynamics of Folklore.* Boston: Houghton Mifflin.

———, and Tacheeni Scott. 1981. Poetic Retranslation and the "Pretty Languages" of Yellowman. In *Traditional Literatures of the American Indian,* ed. Karl Kroeber, pp. 65–116. Lincoln: University of Nebraska Press.

Trevathan, Wenda R. 1987. *Human Birth: An Evolutionary Perspective.* New York: Aldine de Gruyter.

Trible, Phyllis. 1976. Depatriarchalizing in Biblical Interpretation. In *The Jewish Woman: New Perspectives,* ed. Elizabeth Koltun, pp. 217–40. New York: Schocken Books.

Turner, Frederick W., III, ed. 1974. *The Portable North American Indian Reader.* New York: Viking Press.

Turner, Victor, and Edith Turner. 1978. *Image and Pilgrimage in Christian Culture.* New York: Columbia University Press.

Tuzin, Donald F. 1977. Reflections of Being in Arapesh Water Symbolism. *Ethnos* 5:195–223.

Tyler, Hamilton A. 1964. *Pueblo Gods and Myths.* Norman: University of Oklahoma Press.

Tylor, Edward B. 1958 [1871]. *Primitive Culture.* New York: Harper Torchbooks.

———. 1960 [1881]. *Anthropology,* abridged and ed. Leslie A. White. Ann Arbor: University of Michigan Press.

Underhill, Ruth M. 1973 [1938]. *Singing for Power: The Song Magic of the Papago Indians of Southern Arizona.* New York: Ballantine Books.

———. 1979 [1936]. *Papago Woman.* Case Studies in Cultural Anthropology. New York: Holt Rinehart and Winston.

Vaillant, George C. 1966 [1962, 1944]. *Aztecs of Mexico: Origin, Rise, and Fall of the Aztec Nation,* rev. Suzannah B. Vaillant. Baltimore, Maryland: Penguin Books.

Van Over, Raymond, ed. 1980. *Sun Songs: Creation Myths from Around the World.* New York: New American Library.

Volborth, Judith Mountain Leaf (Ivaloo). 1979. Self-Portrait. *Shantih* 4, 2:38.

von Franz, Marie-Louise. 1972. *Patterns of Creativity Mirrored in Creation Myths.* Zurich, Switzerland: Spring Publications.

Walker, Barbara G. 1985. *The Crone: Woman of Age, Wisdom, and Power.* San Francisco: Harper & Row.

Wallace, Anthony F. C. 1958. Dreams and the Wishes of the Soul: A Type of Psychoanalytic Theory Among the Seventeenth Century Iroquois. *American Anthropologist* 60:234–48.

Warner, Marina. 1976. *Alone of All Her Sex: The Myth and the Cult of the Virgin Mary.* New York: Alfred A. Knopf.

Watts, Alan W. 1968. *Myth and Ritual in Christianity.* Boston: Beacon Press.

Weigle, Marta. 1982. *Spiders & Spinsters: Women and Mythology.* Albuquerque: University of New Mexico Press.

———. 1987a. Creation and Procreation, Cosmogony and Childbirth: Reflections on *Ex Nihilo,* Earth Diver, and Emergence Mythology. *Journal of American Folklore* 100:426–35.

———. 1987b. Creation and Procreation: Feminist Notes on Southwestern Emergence Mythology. *New Mexico Folklore Record* 16:1–21.

———, and David Johnson. 1979. *Lightning & Labyrinth: An Introduction to Mythology.* Albuquerque: University of New Mexico, Department of English.

———. 1980. *At the Beginning: American Creation Myths.* Albuquerque: University of New Mexico, Department of English.

West, M. L. 1971. *Early Greek Philosophy and the Orient.* Oxford: Clarendon Press.

Westkott, Marcia. 1986. *The Feminist Legacy of Karen Horney.* New Haven: Yale Univeristy Press.

Westman, Heinz. 1986 [1961]. *The Springs of Creativity.* 2d ed. Wilmette, Illinois: Chiron Publications.

Wheeler-Voegelin, Erminie, and Remedios W. Moore. 1957. The Emergence Myth in North America. In *Studies in Folklore,* ed. W. Edson Richmond, pp. 66–91. Indiana University Publications in Folklore 9. Bloomington: Indiana University Press.

White, Leslie A. 1932. The Acoma Indians. In *47th Annual Report of the Bureau of American Ethnology for the Years 1929–1930,* pp. 17–192. Washington: Government Printing Office.

———. 1962. *The Pueblo of Sia, New Mexico.* Bureau of American Ethnology Bulletin 184. Washington: Government Printing Office.

Witherspoon, Gary. 1977. *Language and Art in the Navajo Universe.* Ann Arbor: University of Michigan Press.

Wolf, Eric. 1972 [1958]. The Virgin of Guadalupe: A Mexican National Symbol. In *Reader in Comparative Religion: An Anthropological Approach.* 3d ed., ed. William A. Lessa and Evon Z. Vogt, pp. 149–53. New York: Harper & Row.

Wroth, William. 1982. *Christian Images in Hispanic New Mexico.* Colorado Springs, Colorado: The Taylor Museum of the Colorado Springs Fine Arts Center.

Wyman, Leland C. 1970. *Blessingway: With Three Versions of the Myth Recorded and Translated from the Navajo by Father Berard Haile, O.F.M.* Tucson: University of Arizona Press.

———. 1973. *The Red Antway of the Navaho.* Navajo Religion Series vol. 5. Santa Fe, New Mexico: Museum of Navaho Ceremonial Art.

Permissions

Brigitte Jordan, from *Birth in Four Cultures: A Crosscultural Investigation of Childbirth in Yucatan, Holland, Sweden and the United States* (Montreal: Eden Press Women's Publications, 1980). By permission of the publisher.

George Lakoff and Mark Johnson, from *Metaphors We Live By,* by George Lakoff and Mark Johnson. Copyright © 1980 by The University of Chicago. By permission of University of Chicago Press.

Richmond Lattimore, from Aeschylus, *Oresteia,* translated and edited by Richmond Lattimore. Copyright © 1953 by The University of Chicago. By permission of University of Chicago Press.

Richmond Lattimore, from *Hesiod* translated and edited by Richmond Lattimore. Copyright © 1959 by The University of Michigan. By permission of University of Michigan Press.

Emily Martin, from *The Woman in the Body,* by Emily Martin. Copyright © 1987 by Emily Martin. Reprinted by permission of Beacon Press.

Erich Neumann, from Erich Neumann, *The Great Mother,* trans. Ralph Manheim, Bollingen Series 47. Copyright 1955, © 1983 renewed by Princeton University Press.

Rosalind Pollack Petchesky, "Fetal Images: The Power of Visual Culture in the Politics of Reproduction," *Feminist Studies* 13 (1987): 271, 277. By permission of the publisher.

Barbara Corrado Pope, from "Immaculate and Powerful: The Marian Revival in the Nineteenth Century," by Barbara Corrado Pope, in *Immaculate and Powerful,* ed. Atkinson, Buchanan, and Miles. Copyright © 1985 by Clarissa W. Atkinson, Constance H. Buchanan, and Margaret R. Miles. By permission of Beacon Press.

Carol H. Poston, from "Childbirth in Literature," by Carol H. Poston. This article is reprinted from *Feminist Studies,* volume 4, no. 2 (June 1978): 18–31, by permission of the publisher Feminist Studies, Inc., c/o Women's Studies Program, University of Maryland, College Park, MD 20742.

William K. Powers, from *Sacred Language: The Nature of Supernatural Discourse in Lakota,* by William K. Powers. Copyright © 1986 by the University of Oklahoma Press. By permission of the publisher.

James B. Pritchard, ed., *Ancient Near Eastern Texts: Relating to the Old Testament,* 3rd ed. with Supplement. Copyright © 1969 by Princeton University Press. Excerpts reprinted with permission of Princeton University Press.

Paul Radin, from *Monotheism among Primitive Peoples* (Basel: Ethnographi-

Judith Mountain Leaf (Ivaloo) Volborth, "Self-Portrait." Reprinted by permission of *Shantih* © 1979 and Irving Gottesman.

Marie-Louise von Franz, from *Patterns of Creativity Mirrored in Creation Myths* (Zurich, Switzerland: Spring Publications, 1972). By permission of Spring Publications, Dallas, Texas.

Marina Warner, from *Alone of All Her Sex: The Myth and the Cult of the Virgin Mary,* by Marina Warner. Copyright © 1976 by Marina Warner. By permission of Alfred A. Knopf, Inc.

Gary Witherspoon, from *Language and Art in the Navajo Universe,* by Gary Witherspoon. Copyright © 1977 by The University of Michigan. By permission of University of Michigan Press.

Index

Abbreviations: coll. = collector; inf. = informant; NT = New Testament; OT = Old Testament

Abraham (OT), 85
Abyssinian woman (inf.), 150–51
accretion creation, 6, 22
Acoma Pueblo Indian, 91, 214–19, 255
Adam (OT), 60, 133, 134, 252
Aeschylus, cited, 117, 137
Agra of Mbeban (inf.), 177
Agʼttin·qeu (inf.), 227–28
Ahkeah, Sam (inf.), 220–21
alchemy, 69, 97, 102–7, 110, 137, 159, 163, 187, 256–57
Alexander, Hartley Burr, cited, 42–43
Algonkin Indian, 45
allegory, 140–41, 143, 187, 256
Allen, Paula Gunn, cited, 26, 89, 119–20, 248; poem, 32
Allen, Sally G., cited, 104–5, 107, 137
Amlodhi (Icelandic), 257–58
Andry, Nicholas, cited, 100
angels, 109, 169
animism, 7, 43, 49–51, 52, 80
Annunciation, 79, 253–54
anthropogony, 51–52, 66, 132, 160–61
Apollo (Greek), 117, 137
Apollodorus, cited, 184
Apollonius of Rhodes, cited, 132
Arachne (Greek), 183
Arapaho Indian, 19
architecture, 11–13
Aristotle, cited, 5, 75–76, 79, 85, 98, 107, 155
art, 7, 8, 10, 21, 22, 41, 42, 43, 70, 97, 98, 111, 113, 119, 124, 134, 135, 183–84, 185–87, 255. See also weaving
Artemis (Greek), 88, 254
Assumption, 86, 91
Athena (Greek), 36, 82–83, 134, 137, 162, 183, 254–55
Atum (Egyptian), 73, 74
Australia, 4
autochthony, 53, 154
Awonawilona (Zuni), 4, 82–83, 208, 254
Aztec Indian, 55–56, 77, 89, 123, 251, 258

Babylonia, 4, 6, 13, 73, 139, 252, 253
Bachelard, Gaston, cited, 256
Bachofen, Johann Jakob, cited, 57–59
Barbelo (Phibionite), 75
Barnes, J. A., cited, 117
Barthes, Roland, cited, 42, 43, 108–10, 184–87
Bergren, Ann L. T., cited, 35–36, 134–35
Bettelheim, Bruno, cited, 132–33, 162
Bierhorst, John (trans.), 56, 251
bird soul, 68–69, 252
birth. See parturition
Birth Project, The. See Chicago, Judy
birth talk, 164–65, 166–67, 169, 242. See also gossip
black madonna, 88–89. See also Virgin Mary
blind brother creation, 6, 33
Boas, Franz, cited, 4, 5, 51, 173, 187, 219, 262
Boehm, Felix, cited, 8
Bogoras, Waldemar (coll.), 227–28
Boscana, Geronimo, Father, cited, 203, 204, 205
Bowler, Peter J., cited, 255
brain, 51, 75, 101, 105, 107–11, 134
Brandon, S. G. F., cited, 74, 123–24
Breasted, James, cited, 250
breath, 5, 7, 24, 25, 27, 29, 51, 75, 77, 82, 117, 132, 165, 193, 197, 247
Brinton, Daniel G., cited, 44–45
Bruyn, Bartel (artist), 79, 253
Buck, John and Joshua (inf.), 192
Buddha (Far Eastern), 77, 259
Bunzel, Ruth L., cited, 97, 119, 207, 254, 255
Bynum, Caroline Walker, cited, 257

cabalistic myth, 107
Calisher, Hortense, cited, 130
Callaway, Helen, cited, 125
Cantarella, Eva, cited, 183
Canto, Monique, cited, 140–41
Caputi, Jane, cited, 160, 164, 259, 261
Carson, Rachel, cited, 139

cat's cradle, 29, 30
Ceres (Roman), 88, 110
Cerus (Roman), 110
cesarean birth, 157
Chamberlain, Mary, cited, 154, 156–57
chaos, 4, 5, 6, 11, 14, 27, 97, 102, 114, 119, 139, 163, 190, 203, 252
Chaos (Greek), 3, 5, 65, 107
Chicago, Judy (artist), iv, 169; cited, xi, 258
Chief Luther Standing Bear, cited, 138
childbirth. *See* parturition
childbirth metaphor, 126, 128–29, 130–31
China, 6, 45, 102
Christianity, 46, 81, 84, 86, 91, 172, 252
Chronus (Orphic), 107, 248
Chthonia (Greek), 20, 248
Chuckchee, 126–27, 227–31
Clark, Alice, cited, 160
Clarke (inf.), 190–91
Clifton, Lucille, poem, 167, 169
Coatlicue (Aztec), 55–56, 77, 251
Cohen, Percy S., cited, 50
Colum, Padraic, cited, 151, 153
conception, 65, 72, 75, 77–82, 191, 193, 211, 257
Cooke, Rose Terry, poem, 21–22
Copper Eskimo, 250
copulation. *See* intercourse
cosmogonic myth, 9, 10, 13, 14, 43, 51, 83, 102, 144, 169, 170, 175, 190; classification of, 5–7; defined, 3–5. *See also* creation myths and motifs
Count, Earl W., cited, 67
couvade, 125, 132–34, 167, 176, 191, 233
Coyote (trickster), xii, 55, 68, 161, 170, 180–81, 219, 223, 225, 250
creation myths and motifs. *See* accretion; blind brother; cosmogonic myth; *Deus faber;* dream; egg; emanatistic; emergence; *ex nihilo;* sacrifice; spider; two creators; world parent
Cronos (Greek), 132, 134, 135
Culler, Jonathan, cited, 185
Cuna Indian, 155
Curtin, Jeremiah, cited, 153, 262
Curtis, Edward S. (coll.), 181
Cushing, Frank Hamilton (coll.), 4–5, 82, 111, 114, 117, 129, 142, 154, 205–8

Dakota Indian, 45
Daly, Mary, cited, 87, 160, 164, 261

Dante, 119, 134
Davidson, H. R. Ellis, cited, 261
de Beauvoir, Simone, cited, 59, 91, 111, 114, 119
de Bry, Johann Theodore (engraver), 3, 41, 55, 249
De Forest, J. W., cited, 130
de Rochfort, Charles, cited, 132
de Santillana, Giorgio, cited, 257–58
death, 21, 49, 52, 53, 55, 57, 61, 89, 91, 125, 143, 151, 152, 162, 166, 183, 188, 189, 194, 245, 248, 251, 252
defecation, 6, 20, 23, 55, 67, 68, 113, 127–28, 167, 227, 229, 230, 254. *See also* flatus
Delaney, Carol, cited, 81, 84–85, 99–100
Delaware Indian, 11, 13, 44
Dellenbaugh, Anne G., cited, 131–32, 138–39, 258–59
Deus faber creation, 6, 7, 13, 20, 22, 66, 133, 180–81, 190, 227, 247
Devil (Christian), 68
dialogue, 172–74; Platonic, 140, 143, 155
Diana (Roman), 41, 88
Diodorus of Sicily, cited, 117
Diotima (Mantinean wise woman), 7
Doña Juana (inf.), 149, 237–46
Doria, Charles, cited, 5
Dorsey, J. Owen, cited, 142
Dorson, Richard M., cited, 44–45, 249
dove, 65, 79, 247, 252
dream creation, 7, 24, 26, 182
dream(ing), 5, 9, 10, 50, 68, 80, 139, 151–52, 171, 182, 186, 191, 199, 235, 253, 255, 257
DuBois, Constance Goddard (coll.), 203
Dundes, Alan, cited, xi, xiii, 8, 19–20, 21, 22–23, 66–67, 115, 132, 133–34, 153, 162, 165–66, 227, 254
Dupuis, Charles, cited, 257

earth, 6, 7, 19, 22, 42, 49, 51–52, 57, 59, 65, 68, 88, 91, 97, 102, 107, 108, 123, 125, 138, 139, 140, 164, 180, 181, 182, 183, 188, 201, 237, 248, 249
earth-diver creation, xi, 6, 7, 20, 65, 67–70, 79, 125, 191, 201, 252, 259
earth-goddess, 20, 55–56, 73, 89, 117, 161, 162, 250
earth mother, iv, 43, 49, 51, 52–53, 55, 61, 67, 71, 72, 81, 91, 93, 103, 117, 119, 123, 154, 187, 189, 203, 204, 205, 208, 209, 211, 251, 253, 254, 256

Earthmaker, Papago, 14; Winnebago, 48
Ecclesiasticus, Book of, 83
egg creation, iv, xi, 6, 7, 20, 65, 101–7, 111, 256, 257. *See also* ovum
Egypt, 36, 57, 71, 73, 91, 102, 117
Ehrenreich, Barbara, cited, 156
Einstein, Albert, 108–10, 111
Ekoi, 177–80
Eliade, Mircea, cited, 3–4, 5–6, 10–11, 13, 23, 52, 61, 67–68, 69, 72, 80–81, 103–4, 149–50, 175, 251, 253
Ellis Chips (inf.), 23
Elohim (OT), 3, 10, 25, 176, 180, 247
emanatistic creation, 51–52, 187, 190, 251
embryo(logy), 75, 87, 102, 103, 111, 255, 260
emergence creation, 6, 7, 9, 27, 93, 117, 119, 125–26, 129–30, 139–45, 154, 157, 214, 217, 218, 219, 224, 226, 233
Emerson, Ralph Waldo, cited, 163, 261–62
Engelsman, Joan Chamberlain, cited, 83–84
English, Deirdre, cited, 156
Epiphanius, Saint, cited, 74, 253
Eros (Greek), 3, 5, 107, 137
Estonia, 102, 248
Eurynome (Pelasgian), 65, 252
Eve (OT), 60, 133, 252, 259
ex nihilo creation, 3, 5, 6, 7, 10, 19, 24–25, 48, 71, 110, 125, 173, 182
Exodus, Book of, 150

Farnham, Marynia F., cited, 76
Fátima, 86
fetus, 85, 98, 107, 113, 115, 117, 129, 157, 233
Finland, 67, 68, 102
flatus, 165, 166, 167, 254. *See also* defecation
Fletcher, Alice C. (coll.), 107–8, 175, 257
Fludd, Robert, cited, 3, 41, 43, 55, 247, 249
Forde, C. Daryll, cited, 214
Frazer, James George, Sir, cited, 66
Freud, Sigmund, cited, 23, 30–31, 66, 70–71, 127–28
Friedman, Emanuel, cited, 129
Friedman, Susan Stanford, cited, 126, 138
Friedrich, Paul, cited, 254–55
Frobenius, Leo, cited, 150–51
Fromm, Erich, cited, 8
Fuller, Nancy, cited, 149, 169, 237–46

Gaia (Greek), 3, 5, 42, 52, 61, 73, 135, 203

Genesis, Book of, 3, 5, 10, 14, 60–61, 69, 132, 133–34, 172, 173, 174, 180, 252
genitals, 31, 75, 113, 159, 188, 227. *See also* penis; vulva
gia (Tewa Pueblo Indian), 91, 93
Gill, Sam, cited, 14–15, 129, 203, 207–8, 219, 250–51, 253
Giotto, cited, 134
Gishin Biye' (Guisheen Bige) (inf.), 27, 29
Gnosticism, 74, 79, 109
Goethe, 153, 262
gossip, xi, xii, 152, 164–69, 176, 238
gossips, 150, 157, 159–63, 164, 175, 238, 240, 243
Grahn, Judy, poem, 176
Graves, Robert, cited, 65, 79, 252
Gray, C. Buchanan, cited, 46
Greece, Classical, 3, 5, 20, 35–36, 57, 65, 66, 71, 73, 102, 105, 114, 132, 137, 149, 172, 183–84
Greenland, 102, 231
Griffin, Susan, cited, 167
Grillot de Givry, Emile, cited, 41, 247
Guadalupe, Our Lady of, 88–89, 91
Gunn, John M., cited, 25, 218, 248
gynaeceum, 42, 141, 187
gypsy, 71

H.D., cited, 138
Haile, Berard, O.F.M. (coll.), 27, 144
Hale, Horatio (coll.), 190
Hall, Manly Palmer, cited, 76–77, 107
Handy, E. S. Craighill (coll.), 101
Harrington, M. R., cited, 44
Harris, Marvin, cited, 49–50, 56
Harrison, Jane Ellen, cited, 114, 161–62
Harrison, Michael, M.D., cited, 115
Harvey, William, cited, 99, 100–101
Hastin Tlo'tsi hee (inf.), 129, 160–61, 219, 220–21
Hawaii, 14, 102, 203
Hebrews, Book of, 83
Hellbom, Anna-Britta, cited, 101–2, 105, 107
Hermes Trismegistus (alchemy), 107, 256–57
Herodotus, cited, 36
Hertz, Robert, cited, 125
Hesiod, cited, 3, 5, 61, 132, 134–35, 140, 161, 202–3, 253, 261
Hewitt, J. N. B. (coll.), 70, 192–94, 195
hierogamy, 5, 7, 20, 42, 61, 71, 72, 203. *See also* world parent creation

Hinsley, Curtis, cited, 206
Holy Ghost (Christian), 79, 247, 254
Homer, 140, 252
Horney, Karen, cited, 8–9
Horowitz, Maryanne Cline, cited, 98
Hubbs, Joanna, cited, 104–5, 107, 137
Hultkrantz, Åke, cited, 19, 51, 71, 72, 249, 250
Hungarian-Vogul, 252–53
Hupa Indian, 13
Huron Indian, 190–91
Huxley, Francis, cited, 260

Iatiku (Keresan Pueblo Indian), 89, 91, 139, 217, 219
Immaculate Conception, 67, 86–87
Indian, East, 4, 6, 10–11, 102
Indo-European, 51–52, 249
Indra (Indian), 11
initiation, 131, 133, 151, 162, 165–66, 167, 176, 183, 206
Inktomi (Lakota), 33, 35
intercourse, 7, 65, 69, 72, 74, 76, 80, 84–85, 131, 137, 162, 227, 231, 252, 253
Io (Maori), 81, 254
Iroquois Indian, 70–71, 190–202, 250
Isaiah, Book of, 164
Isis (Egyptian), 57, 88
Islam, 46, 81

James, G. W. B., cited, 135
Japan, 102
Jesus Christ (NT), 74, 79, 84, 87, 88, 153, 163, 247, 250, 257
Jewish, 46, 81, 83
Job, Book of, 13, 174, 180
John, Book of, 5, 83, 84
John, First Epistle of, 75
Johnson, Mark, cited, 8
Johnson, Samuel, cited, 59, 159–60
Jones, Ernest, cited, 165–66, 254
Jong, Erica, cited, 113
Jonson, Ben, cited, 103–4
Jordan, Brigitte, cited, 149, 160, 166–67, 169, 237–46
Jove (Roman), 77
Joyce, James, cited, 135
Juan Dolores (inf.), 22
Judd, Neil M., cited, 192
Judeo-Christian, 3, 5, 60, 83–84, 150
Jung, Carl G., cited, 53, 55, 71, 97, 104, 105

Jungian interpretation, 6, 9–10, 70–71, 104–5, 113

Kagaba Indian, 42, 47, 48, 49, 249, 250
Karok Indian, 13
Kato Indian, 173
Keresan Pueblo Indian, 25–26, 89
Kittay, Eva Feder, cited, 135, 138, 155
Kitzinger, Sheila, cited, 128
Köngäs, Elli Kaija, cited, 68–69
Kramarae, Cheris, cited, 251
Kramer, Samuel Noah, cited, 259
Kris, Ernst, cited, 134
Kroeber, A. L. (coll.), 180–81
Kroeber, Henriette Rothschild (coll.), 22
Kubrick, Stanley. See 2001: A Space Odyssey
Kurz, Otto, cited, 134

La Flesche, Francis (coll.), 107–8, 175, 257
labor, 98, 129, 157, 164–65, 176, 243–44, 260
Labouré, Catherine, 86
Laguna Pueblo Indian, 19, 26, 218, 219, 247–48
Lakoff, George, cited, 8
Lakota Indian, 23, 33, 35, 141–42
Landes, Ruth, cited, 151–52
Lang, Andrew, cited, 47–48
Leach, Edmund, cited, 255
Lenardon, Robert J., cited, 5, 107, 114, 184
Lenowitz, Harris, cited, 5
Lepcha, 250
Lerner, Gerda, cited, 60–61, 72–73, 81–82
Lévi-Strauss, Claude, cited, 154, 155, 251
LeVine, Robert A., cited, 253
Leviticus, Book of, 159
Libavius, cited, 97
Lincoln, Bruce, cited, 51–52
Little Red Riding-Hood, 127
Llewellyn, Martin, poem, 100–101
Lockhart, Russell A., cited, 256
logos, 25, 76, 84, 153, 173, 247
Long, Charles H., cited, 6
Lourdes, 86–87
Lubbock, John, cited, 56–57, 59
Luckert, Karl W., cited, 143–44
Luiseño Indian, 202–5
Lundberg, Ferdinand, cited, 76
Luomala, Katharine, cited, 14

MacCormack, Carol P., cited, 251
MacMurray, J. W., Major (coll.), 49

Macrobius, cited, 134
magic mill, 108, 257–58
Maidu Indian, 173
Maier, Michael, cited, 104, 107, 137, 256
Mallius, Lucius, cited, 134
Mami (Assyrian), 73
Man-never-known-on-earth (Wichita), 49
Manus, 175–76
Maori, 81, 255–56
Marduk (Babylonian), 139, 252
Maria Chona (inf.), 262
Maria Prophetissa, cited, 105
Martin, Emily, cited, 129, 131, 157
masturbation, 6, 72, 73–74, 105, 162
maternity, xi, 58–59, 86, 163
matriarchy, 57–59, 85, 159, 161
Matthew, Book of, 42, 84
Matthews, Washington, cited, 126, 154–55, 225
Maud, Ralph, cited, 187, 250
Maya, Quiché, 172–74; Yucatan, 149, 166–67, 237–46
Mayahuel (Aztec), 258
McNeley, James Kale, cited, 27, 29
Mead, Margaret, cited, 175–76, 262
medical science, 115, 117, 128, 129, 156, 157, 162, 164–65, 166, 237, 246, 261
Meltzer, David, cited, xii–xiii, 150–51
menstruation, 75, 85, 98, 130, 141, 171, 253
Merchant, Carolyn, cited, 53, 249, 256
Mercurius (alchemy), 97, 104
Mesa Verde National Park, 220–21
metis, 35–36, 135, 183, 255
Metis (Greek), 36, 135, 183
Michelangelo, cited, 134
midwifery, xi, xii, xiii, 14, 128, 149, 150, 153–57, 160, 175, 176, 227, 233, 237–46, 260, 261, 262; taboo against, 232
Miller, Henry, cited, xi, 70
Miwok Indian, Pohonichi, 68
monotheism, 7, 24, 43, 44–48, 60, 81, 85, 250
moon, 23, 41, 51, 55, 57, 65, 89, 91, 97, 104, 113, 119, 249, 252, 254, 256
Moon, Sheila, cited, 9
Mooney, James, cited, 49
Moore, Henry, cited, 97
Moore, Remedios W., cited, 126
Mor, Barbara, cited, 113
Morford, Mark P. O., cited, 5, 107, 114, 184
Moses (OT), 133, 150

Müller, Max, 44, 249
Mundurucú Indian, 152
mundus, xi, 11, 150, 152, 169, 175, 176
Murphy, Yolanda and Robert F., cited, 152
mythos, xi, 149–50, 153, 169, 175, 176

Nâlungiaq (inf.), 123, 231–32, 233–35
Nambicuara, 250
naming, 14, 26, 35, 60, 74, 82, 164, 233, 248
Nammu (Sumerian), 73
Naotsete (Naotsiti) (Keresan Pueblo Indian), 19, 26, 33, 217, 219
Naranjo, Tito, cited, 91, 93
nature, 7, 19, 20, 30, 31, 41, 42, 43, 48, 53, 55, 56, 57, 58, 103, 104, 139, 185
Navajo Indian, xii, 9, 27–32, 55, 117, 129, 143–44, 160, 219–27
Needham, Jacob, cited, 99, 117
Netsilik Eskimo, 123, 128, 231–37
Neumann, Erich, cited, 113, 119, 159, 253–54, 259
Newall, Venetia, cited, 102–3
Ninhursag (Sumerian), 259
Nkamtcinê'lx (inf.), 187
Noah (OT), 115
Nun (Egyptian), 73

O'Bryan, Aileen (coll.), 117, 160, 220–21
Odysseus (Greek), 162, 183
Oedipus (Greek), 154
Oglala Sioux Indian, 142, 144
Ojibwa Indian, 151–52
Okanagan Indian, 51, 250
Old-One, Okanagan, 51; Thompson Indian, 187–89
old wives' tales, 153–54, 156–57, 261
Older (Elder)-Brother (Papago), 22, 170
Omaha Indian, 107–8, 257
Onians, Richard Broxton, cited, 75, 256
Onondaga Indian, 191–202
origin myth, 4, 144, 207
Orpheus (Greek), 107, 151, 183
Ortner, Sherry B., cited, 251
Osage Indian, 175, 257
Otto, Rudolf, cited, 149–50, 260
Ouranos (Greek), 5, 73, 132, 135, 203
Ovid, cited, 77, 114, 183–84
ovum, 77, 99, 100, 258

Pagels, Elaine, cited, 252
Pandora (Greek), 161–62, 261

Papago Indian, 14–15, 22, 169–72
Paracelsus, cited, 69
Paris, France, 86
parthenogenesis, 6, 42, 71, 72, 73, 85, 87, 131–32, 138–39, 162, 176, 186, 193, 253, 258–59
parturition, xi, 7, 14, 42, 43, 85, 123–33, 135, 140, 145, 149, 150, 151, 153, 155, 160, 167, 171–72, 176, 191, 198, 202, 229, 232–33, 257, 259, 260
paternity, 58–59, 84–85, 132
patriarchy, 57, 59, 61, 105, 135, 161, 162
Pawnee Indian, 48
Pelasgian, 65
Penelope (Greek), 36, 183
penis, 69, 72, 74, 123, 133, 165, 166, 237, 254
penis envy, 8–9, 31, 135
Petchesky, Rosalind Pollack, cited, 115, 117
Peterson, Gayle, cited, 131
Petrarch, cited, 134
Phanes (Orphic), 107, 162
Pherekydes, cited, 20, 248
Phibionite, 74–75, 253
Philo, cited, 84
Philomela (Greek), 36, 183–84
philosopher's stone, 102–3, 104, 105, 110
Philosophia, 119. See also Wisdom
Phipps, William E., cited, 133
Phoenicia, 102
Pima Indian, 248
Plato, cited, 7, 140, 142–43, 155, 247, 262
Pliny, cited, 252
Plutarch, cited, 114
Polynesia, 4, 71, 101, 102
Pope, Barbara Corrado, cited, 86–87, 88
Popol Vuh (Quiché Mayan), 172–74
Poston, Carol H., cited, 128, 130–31
Potter, Charles Francis, cited, 154
Powers, Marla N., cited, 141–42, 144
Powers, William K., cited, 23, 35
Preuss, Konrad Theodor (coll.), 24, 42, 47, 182
procreation, xi, 5, 7, 43, 59, 60, 81, 85, 103, 126, 138, 141, 162, 163, 175
Prometheus (Greek), 66
Proverbs, Book of, 83
Psalms, Book of, 164
psyche (soul), 10, 75, 80–81, 105, 256. See also animism
psychoanalytic interpretation, 8–9, 19–20, 66–67, 68, 69, 132–33, 252–53, 254
Ptah (Egyptian), 74

Purce, Jill, cited, 110–11
Purley, Anthony F., cited, 19, 247–48

Quetzalcoatl (Aztec), 55, 174, 251

Radin, Paul, cited, 24–25, 45–46, 47–48, 49, 181–82, 249–50
Rasmussen, Knud (coll.), 123, 128, 231–32, 233–34
Raven (Chuckchee), 126–27, 227, 228–31
Re (Egyptian), 73–74
Red-Arm (inf.), 51, 250
Reichard, Gladys A., cited, 31–32, 143
Reichel-Dolmatoff, Gerardo, cited, 250
reproductive technology, 163, 257. See also test-tube baby
Revelation, Book of, 83
Rhea (Greek), 88, 132, 134, 135
Rich, Adrienne, poem, 24
Richardson, Herbert W., cited, 162–63
Rig Veda, 11, 248
Róheim, Géza, cited, 68, 69, 252–53
Roman Catholicism, 14, 84, 215, 219
Rome, 11, 105, 110
Rooth, Anna Birgitta, cited, 6, 19, 33, 71–72, 125–26
Ruether, Rosemary Radford, cited, xiii, 87–88, 251

sacrifice creation, 6
Saint Augustine, 88, 119
Saint Thomas Aquinas, cited, 155
Sambia, 253
Sanday, Peggy Reeves, cited, 250
Sanskrit, 45, 105, 249
Santa Ana Pueblo Indian, 218
Santa Clara Pueblo Indian, 91, 93
Scandinavia, 6, 154
Scarberry, Susan J., cited, 248
Schafer, R. Murray, cited, 165
Schmidt, Wilhelm P., Father, cited, 250
sea, 3, 6, 14, 50, 57, 58, 67, 68, 73, 77, 79, 81, 82, 97, 108, 139, 151, 173–74, 180, 181, 190, 191, 200, 205, 208, 236, 257, 259
Seligmann, Kurt, cited, 137, 256–57
Semang, 250
semen, 69, 73, 74, 75, 76–77, 98, 99, 100, 107, 253, 256, 258
Seneca Indian, 193–94
serpent, 10–11, 51, 55, 60, 65, 71, 73, 89, 114, 170, 171, 172, 174, 205, 252

shamanism, 56, 65, 68, 123, 155, 187, 233, 235, 236–37, 248, 252
Shilluk, 250
Silent Scream, The, 115
Silko, Leslie Marmon, epigraph, *Ceremony,* 26
Simpson, Michael, cited, 183–84
singing, 26, 27, 33, 120, 152, 169, 170, 180, 235
Sioux Indian, 138
Sjöö, Monica, cited, 113
sky, 7, 41, 42, 44, 45, 71, 72, 73, 101, 102, 107, 108, 117, 119, 137, 151, 174, 182, 186, 193, 194, 248, 249, 252–53
sky father (god), 20, 43, 67, 71, 72, 73, 117, 119, 208, 209, 254
Smohalla (inf.), 49
Socrates, 7, 140, 141, 142, 143, 155
Sokol, Robert, M.D., cited, 157
Soma (Indian), 11
Somadeva, cited, 105, 107
Sophia. *See* Wisdom
Soubirous, Bernadette, 86–87
Spacks, Patricia Meyer, cited, 160
Speck, Frank G., cited, 11–12
speech, 5, 29, 36, 74, 81, 100, 138, 164, 183, 220, 225
Speert, Harold, M.D., cited, 149, 260
Spender, Dale, cited, 251–52
spider creation, iv, 6, 19–26, 33, 157, 218
spider web, 19–20, 22–23, 27, 29, 183, 211, 248
Spider Woman, Chuckchee, 227, 230; Keresan Pueblo Indian, 19, 25, 26, 32, 214, 248; Navajo, 27, 29–30, 117, 223, 226
Spurway, Helen, cited, 258–59
Stephen, Alexander M. (coll.), 29
Stevens, Fred (artist), 55
Stevenson, Matilda Coxe, cited, 82, 207, 254
Stirling, Matthew W. (coll.), 214–15
stork, 66, 81
storytelling, xii, 26, 140, 166, 167, 170–71, 177–78, 221, 235, 240
Suarez, Francisco, cited, 79
Sumer, 73, 259
sun, 43, 45, 50, 55, 57, 60, 65, 77, 80, 91, 97, 104, 119, 137, 138, 143, 154, 160, 203, 204, 210, 211, 213, 214, 217, 249, 253, 254, 256, 257
supreme deity, 7, 11, 25, 26, 44–49, 50, 55, 81, 187
Swanson, Guy E., cited, 250

Swanton, John R., cited, 65
Swentzell, Rina, cited, 91, 93

Ta'aroa (Polynesian), 101
Taikó-mol (Yuki), 180–81
Talbot, Percy Amaury (coll.), 177
Tedlock, Dennis, cited, 5, 172–74, 207, 254
Teit, James A. (coll.), 51, 187–88, 250, 251
test-tube baby, 105, 163. *See also* reproductive technology
Tezcatlipoca (Aztec), 55, 251
theogamy, 79
thinking, 6, 7, 25, 26, 27, 29, 30, 82, 89, 109
Thompson, Stith, cited, 4, 5, 77, 80, 108
Thompson Indian, 187–90, 251
Thought (Thinking, Prophesying) Woman (Keresan Pueblo Indian), 19, 25, 26, 32–33, 89, 120, 208, 214–18, 248
thunder, 80, 82, 164, 165, 166, 211
Tiamat (Babylonian), 6, 73, 138–39, 259
Timothy, First Letter of Paul to, 153
Tirawa (Pawnee), 48
Titian, 91
Tiwai Paraone (inf.), 254
Tlazolteotl (Aztec), 123
Toelken, Barre, cited, xii, 30, 31, 144
Tonantzin (Aztec), 89
Tooth (Onondaga), 195, 198, 199
tree, of knowledge, 60; of life, iv, 169; of light, 194; magic, 80; world, 154. *See also* Tooth; Yggdrasill
Treichler, Paula, cited, 251
Trevathan, Wenda R., cited, 262
trickster, 32, 35, 37, 43, 55. *See also* Coyote; Inktomi
Truchas Master (artist), 93
Tuareg, 250
Tuggle, W. O. (coll.), 253
Tuzin, Donald, cited, 227
two creators creation, 6, 7, 33, 173
2001: A Space Odyssey, 115, 162, 163
Tyler, Hamilton A., cited, 25
Tylor, Edward B., Sir, cited, 49–51, 132; mentioned, 56

Uitoto Indian, 24, 181–82
Underhill, Ruth (coll.), 170–72
Uretsete (Utctsiti) (Keresan Pueblo Indian), 19, 26, 33, 89, 219
urination, 6, 36, 127, 144, 227, 229–30

vagina, 130, 153, 157, 166, 167, 212, 241
Venus (Roman), 137
Venus of Lespugue, 113
Vesalius, Andreas, cited, 133
Vico, 153
Virgin Mary (Christian), 41, 67, 79, 84, 85–89, 91, 119, 165, 254
virginity, 79, 85, 86
Volborth, Judith Mountain Leaf (Ivaloo), poem, 37
von Baer, Karl Ernst, 99
von Dechend, Hertha, cited, 257–58
von Franz, Marie-Louise, cited, 6, 9–10, 20, 70–71, 105
von Leeuwenhoek, Anton, cited, 99
vulva, 73, 153, 166

Wakoⁿ'da (Omaha), 107
Warner, Marina, cited, 79, 85–86, 91
Watts, Alan, cited, 14, 83, 109, 150, 169
weaving, 20, 23, 29, 30–32, 36–37, 159, 177, 178, 183–84, 211, 248
Wells, H. G., cited, 100
Westman, Heinz, cited, 10
Wheeler-Voegelin, Erminie, cited, 67, 126
White, Leslie A. (coll.), 32–33, 139
Whitman, Walt, poem, 20–21
Wichita Indian, 49
Williams, Tennessee, cited, 128
Wilson, John A., cited, 74
wind, 13, 27, 29, 51, 65, 80, 82, 97, 161, 164, 165, 174, 176, 226, 252, 256

Winnebago Indian, 48
Wisdom (Greek, Judeo-Christian), 7, 83–84, 119, 254, 255
witch(craft), 55, 123, 143, 156, 225, 236
Witherspoon, Gary, cited, 27, 31–32, 219–20
Wolf, Eric, cited, 88–89
womb, 7, 14, 53, 58, 61, 69, 73, 79, 81, 87, 91, 93, 98, 100, 103, 104, 105, 107, 111–20, 126, 129–30, 135, 137, 138, 141, 162, 163, 208, 210, 212, 257, 259
womb envy, 8, 227
word, 5, 6, 83, 153, 167, 180, 199, 233, 235, 236, 247, 255, 256. *See also* naming; speech
world parent creation, 6, 67, 71–72, 253. *See also* hierogamy

Yahweh (OT), 84, 134, 176, 249, 252
Yellowman (inf.), xii, 144
Yggdrasill (Scandinavian), 154, 159
Ymir (Scandinavian), 6
Yoruba, 71
Yuchi Indian, 253
Yuki Indian, 180–81
Yuma Indian, 71
Yurok Indian, 13

Zeus (Greek), 20, 42, 45, 134, 135, 137, 161, 162, 248
Zia (Sia) Pueblo Indian, 25, 32–33, 218
Zuni Pueblo Indian, 4–5, 71, 82, 97, 111, 114, 117, 118, 129–30, 142, 154, 205–14, 254